HASHIMOTO'S TRIGGERS

ELIMINATE YOUR THYROID SYMPTOMS
BY FINDING AND REMOVING YOUR
SPECIFIC AUTOIMMUNE TRIGGERS

ERIC M. OSANSKY–DC, CCN, CNS, IFMCP

Hashimoto's Triggers: Eliminate Your Thyroid Symptoms by Finding and Removing Your Specific Autoimmune Triggers

By Eric M. Osansky, DC, MS, CCN, CNS, IFMCP

Copyright ©2018

Printed in the United States of America

Natural Endocrine Solutions
10020 Monroe Road Ste #170-280
Matthews, NC 28105
www.NaturalEndocrineSolutions.com

ISBN: 978-0-692-98949-4

Cover and interior design by Adina Cucicov

A Word Of Caution To The Reader

Your Free Bonus Gifts

As a small token of thanks for buying this book, I'd like to offer two free bonus gifts exclusive to my readers:

* Bonus #1: The Hashimoto's Triggers FREE Video Training Series
* Bonus #2: The Hashimoto's Triggers FREE Action Plan Checklist

You can download your free gifts here:
http://www.naturalendocrinesolutions.com/freegift

Dedication

I dedicate this book to those people with Hashimoto's thyroiditis who are sick and tired of dealing with their symptoms and are looking to detect and remove their specific autoimmune triggers.

Acknowledgements

First of all, I'd like to thank my family for putting up with me while writing this book. This includes my wife Cindy for her continued love and support while writing this book, along with my two daughters Marissa and Jaylee.

Second, I'd like to thank my staff Kate and Carson for their help and support during this process.

And finally, I'd like to commend all of the people with Hashimoto's who are open minded enough to look for a natural treatment solution.

TABLE OF CONTENTS

PLEASE READ THIS FIRST

IN THE SPRING OF 2008, I was walking around a Sam's Club and came across an automated blood pressure machine. I decided to take my blood pressure, which was normal, but my heart rate was elevated. This was the beginning of my journey with Graves' disease.

Just as is the case with Hashimoto's thyroiditis, Graves' disease is an autoimmune condition involving the thyroid gland. The difference is that Graves' disease involves thyroid stimulating immunoglobulins, and the immune system attacks the TSH receptors, which, in turn, leads to an excess production of thyroid hormone.

Hashimoto's thyroiditis is characterized by elevated thyroid peroxidase and/or thyroglobulin antibodies. When someone has these antibodies this means that the immune system is damaging the thyroid gland, which, over time, can lead to a decreased production of thyroid hormone.

While Graves' disease and Hashimoto's cause different symptoms, what they have in common is that they both are autoimmune thyroid conditions. The reason why they result in different symptoms is because they affect the thyroid gland in a different way. It's also worth mentioning that some people with Hashimoto's will also have the antibodies for Graves' disease.

However, regardless of whether someone has the antibodies for Hashimoto's, Graves' disease, or both, it's important to understand that an environmental trigger is a necessary component of these and other autoimmune conditions, and while different autoimmune conditions can have different triggers, there is a lot of overlap when it comes to autoimmune triggers.

For example, I work with patients who have Graves' disease and Hashimoto's, and, over the years, I've noticed that stress and H. pylori are more common triggers in those people with Graves' disease, whereas Blastocystis hominis seems to be a more common trigger in those with Hashimoto's. However, stress and H. pylori can still be triggers in those with Hashimoto's, and Blastocystis hominis can be a trigger of Graves' disease.

Endocrinologists Are Not Immune System Specialists

I realize that not everyone reading this book has seen an endocrinologist for their condition. However, many people with Hashimoto's do see an endocrinologist. Nevertheless, whether someone sees an endocrinologist or a general medical practitioner, in most cases the result is the same: a prescription for thyroid hormone replacement. However, what you need to understand is that most medical doctors, including endocrinologists, don't focus on the immune system.

Endocrinologists focus on the endocrine system, and while the thyroid gland is part of this system, you need to remember that Hashimoto's is primarily an immune system condition. Therefore, it shouldn't be surprising that endocrinologists will focus on balancing the hormones. We also need to keep in mind that most medical doctors don't do anything to address the underlying cause of chronic health conditions.

Are You More Knowledgeable Than Your Medical Doctor?

Without question, medical doctors go through extensive training while in medical school, and they do an excellent job when it comes to emergency care. For example, if you had an acute case of appendicitis and suspected that your appendix was getting ready to rupture, it would be a very good idea to visit a medical doctor. However, for those who have a chronic health condition, whether it be an autoimmune condition or a different condition such as cancer, most medical doctors won't do anything to address the actual cause of the condition.

With regards to improving one's overall state of health, many nonpractitioners are more knowledgeable than the average medical doctor. This might sound like a crazy claim to make, but the truth is that most medical doctors don't teach their patients to improve their health through dietary and other lifestyle factors. Thus, it shouldn't be surprising that many nonhealthcare professionals are more knowledgeable than medical doctors about dietary and lifestyle factors. If you're not currently in this position, you will be after you finish reading this book.

Why Would the Immune System Attack the Thyroid Gland?

One of the oversimplified concepts in the world of autoimmunity is that the body attacks our own tissues. The truth is that in a healthy environment our body is smart enough to distinguish self (our own cells) from nonself (foreign material). The problem is that, over the last century, we've been exposed to more and more chemicals through the food we eat, the water we drink, the air we breathe, and the products we use (i.e., body creams, shampoos, and toothpaste). This, in turn, has caused dysregulation of our immune system and a loss of immune tolerance, and it's one of the main factors behind the increased incidence of autoimmune conditions such as Hashimoto's.

Another thing to keep in mind is that some of these triggers (i.e., environmental chemicals and pathogens) can directly bind to the thyroid gland. In this situation, the immune system isn't randomly trying to destroy its own tissues, but due to the chemical or infection that's bound to the thyroid gland, it recognizes the thyroid gland as being nonself and attacks it. The same concept applies to other autoimmune conditions, and testing is available that evaluates the immune system response to certain chemicals and pathogens, which I discuss in section three.

Thus, for those who think it's a ridiculous concept for the immune system to attack the thyroid gland, there's some truth behind this. However, without question, we live in a world that's much more toxic than in the past, and to think that this unhealthy environment would have no impact on our immune system and overall health is equally ridiculous.

How to Detect and Remove Your Specific Autoimmune Triggers

In section one of this book, I try to provide you with a good understanding of why you developed Hashimoto's in the first place. Although I'm confident that you'll find section one to be interesting regardless of whether you have a basic or a more advanced knowledge of Hashimoto's, I admit that the majority of people who purchase this book will be doing so for the information that is in section two, three, and four. Section two consists of arguably the most comprehensive information on the triggers of Hashimoto's available in any book. After reading this section, you'll have an excellent knowledge of the different triggers of Hashimoto's.

However, while it's important to understand all of the different triggers of Hashimoto's, it is, of course, just as important to find and remove your specific triggers. This is where sections three and four will help you. Section three focuses on helping you detect your specific autoimmune triggers, while section four will show you how to remove your autoimmune triggers and achieve a state of overall optimal health. Although I discuss nutritional supplements and herbs (and give suggested doses), I also include a lot of information on using healthy whole foods to improve your health.

How Is This Book Different From Others?

No shortage of books exists on Hashimoto's thyroiditis, so you might be wondering what separates this book from others out there? While there are some excellent books on Hashimoto's, this one includes the most comprehensive information on the different triggers. In addition, I don't hold back any information in section three and four, as after going through these sections you'll know how to find and remove your specific triggers.

In addition, this book has more research than most other books on Hashimoto's thyroiditis. While I try to include plenty of research to support the relationship between certain triggers and Hashimoto's, I try to present both sides of the story by discussing some research studies that try to disprove the link between certain triggers and thyroid autoimmunity. While this book has a lot of scientific references, it also includes some theories as well.

No Recipes?

One of the downsides of this book is that it doesn't include any recipes because 1) I wanted to include as much content as possible to help you identify and remove your specific triggers, and 2) plenty of other resources are available elsewhere if you're interested in recipes. While it seems that most health-related books include recipes these days, this isn't a recipe book. If your primary interest is in having recipes then this book isn't the right one for you, although if you want to know where to get recipes that are suitable for those with Hashimoto's please visit **www. naturalendocrinesolutions.com/recipes**.

How to Get the Most out of This Book

The most likely reason why you purchased this book is because you were interested in finding your specific autoimmune triggers. Because of this, you might be tempted to skip over section one and start with section two. However, even if you consider yourself to have a great deal of knowledge about thyroid autoimmunity, I would still recommend that you read section one. However, if you're eager to jump into the triggers section (followed by sections three and four), at the very least, I would read the chapter highlights of each of the individual chapters of section one.

The fifth section of this book focuses on some of main questions people with Hashimoto's have. I've been working on this book for a few years, and in 2016 I started surveying my email list to find out some of the main questions and concerns people have with regards to Hashimoto's, which is how I came up with most of the questions in section five. A few questions weren't asked by those people I surveyed, but instead were questions I thought were important to bring up.

For those who have a basic knowledge of Hashimoto's, although I try to make the information easy to understand, you still might find some of the material to be somewhat advanced. This is especially true with the information in section one. Keep in mind that you don't need to have a comprehensive understanding of the immune system to benefit from this book. However, I still think it's beneficial to have some knowledge of the immune cells, and while some of the information might go over your head, the more you're exposed to it the more you'll retain it.

I'd like to thank you again for investing in this book, and you can now proceed to Chapter 1!

• SECTION ONE

UNDERSTANDING THE AUTOIMMUNE
COMPONENT OF HASHIMOTO'S

IN THIS SECTION, I try to provide you with a good understanding of why you developed Hashimoto's in the first place. In Chapter 1, I discuss some of the different genetic markers involved, as well as the importance of regulatory T cells and immune tolerance in helping to prevent autoimmunity. I also discuss the autoimmunity timeline. In Chapter 2, I briefly discuss antecedents, triggers, and mediators, and how to use nutrients and herbs to modulate the immune system.

Chapter 3 focuses on the immune gut connection, where I talk in detail about leaky gut syndrome, and differentiate between direct triggers and leaky gut triggers. I also discuss the importance of having a healthy microbiome. Chapter 4 focuses on the hygiene hypothesis, and how being too sanitary can be a factor in autoimmunity.

CHAPTER 1

THE AUTOIMMUNE TIMELINE: HOW HASHIMOTO'S DEVELOPS

WHEN SOMEONE IS DIAGNOSED with Hashimoto's thyroiditis or any autoimmune condition for the very first time, they are frequently in a state of disbelief. However, when you consider that autoimmune conditions are more prevalent than heart disease and cancer and that, according to the National Institute of Allergy and Infectious Diseases, there are more than 80 different types of diagnosed autoimmune conditions[1] and dozens of other conditions are suspected as being an autoimmune condition as of the writing of this book, then it shouldn't be surprising that so many people develop Hashimoto's.

The focus of this book is on detecting and removing the triggers of Hashimoto's. Doing this is necessary in order to reverse the autoimmune component and get the person into a state of remission. One question you might have is "why do some people develop Hashimoto's thyroiditis, and not a different autoimmune condition such as multiple sclerosis or rheumatoid arthritis?" I'll go ahead and answer this question without trying to make it too complex, and then I'll expand on it shortly.

Autoimmunity happens when the body doesn't recognize its own cells and tissues as self, which, in turn, leads to an immune response against these cells and tissues. As I mentioned in the introduction, under a healthy environment, our body is smart enough to distinguish self from nonself. However, certain factors result in immune system dysregulation and a loss of immune tolerance, which can cause the immune system to mistakenly attack the thyroid gland, which, in turn, can result in elevated thyroid autoantibodies on a blood test.

The two main types of autoantibodies in Hashimoto's are thyroglobulin antibodies and thyroid peroxidase (TPO) antibodies. Thyroglobulin is a protein produced by the thyroid gland. Thyroid peroxidase in an enzyme that plays an important role in the formation of thyroid hormone.

What happens is that, over time, the immune system can cause extensive damage to thyroglobulin and/or thyroid peroxidase, which reduces the thyroid gland's ability to produce adequate amounts of thyroid hormone. Over a prolonged period, if the trigger isn't removed and the autoimmune response isn't suppressed, then the person with Hashimoto's will have decreased production of thyroid hormone, and as a result, thyroid hormone replacement will usually be recommended.

Can Hashimoto's Thyroiditis Be Cured?

When I discuss reversing the autoimmune component of Hashimoto's, some will wonder if I'm suggesting that Hashimoto's thyroiditis can be cured. The truth is that while I have used the word "cure" in the past, and while some other natural healthcare professionals discuss curing Hashimoto's thyroiditis, we do need to keep in mind that there is a genetic component. While it is true that lifestyle and environment are even greater factors in the development of autoimmune conditions, we still can't dismiss the genetics behind these conditions.

Thus, my goal isn't necessarily to "cure" Hashimoto's but, instead, to try to help those with this condition get into a state of "permanent remission." Although this can be challenging, many people will be able to reverse the autoimmune component if they follow the advice given in this book. Even those who don't achieve a state of "permanent remission" should still experience a tremendous improvement in their health.

Why Do Some People Develop Hashimoto's And Not a Different Autoimmune Condition?

As I mentioned earlier, many different autoimmune conditions exist. Why does autoimmunity develop, and what factors determine whether someone will develop an autoimmune thyroid condition such as Hashimoto's, or another autoimmune condition such as rheumatoid arthritis or multiple sclerosis? Well, there is something called the triad of autoimmunity, which is also known as the 3-legged stool of autoimmunity. These three factors will determine whether someone will develop an autoimmune condition.

First, a genetic predisposition is required. Second, there needs to be some type of environmental trigger, such as a food allergen, environmental toxin, infection, or trauma. Even stress can potentially be a trigger of autoimmunity.

In addition, there is strong evidence that a third factor is required to develop an autoimmune condition, which is hyperpermeability of the intestinal barrier. This process is also known as a leaky gut, and I'll use the terms *leaky gut* and *increase in intestinal permeability* interchangeably throughout this book. As of now, this is still a theory, although it makes a lot of sense, and I will talk about a leaky gut in greater detail in Chapter 3. I will say that I have had some patients with elevated thyroid autoantibodies test negative for an increase in intestinal permeability (a leaky gut) using either the classic lactulose-mannitol test, or the Intestinal Antigenic Permeability Screen (Array #2) from Cyrex Labs.

In other words, some of my patients with elevated thyroglobulin antibodies and/or thyroid peroxidase antibodies tested negative for a leaky gut. While neither of the tests I mentioned are 100% accurate in confirming the presence of a leaky gut, it's also possible that not everyone with an autoimmune condition has an increase in intestinal permeability. Although I don't test all of my patients for a leaky gut, I have tested numerous patients over the years, and I have found that most people with Hashimoto's test positive for a leaky gut.

The Role of Human Leukocyte Antigen (HLA) In Autoimmunity

I will try to keep most of this book easy to understand, but the next few paragraphs might be somewhat advanced for some people. Different autoimmune conditions will have different types of genetic markers, and something called human leukocyte antigen (HLA) is a gene complex that consists of different cell-surface proteins, which, in turn, help regulate the immune system.

To make it easier to understand, I'm going to refer to these cell-surface proteins as "genetic surface markers." It's important to understand that someone who has Hashimoto's will have different genetic surface markers than someone else who has a different autoimmune condition, such as multiple sclerosis. Some people have the genetic surface markers for multiple autoimmune conditions, which is why some people will develop more than one of these conditions.

What makes this complex is that an autoimmune condition can have more than one genetic surface marker, which, in turn, predisposes the person to develop multiple autoimmune conditions. However, some autoimmune conditions share the same surface markers. It's also important to understand that these genetic surface markers aren't just a factor in autoimmune conditions, but in other chronic health conditions as well, such as cancer.

Regarding autoimmunity, people with certain HLA types are more likely to develop an autoimmune condition. However, just having a specific HLA genetic surface marker doesn't mean that the person will develop autoimmunity.

For example, some people reading this may be familiar with the HLA markers associated with celiac disease, which are HLA-DQ2 and HLA-DQ8. If someone has one or both of these markers, it doesn't necessarily mean that they will develop celiac disease. This is true even if they consume gluten, which is the environmental trigger associated with celiac disease. Thus, what this tells us is that having a genetic marker and being exposed to an environmental trigger doesn't always lead to autoimmunity. As mentioned earlier, you also need to have a leaky gut, which is associated with a decrease in regulatory T cells and a loss of immune tolerance, which I'll discuss in this chapter.

I personally dealt with Graves' disease, which is an autoimmune thyroid condition characterized by the genetic surface marker HLA-DR3. However, with Hashimoto's, there has been some controversy with regards to what the primary genetic surface marker is[2,3], although HLA-DR3 and HLA-DR5 seem to be associated with this condition. Either way, unlike celiac disease, where gluten is the trigger, there is no specific trigger that has been associated with all cases of Hashimoto's, as it appears that numerous factors can trigger the autoimmune response in this condition.

Another thing to keep in mind is that some autoimmune conditions can share the same genetic surface marker. I mentioned how the surface marker HLA-DR3 is present in Graves' disease and Hashimoto's, and it is present in Sjögren's syndrome and systemic lupus erythematosus.[4]

The Importance of Regulatory T Cells in Preventing Autoimmunity

While the last few paragraphs might have been difficult for some people to understand, hopefully what is clear at this point is that factors other than genetics and environmental triggers will determine whether someone will develop an autoimmune thyroid condition, or any other autoimmune condition for that matter. One of these factors is something called regulatory T cells (Tregs), as these are immune cells that help prevent autoimmunity from developing. I'm going to briefly discuss Tregs here, and then I'll discuss them in greater detail in Chapter 2.

If someone has a healthy immune system, they will have plenty of Tregs, which will help prevent them from developing an autoimmune condition. However, over a period of months and years, if someone eats a poor diet, is constantly stressed out, doesn't get quality sleep each night, and/or has a high toxic load, then this will lead to a decrease in Tregs, and will increase the likelihood of the person developing autoimmunity. Other factors can lead to a decrease in Tregs as well.

So a very likely scenario is that someone has a genetic predisposition for Hashimoto's, but, despite being exposed to numerous environmental triggers, they don't develop this autoimmune thyroid condition unless their body reaches a point where there isn't enough Tregs present to keep autoimmunity in check. Certain factors can potentially affect the number of Tregs such as stress, a chronic infection, exposure to environmental toxins, a leaky gut, mitochondrial dysfunction, and deficiencies in nutrients such as vitamin A and vitamin D. Autoimmunity is very complex, and, as I mentioned earlier, we still don't know a lot about autoimmune conditions.

While Tregs help keep autoimmunity in check, Th17 cells drive the autoimmune process. Th17 cells are one of the predominant proinflammatory cell types and they produce Interleukin 17 (IL-17), which further drives the inflammatory process. Numerous studies specifically show a correlation between increased Th17 levels and the pathogenesis of Hashimoto's thyroiditis.[5,6,7] The good news is that taking steps to increase Tregs can shut down the production of Th17 cells.

What Is Immune Tolerance?

Hopefully, you have a better understanding of the importance of Tregs in preventing autoimmunity. And if someone already has an autoimmune condition, which describes most people reading this book, then they will want to take measures to increase Tregs in order to help suppress the autoimmune response. I'll further discuss how to increase Tregs in the next chapter. What I'd like to discuss now is immune tolerance.

Remember that the goal of the immune system is to protect us against foreign substances and invaders, such as infections. The immune system also assists in repair when there is an injury, and it will also destroy any abnormal cells that are created. However, another big challenge of the immune system is to differentiate self from nonself. When the immune system is unable to do this, then autoimmunity can develop.

It's quite amazing when you think about it, as not only is the immune system designed not to attack our own tissues but also, under normal conditions, it won't mount an immune response against food proteins, and it won't attack our commensal or good bacteria. Immune tolerance begins upon being born, as the infant acquires good bacteria from the mother during the birth process (for those who are born via a natural birth); breastfeeding also plays a big role. This doesn't mean that immune tolerance doesn't develop in those who are born via a C-section and/or aren't breastfed, but being born via a vaginal birth and being breastfed both play very important roles in the activation of Tregs.

Oral Tolerance vs. Central Tolerance

Oral tolerance and central tolerance are two different mechanisms preventing us from developing autoimmunity. Oral tolerance plays a key role in preventing our immune system from attacking dietary proteins. Also, the Tregs I just discussed play a big role in preventing our immune system from reacting to food antigens, as well as from attacking the commensal bacteria. I mentioned breastfeeding earlier, which helps the baby to develop oral tolerance, although other factors can also activate Tregs earlier in life.

However, having a decrease in Tregs can cause a loss of oral tolerance. This loss of oral tolerance can set the stage for an increase in intestinal permeability, which, in turn, can lead to food sensitivities. I'll discuss food sensitivities in Chapter 23, and while food sensitivities won't always lead to autoimmunity, having a loss of oral tolerance can increase the likelihood of certain foods becoming an autoimmune trigger.

What is the difference between oral tolerance and central tolerance? Well, there definitely are similarities between these two mechanisms, as both oral and central tolerance helps to protect us against foreign antigens. However, oral tolerance is more dependent on Tregs, while central tolerance is more dependent on the function of the thymus.

T-cell development occurs in the thymus, and many of these T cells will respond to foreign proteins (i.e., bacteria) but not to our own tissues and bacteria. However, some T cells are autoreactive and, as the name implies, will attack our own tissues. Fortunately, they are normally eliminated in the thymus. However, sometimes, they can "escape" the thymus and get into the circulation, and then it is up to the Tregs to suppress these auto-reactive T cells.

Another way that autoimmunity can occur is when someone is low in Tregs and develops a loss of oral tolerance. So while oral tolerance is more dependent on Tregs, these cells are also important for preventing a loss of central tolerance.

Both oral and central tolerance are forms of immune tolerance. Thus, when someone has a loss of immune tolerance, the immune system becomes confused and can not only attack dietary proteins and the commensal bacteria but also our own tissues. Either a loss of oral or central tolerance is necessary to cause an autoimmune condition such as Hashimoto's.

Understanding the Autoimmunity Timeline

In addition to understanding what factors can lead to the development of an autoimmune condition such as Hashimoto's, it is also beneficial to understand the autoimmunity timeline. After all, most chronic health conditions take many years to develop. Then, when they do develop, it can take many more years for symptoms to manifest. So let's look at the different stages of autoimmunity:

Stage #1: Pre-autoimmunity. This is the most critical time to prevent an autoimmune condition from developing. As I already mentioned, having a genetic predisposition and being exposed to an environmental trigger usually won't cause an autoimmune condition without other factors being present. I also mentioned that there is strong evidence that a leaky gut needs to be present. In addition, a decrease in Tregs and a loss of immune tolerance are necessary factors in the development of autoim-munity. However, what's important to understand is that it usually takes years for people to develop a leaky gut and a loss of immune tolerance.

Thus, the pre-autoimmune stage is essentially when, over time, a person's body becomes more susceptible to developing autoimmunity. During this stage, they will develop a leaky gut, a decrease in Tregs, and a loss of immune tolerance. Of course, many other factors can have a negative effect on your health and lead to a leaky gut and a loss of immune tolerance such eating a poor diet consisting of a lot of refined foods and sugars, consuming common allergens such as gluten and dairy, being exposed to prolonged chronic stress, getting insufficient sleep for many months or years, toxic overload, an acute or chronic infection, etc.

Although being exposed to an environmental trigger is necessary for the development of autoimmunity, please remember that, in most cases, if someone has a genetic marker for an autoimmune thyroid condition such as Hashimoto's, a single exposure to an environmental trigger usually isn't going to cause autoimmunity. After all, most people deal with chronic stress these days, and everyone is exposed to environmental toxins.

However, if someone eats a poor diet daily, is stressed out, has toxic overload, etc., then over a prolonged period, this can cause an increase in intestinal permeability, along with a decrease in Tregs and a loss of immune tolerance, which can set the stage for autoimmunity. Thus, perhaps the best way to think of it is that we're all exposed to many "environmental triggers," but other factors are necessary in order for someone to develop an autoimmune condition.

Stage #2: Silent autoimmunity. In this stage, the autoimmune process has already started. However, there has been very little or no tissue damage (i.e., to the thyroid gland), and, therefore, no symptoms are present, and the basic thyroid panel results are negative at this point (i.e., normal TSH and thyroid hormone levels). This is what happens with just about all autoimmune conditions. However, the duration of this stage will vary greatly depending on the type of autoimmune condition.

For example, if someone has elevated thyroglobulin antibodies, then there is a good chance that, over time, the immune system will cause damage to the thyroid gland. If nothing is done to address the autoimmune component, then the damage can be so extensive that the person might reach the point where they need to take thyroid hormone replacement.

However, the person with Hashimoto's can be in the "silent" stage for many years because, when dealing with autoimmune conditions that involve tissue damage (i.e., Hashimoto's, multiple sclerosis), the tissue damage can be minimal for many years. In some cases, it can take a long time for the person to develop symptoms, which I'll discuss next in stage #3.

Stage #3. Symptoms are present with some tissue damage. Although stage #2 might involve some tissue damage, it's minimal, but stage #3 is when this damage reaches the point where the person begins to experience symptoms. Once again, it can take many years for this to happen. Here are some of the common symptoms associated with Hashimoto's:

- Fatigue
- Cold hands and feet
- Weight gain
- Brain fog
- Hair loss
- Constipation
- Insomnia
- Dry skin

Thus, what will frequently happen is that, due to tissue damage to the thyroid gland, the person with Hashimoto's will begin to experience some of the symptoms I just listed. Thus, they might visit their general medical practitioner, who will run a thyroid panel, and, at this point, the TSH might be elevated, or it still might look fine.

You shouldn't rely on the TSH alone, but, unfortunately, this still is what frequently happens at many medical doctor's offices. Thus, if the TSH is within the lab reference range, regardless of how the person feels, they might be told that everything is fine, since the thyroid markers are within the "normal" reference range. However, a competent doctor will run a more comprehensive panel, which not only evaluates the thyroid hormone levels (usually normal during stage #3) but also looks at the thyroid antibodies, in this case, the thyroid peroxidase antibodies and thyroglobulin antibodies.

Just keep in mind that for some people with Hashimoto's, the thyroid antibodies will show up as negative on a blood test. Thus, it's important to understand that negative thyroid peroxidase and thyroglobulin antibodies don't always rule out Hashimoto's. If Hashimoto's is suspected yet both of these thyroid antibodies are negative, getting a thyroid ultrasound can provide some valuable information, although some sources claim that the most accurate method of diagnosing Hashimoto's thyroiditis is through a biopsy and histologic study.[8,9] In other words, getting a biopsy of the thyroid gland can help with the diagnosis of Hashimoto's in the absence of positive thyroid antibodies, although I can't say this is something that I commonly recommend.

Stage #4. Symptoms are present and there is greater tissue loss. This is the "final" stage of autoimmunity, as it's when the person's symptoms will usually worsen, there is greater tissue loss, and the thyroid blood tests are positive. Although some people might be diagnosed with an autoimmune thyroid condition in stage #3, many people with Hashimoto's won't be diagnosed until they reach stage #4 because the symptoms of Hashimoto's can't be measured.

In other words, if someone with Hashimoto's is in stage #3 and presents with negative blood tests, yet they are experiencing symptoms related to Hashimoto's such as fatigue and brain fog, these aren't considered to be objective findings, as such symptoms are only perceived by the patient. However, if someone is in stage #3 and has negative blood tests, often-times, doing a good case history and conducting a thorough examination can help determine if they have a thyroid imbalance. However, this isn't always the case, and, unfortunately, many medical doctors won't further evaluate the health of the thyroid gland if all of the blood tests look good to them.

Why Do Some People Have More Extreme Symptoms Than Others?

One question you might have is why some people with Hashimoto's experience more severe symptoms than others. Well, one reason is because different people will have different triggers, which can lead to different symptoms. For example, if someone's trigger was an infection, then this person might experience not only hypothyroid symptoms due to the damage caused to the thyroid gland but also other symptoms caused by the infection. And the type of symptoms depends on the infection, as someone with Lyme disease will usually present with different symptoms compared to someone who has an H. pylori infection.

Another overlooked factor is that different people will have different nutrient deficiencies, which can also cause different symptoms. Environmental toxins are also a factor, and while everyone is exposed to environmental toxins, some people are exposed to a much greater amount than the average person and others might have challenges eliminating toxins from their body.

Chapter Highlights:

- Autoimmunity happens when the body doesn't recognize its own cells and tissues as self.
- The triad of autoimmunity includes: 1) a genetic predisposition, 2) an environmental trigger, and 3) a leaky gut.
- Different autoimmune conditions will have different types of genetic markers.
- Regulatory T cells are immune cells that help prevent autoimmunity from occurring.
- While both oral and central tolerance helps to protect us against foreign antigens, oral tolerance is more dependent on regulatory T cells, while central tolerance is more dependent on the function of the thymus.
- Either a loss of oral or central tolerance is necessary to cause an autoimmune condition such as Hashimoto's.
- The four stages of the autoimmunity timeline include: 1) pre-autoimmunity, 2) silent autoimmunity, 3) symptoms present with some tissue loss, and 4) symptoms present with greater tissue loss.

· CHAPTER 2 ·

ANTECEDENTS, TRIGGERS, AND
MEDIATORS OF HASHIMOTO'S

THE INSTITUTE FOR FUNCTIONAL Medicine focuses a great deal on antecedents, triggers, and mediators, as addressing these three factors are essential for anyone looking to get into remission and achieve a state of optimal health. This is especially true for triggers and mediators, although we can't ignore the antecedents. In this book, I dedicate an entire section to the different triggers of Hashimoto's, but I'm going to briefly discuss triggers in this chapter, along with the role of antecedents and mediators.

1. Antecedents. With regards to Hashimoto's, or any other chronic health condition, think of an antecedent as a predisposing factor to your condition. It can be a factor that is congenital in nature, or something acquired early in life. For example, being exposed to an environmental toxicant in utero would be one example of an antecedent. Other examples include if you were born via a C-section, weren't breastfed as a baby, and/or received many antibiotics as a child. All of these factors can set the stage for an autoimmune thyroid condition such as Hashimoto's; thus, they would be classified as being antecedents.

Why bother looking at the antecedents if you can't change them? After all, if you had been exposed to an environmental toxicant in utero or were born via a C-section, you can't go back in time and change these factors.

Well, even though you can't turn back time, being aware of the antecedent can still provide some important information.

For example, if someone received antibiotics frequently during childhood, then there is a good chance that this caused intestinal dysbiosis, and perhaps an increase in intestinal permeability (a leaky gut). If these factors were never addressed, then this can be the main factor that made the person susceptible to developing Hashimoto's.

Another example involves the person having a specific genetic polymorphism (a common genetic defect). While this can't be reversed, identifying the polymorphism can help determine what type of nutritional support the person may need. Some people reading this may have an MTHFR C677T genetic polymorphism, which can affect the metabolism of folate, which, in turn, can cause a number of different problems. While you can't reverse an existing MTHFR polymorphism, you can take nutritional support to help with this genetic defect.

While you can't do anything to reverse genetic polymorphisms, you can take measures to improve methylation through diet and supplementation. I'll provide a personal example, as I am homozygous for the MTHFR C677T gene. In the past, this resulted in elevated homocysteine levels, which in turn is a cardiovascular risk factor. While I can't reverse the C677T mutation, I take nutritional support to keep homocysteine at a healthy level.

2. Triggers. According to the textbook for The Institute for Functional Medicine, a trigger is defined as "anything that initiates an acute illness or the emergence of symptoms."[10] Although genetics play a role in Hashimoto's, not everyone who has a genetic predisposition will develop this condition. There needs to be some type of trigger that leads to the initiation of the autoimmune process.

Many factors can trigger an autoimmune response, and I'll be discussing these factors in greater detail in the second section of this book. Some potential triggers of thyroid autoimmunity include food allergens such as gluten or dairy, pathogens such as H. pylori or Epstein-Barr, certain environmental toxins (e.g., mercury), overtraining, and even stressful life events.

How does someone find out what specifically is triggering their condition? Is it possible for them to have multiple triggers? I'll answer the second question first, as, no doubt, it is possible for someone to have multiple autoimmune triggers.

For example, someone can be dealing with chronic stress and an infection. Either one of these can result in autoimmunity. The prolonged chronic stress might have made the person more susceptible to getting an infection by decreasing secretory IgA, which serves as a form of protection. The infection, in turn, can cause a leaky gut. These factors combined caused a decrease in regulatory T cells and a loss of immune tolerance, which triggered an autoimmune response, thus leading to the development of Hashimoto's. In order for this person to restore their health, they need to not only remove the infection and heal the gut but also improve their stress-management skills as well.

Sticking to the topic of healing the gut, a leaky gut is a factor in autoimmune conditions such as Hashimoto's. I'll discuss in greater detail Hashimoto's and the immune-gut connection in Chapter 3, but if you have read articles and other books that discuss autoimmunity, then you may be aware that approximately 70% to 80% of the immune cells are located within the gut. Thus, one can't have a healthy immune system without having a healthy gut.

How someone finds out what factor or factors are responsible for triggering the autoimmune response usually involves a combination of taking a good health history and doing the proper testing. For example, if someone traveled outside of the country, developed gastrointestinal symptoms, and later was diagnosed with Hashimoto's, one might suspect that a parasitic infection was the potential trigger.

Obviously, there is also a chance that another factor triggered the autoimmune response, but, in this scenario, it would still be a good idea to do some testing for parasites. This is especially true if the person were still experiencing gastrointestinal symptoms at the time of the testing. In section three, I'll discuss how to detect triggers through both a thorough health history and testing.

3. Mediators. A mediator is anything that perpetuates the symptoms caused by the trigger, and it can cause damage to the tissues of the body. For Hashimoto's, a good example of a mediator is a proinflammatory cytokine. As the name implies, proinflammatory cytokines promote inflammation.

For example, if someone with a genetic predisposition to Hashimoto's has a gluten sensitivity and eats some wheat bread, the gluten can cause an increase in proinflammatory cytokines, which are involved in the inflammatory process. The cytokines and inflammation can be seen as mediators.

In this scenario, even when the trigger, gluten, has been removed from the diet, the inflammation will still remain for a while.

Why Removing the Trigger Alone Usually Won't Eliminate the Inflammation

Although there are other types of mediators, because inflammation is a factor with everyone who has Hashimoto's, I want to focus more on this here. Something called Nuclear Factor Kappa B (NF-kB) is a transcription factor that plays a role in the inflammatory process. When someone gets exposed to an autoimmune trigger, this, in turn, will activate proinflammatory cytokines.

These cytokines promote inflammation. While the activation of NF-kB is a normal process, what occurs with autoimmunity is the chronic activation of NF-kB. Thus, you have a vicious cycle that perpetuates the inflammation, even after the autoimmune trigger has been removed.

As a result, it is necessary to downregulate NF-kB. This can be accomplished through diet, stress management, and taking certain nutrients and herbs. For example, although vitamin D is known for the role it plays in bone health by increasing the intestinal absorption of calcium, it is also important in modulating the immune system. Vitamin D can help inhibit NF-kB.[11,12] This is yet another reason why anyone with Hashimoto's needs to make sure they have healthy levels of vitamin D, which should be at least 50 ng/ml (125 nmol/L), and between 60 and 80 ng/ml would be even better.

Turmeric is a wonderful herb with the active compound curcumin, which can help inhibit NF-kB.[13,14,15] However, you should keep a few things to keep in mind about turmeric. First, turmeric is poorly absorbed. Thus, if you plan on eating turmeric or take a turmeric supplement, then you need to combine it with other substances to enhance its absorption. Piperine, which is an alkaloid that is responsible for the pungency of black pepper, can greatly increase the bioavailability of curcumin in humans.[16,17]

Another option is to combine turmeric with a liposome or phospholipid complex. This involves combining turmeric with a source of fat, which can also increase its absorption.[18] As for the dosage of turmeric one should take, I usually recommend between 500 to 2,000 mg/day to my patients, although higher doses than this can sometimes be beneficial.

Another thing to keep in mind is that black pepper is one of those "gray areas" with regards to autoimmunity. While I've had patients with

Hashimoto's consume black pepper without a problem, some sources suggest that it should be taken with caution.

Green tea also can help reduce inflammation. You probably are aware that green tea is rich in antioxidants, and it can help downregulate NF-kB.[19,20] Green tea has much less caffeine than coffee, as according to the Mayo Clinic, brewed coffee can have anywhere between 95 and 200 mg of caffeine per eight ounces of coffee, whereas green tea will average 24 to 45 mg of caffeine.[21] However, many people with Hashimoto's should avoid caffeine and drink decaffeinated green tea, preferably one that is organic. This is especially true if someone has adrenal problems or is a slow metabolizer of caffeine.

Just keep in mind that decaffeinated green tea has fewer antioxidants than caffeinated green tea,[22] so it probably isn't as effective when it comes to inhibiting NF-kB when compared to caffeinated green tea. However, studies have shown that decaffeinated green tea can still decrease proinflammatory cytokines.[23] Just remember that not all decaffeinated green teas are the same, so you want to use a brand that is careful with the extraction process in order to retain most of the antioxidants.

More About Regulatory T Cells

In addition to downregulating or inhibiting NF-kB, you also want to have an abundance of regulatory T cells (Tregs), which I briefly discussed in Chapter 1. A few different regulatory mechanisms help maintain immune homeostasis and prevent the development of autoimmune thyroid conditions such as Hashimoto's. One of the main components of the immune system that helps to prevent autoimmunity is having an abundance of Tregs.

Tregs are widely regarded as the primary mediators of peripheral tolerance.[24] Tregs originate in the thymus, although they also can be derived from peripheral CD4+ T cells.[25] A healthy immune system will have an abundance of these Tregs. However, autoimmunity not only involves a decrease in Tregs and a loss of immune tolerance, but it also involves an imbalance of the Th1 and Th2 pathways, and an increase in Th17 cells.[26]

While Th17 cells play an important role in getting rid of extracellular bacterial and fungal infections, uncontrolled Th17 activation can play a role in the development of autoimmunity.[27,28] In the previous chapter, I mentioned how evidence shows that an increase in Th17 cells plays a role in the pathogenesis of Hashimoto's.[29,30] Thus, when dealing with someone who has an autoimmune thyroid condition, one of the main goals should be to increase the number and activity of the Tregs, while, at the same time, taking measures to help suppress the Th17 cells.

Decreasing Harmful Th17 Cells Through Nutrients and Herbs

The good news is that the nutrients I just mentioned, which can help downregulate NF-kB (vitamin D, turmeric, and green tea), can also help increase the number of Tregs and decrease Th17 cells. Besides making sure you have healthy vitamin D levels, you can also drink some green tea and take some turmeric regularly.

Other nutrients can also help modulate the immune system in a positive way. These include omega 3 fatty acids[31,32] and probiotics.[33,34] Thus, I have nearly all of my patients with Hashimoto's take a probiotic supplement with well-researched strains, and eat some fermented foods such as sauerkraut, kimchi, and/or pickles. I also recommend a good quality omega 3 fatty acid supplement that is third-party tested for heavy metals and other contaminants, along with a low oxidation level. I usually recommend between 1,000 and 2,000 mg of EPA and between 500 and 1,000 mg of DHA per day.

Research also shows that vitamin A can increase Tregs while decreasing Th17 cells.[35] As of this writing, controversy is brewing about whether medical marijuana should be legalized in all states, but researchers have shown that Δ-9-tetrahydrocannabinol, which is the main psychoactive cannabinoid of cannabis, can modulate the immune system by decreasing Th17 cells, along with interleukin 6.[36] Interleukin 6 (IL6) is a proinflammatory cytokine.

One of the reasons why many of the same nutrients that increase Tregs will also help decrease Th17 cells is because high amounts of Tregs can help decrease Th17 cells and, in some cases, even halt the production of Th17 cells. Fortunately, the reverse isn't true, as large amounts of Th17 cells won't completely shut down the production of Tregs, although it can cause a decrease in Tregs.

A Word of Caution About Taking Nutrients and Herbs to Modulate the Immune System

I mentioned earlier how removing the trigger alone usually won't eliminate the inflammation. However, removing the trigger is important. If this weren't the case, then I wouldn't have written a book that focuses on the triggers of Hashimoto's. Although I spent much of this chapter showing you how to increase Tregs and decrease Th17 cells, taking supplements, such as turmeric and vitamin D, will have minimal impact if you don't remove the autoimmune trigger. However, even after removing the trigger, the inflammatory process might still be present; that's when taking these nutrients and herbs can be beneficial.

Don't Forget About Diet and Stress Management

Although I focused on some of the main nutrients and herbs that can help reduce inflammation, I want to emphasize the importance of eating a diet consisting of whole foods, while at the same time avoiding the allergens that commonly cause inflammation, such as gluten, dairy, and corn. Obviously, there can be other food allergens responsible for this, but gluten, dairy, and corn are three of the main culprits.

In addition, certain foods can also cause an increase in intestinal permeability. As a result, these foods are excluded from an autoimmune Paleo diet. In Chapter 26, I'll further discuss this diet, including the foods that are excluded.

Stress can also be a big factor when it comes to inflammation. Cortisol is considered the most important hormone involved in the stress response. It also plays a big role in controlling inflammation. Thus, if someone has depressed cortisol levels, this will reduce their ability to control inflammation. By the time you're done reading this book, I'm confident that you'll have a pretty good idea of what to do to achieve optimal adrenal health, which includes having healthy cortisol levels.

What Other Mediators Can Be Present Besides Inflammation?

Remember that a mediator is anything that either produces symptoms, or perpetuates the damage to the tissues. In addition to proinflammatory cytokines, other mediators include hormones, neurotransmitters, and free radicals. According to the Institute for Functional Medicine, these are "biochemical" mediators, but they also discuss cognitive and emotional mediators, such as fear of pain or loss, learned helplessness, along with social/cultural mediators.[37]

Chapter Highlights:

- Antecedents, triggers, and mediators play a big role in the development of Hashimoto's.
- Think of an antecedent as a predisposing factor.
- Examples of antecedents include being born via a C-section, not being breastfed, and receiving many antibiotics during childhood.
- Some type of trigger leads to the initiation of the autoimmune response.
- Some potential triggers of Hashimoto's include food allergens, infections, environmental toxins, stress, and trauma.
- A mediator is anything that perpetuates the symptoms caused by the trigger.
- Some examples of mediators include proinflammatory cytokines, hormones, neurotransmitters, and free radicals.
- Although removing the autoimmune trigger is important, doing this alone usually won't eliminate the inflammation.
- With autoimmune conditions such as Hashimoto's, you want to have an abundance of regulatory T cells (Tregs) and attempt to decrease Th17 cells.

CHAPTER 3

HASHIMOTO'S AND THE IMMUNE GUT CONNECTION

M ANY PEOPLE AND POSSIBLY everyone with an autoimmune condition such as Hashimoto's thyroiditis have an increase in intestinal permeability, also known as a leaky gut. A healthy gut is characterized by intact tight junctions, which are a multi-protein complex that forms the main barrier that prevents the passage of large molecules into the bloodstream. While these tight junctions prevent larger molecules from passing into the bloodstream, they allow ions, nutrients, and water to pass through.[38]

These tight junctions can be damaged by different factors, including but not limited to food allergens, infections, and environmental chemicals. This damage to the intestinal barrier allows proteins and other large molecules to pass into the bloodstream where they normally shouldn't be. This, in turn, causes an immune system response, which, when combined with a decrease in Tregs and a loss of immune tolerance, can result in the development of autoimmune conditions such as Hashimoto's.

In fact, there is evidence that all autoimmune conditions involve a disruption of the intestinal barrier. In other words, you can't have an autoimmune condition such Hashimoto's without having a leaky gut. I brought this up in Chapter 1 when I discussed the triad of autoimmunity, which involves a genetic predisposition, an environmental trigger, and a leaky gut.

Dr. Alessio Fasano is the researcher who first proposed this theory. He has done extensive research on intestinal permeability and autoimmunity. In a journal article entitled "Tight Junctions, Intestinal Permeability, and Autoimmunity celiac disease and Type 1 Diabetes Paradigms," Dr. Fasano concluded that "genetic predisposition, miscommunication between innate and adaptive immunity, exposure to environmental triggers, and loss of intestinal barrier function secondary to dysfunction of intercellular tight junctions all seem to be key components in the pathogenesis of autoimmune diseases".[39] In summary, Dr. Fasano discusses how a loss of intestinal barrier function is a key component in the development of an autoimmune condition such as Hashimoto's. This makes a lot of sense when you look at the mechanisms involved.

What Causes a Leaky Gut?

Just as a reminder, I use the words *increase in intestinal permeability* and *leaky gut* interchangeably throughout this book. Before I discuss some of the common causes of a leaky gut, it's important to understand that just because someone lacks gastrointestinal symptoms (i.e., stomach pain, gas, bloating) doesn't confirm that their digestive system is in good health. Although symptoms can frequently be a good indicator of a gut problem, the lack of digestive symptoms doesn't rule out a leaky gut.

For example, gluten is a common allergen, and, as a result, many people who are gluten sensitive will feel significantly better from a symptomatic standpoint when avoiding gluten. However, some people who are sensitive to gluten don't experience any digestive symptoms upon being exposed to gluten. Consuming gluten when they have a sensitivity will still have a negative effect on their gastrointestinal health, as well as other areas of the body.

Research shows that an increase in intestinal permeability occurs after gluten exposure in all individuals, even those who don't have celiac disease.[40] However, while a small amount of gluten may increase intestinal permeability, oral tolerance helps suppress the immune response in most cases. I discussed oral tolerance in Chapter 1. Having oral tolerance explains why a healthy person might be able to consume gluten without a problem, but the excessive exposure to gluten and/or other factors can result in a loss of oral tolerance, which, in turn, can lead to inflammation, food sensitivities, and, eventually, the development of autoimmunity.

Just as a reminder, in order to have oral tolerance you need to have an abundance of regulatory T cells (Tregs). Approximately 80% of these Tregs are located in the gut, so it shouldn't be surprising that having a healthy gut environment is important to have a healthy number of Tregs. Short chain fatty acids (SCFAs) such as butyrate are produced in the intestine, and numerous studies show that they play an important role in increasing Tregs and helping to regulate the Treg/Th17 balance.[41,42]

Other Factors That Can Cause a Leaky Gut

While gluten and other food allergens can cause a leaky gut, other factors can cause this condition. Stress can cause many different problems, including an increase in intestinal permeability.[43] One way chronic stress can accomplish this is by decreasing secretory IgA, which lines the mucosal surfaces of the body, including the gastrointestinal tract. This, in turn, can make the person more susceptible to an infection, which, in turn, can increase gut permeability.

Taking antibiotics will affect the integrity of the gut lining, will usually cause intestinal dysbiosis (an imbalance of the gut flora), and can lead to a leaky gut.[44] NSAIDS can also cause an increase in intestinal permeability.[45] The frequent consumption of alcohol can also lead to a leaky gut.[46] Even exposure to certain environmental toxins can potentially lead to a leaky gut.[47] Thus, as you can see, several different factors can lead to an increase in gut permeability.

What Are Lipopolysaccharides?

Lipopolysaccharides (LPS) are the major components of the cell wall of gram-negative bacteria.[48] Under normal circumstances, they protect the cell membrane. However, when a gram-negative bacteria dies, the LPS of this bacteria is released. LPS can cause many biological effects, such as fever, leukocytosis (high number of white blood cells), iron deficiency, platelet aggregation, thrombocytopenia, and blood clotting disorders.[49] I'm bringing up lipopolysaccharides in this chapter because they can lead to an increase in intestinal permeability.[50,51]

Testing for a Leaky Gut

In Chapter 25 I'll discuss some of the different testing options for a leaky gut. I'll cover the lactulose-mannitol test, along with the Intestinal Antigenic Permeability Screen from Cyrex Labs. Other labs test for zonulin, a protein that regulates intestinal permeability by modulating intercellular tight junctions.[52] Increased zonulin levels usually correlates with dysfunction of the tight junctions and, therefore, an increase in intestinal permeability.[52]

What's the Deal with Positive Autoantibodies and a Negative Leaky Gut Test?

My practice focuses on thyroid and autoimmune thyroid conditions. As a result, I see many people with Hashimoto's. Although I currently don't test most of my patients for the presence of a leaky gut, in the past I ran a decent number of these tests. While some of my patients had obtained the lactulose-mannitol test, most of the time, I recommended the Intestinal Antigenic Permeability Screen (Array #2) from Cyrex Labs.

Many of these test results came back positive, but some came back negative in patients with elevated autoantibodies. As I mentioned earlier, I've also had some patients test negative for the lactulose-mannitol test, even though they had recent elevated thyroid autoantibodies on a blood test.

So what exactly does this mean? Well, this means that either not everyone with an autoimmune condition has a leaky gut or that these intestinal permeability tests aren't 100% accurate. Although the lactulose-mannitol test has a high sensitivity, it still is possible that it can fail to detect an increase in intestinal permeability in some cases. I'm sure the same can be true with the Cyrex Labs testing.

With the Array #2 from Cyrex Labs, if someone has suppressed immunoglobulins, this can cause a false negative result. Thus, before doing the Array #2, it probably would be a good idea to do a separate blood test for serum immunoglobulin A, immunoglobulin G, and immunoglobulin M, as these are the immunoglobulins utilized on the panel. You can get this done at most local labs.

Should You Be Tested for a Leaky Gut?

Based on what I just stated, you might wonder if it is worth spending the money to test for a leaky gut. Many healthcare professionals bypass the testing and assume that everyone with an autoimmune condition has a leaky gut. In other words, they'll put all of their autoimmune patients on a gut repair protocol without doing any testing to confirm the presence of a leaky gut.

Although testing for a leaky gut does have some drawbacks, one also has to consider the benefits. For example, if someone obtains a test for a leaky gut and it comes out positive, this provides a baseline reading. In other words, if someone tests positive for a leaky gut and is put on a gut repair protocol, they can choose to do a follow-up test later as a way of monitoring their progress.

Someone may elect to not do another test if their overall health is improving, but they will only do a retest if they aren't progressing as expected. Obviously, different natural healthcare professionals will take different approaches, and while I currently don't have most of my patients test for a leaky gut, I think that such testing has some value.

How to Heal a Leaky Gut

The good news is that it is possible to heal a leaky gut. I am going to discuss this in greater detail in a Chapter 28, although I'll briefly discuss a few important points here. When trying to heal a leaky gut, the most important thing you need to do is to remove the factor that caused the leaky gut. For example, if you have a gluten sensitivity that caused your leaky gut, then you obviously need to stop consuming gluten.

If you have an infection that caused intestinal barrier dysfunction, then the infection needs to be addressed. Identifying the factor that caused the leaky gut isn't always easy to do, but it's necessary in order to heal your gut. Many people just take supplements, such as L-glutamine, or drink bone broth. While both of these can help with gut healing, the gut won't completely heal if the leaky gut trigger isn't removed.

In addition to removing the "leaky gut trigger," it's also recommended to follow a diet that 1) includes foods that can help heal the gut, and 2) reduces the consumption of compounds that can have negative effects on gut health. I'll discuss in greater detail the autoimmune Paleo diet in Chapter 26, and in Chapter 28, I will also discuss foods and supplements that can assist with gut healing.

Direct Triggers vs. Leaky Gut Triggers

Finding out the factor that caused the leaky gut in the first place can get confusing at times, as the "leaky gut trigger" can be the same as the "direct" environmental trigger, although this isn't always the case. For example, for those who have celiac disease, gluten is not only the environmental trigger, but gluten also has been shown to cause an increase in intestinal permeability in everyone, regardless of whether or not they have a sensitivity to gluten. Thus, with celiac disease, gluten is both the "direct" environmental trigger and the "leaky gut" trigger.

However, in some situations, the leaky gut trigger might differ from the environmental trigger. For example, someone with a genetic predisposition to developing Hashimoto's might have a history of taking antibiotics, which can cause a leaky gut. Thus, this person has a genetic predisposition and a leaky gut, but the autoimmune process hasn't started yet, since they haven't been exposed to an environmental trigger. Then, one day, this person is infected with Yersinia enterocolitica, which, in this case, is the environmental trigger, and they develop thyroid autoantibodies. Thus, in this example, the antibiotics were the "leaky gut trigger," but not the environmental trigger.

Differentiating Between the Environmental Trigger and Leaky Gut Trigger

The truth is that it can be challenging to differentiate between the environmental and leaky gut trigger. In the example I just gave, while the excessive use of antibiotics might have caused the leaky gut, it's also possible that the infection (Yersinia enterocolitica) caused the leaky gut. Thus, while gluten is both the environmental trigger and the leaky gut trigger in celiac disease, it's probably safe to say that, in many cases of Hashimoto's, the environmental trigger and the leaky gut trigger are also the same, although this isn't always the case. Hopefully, you don't find this to be too confusing, but the overall point is that the ultimate goal should be to remove anything that can be either an environmental trigger, a leaky gut trigger, or both.

What Should You Do if You Test Negative for a Leaky Gut?

If you have elevated thyroid antibodies (i.e., thyroid peroxidase and/or thyroglobulin antibodies), and you choose to order an intestinal permeability test, what should you do if you test negative for a leaky gut? Should you assume that the test is accurate and not provide any gut repair support? Although I don't recommend leaky gut testing as frequently as I used to, if someone with Hashimoto's orders such a test and the results are negative, then I still would recommend that they support their gut. Even if they don't have a leaky gut, it's not going to hurt to take measures to improve the health of their gut.

What Is The Microbiome?

Although the primary focus of this chapter is on the connection between having a leaky gut and autoimmunity, I think it's important that you have a basic understanding of the human microbiome. The microbiome is composed of bacteria, archaea, viruses, and eukaryotic microbes that reside in and on our bodies, and these microbes can have a profound impact on our physiology.[53] Healthy adult humans each typically harbor more than 1,000 species of bacteria, and the microbiota of the gut is more diverse when compared to other areas of the body.[53] Unfortunately, many people have their gut microbiota disrupted by eating a poor diet, being exposed to environmental toxins, and taking antibiotics. While these factors can also lead to an increase in intestinal permeability, having a disrupted microbiome can also be a factor in autoimmunity.

In Chapter 1, I discussed immune tolerance, as the immune system plays a key role in eliminating harmful pathogens while, at the same time, tolerating our self tissues, along with the food we eat and the good bacteria in our gut. However, having an unhealthy microbiome can lead to a loss of immune tolerance, which can set the stage for a condition such as Hashimoto's. One of the main reasons for this is because the gut microbiota play a role in the development of T helper cells, which include not only Th1, Th2, and Th17 cells but also Tregs.

I mentioned earlier how factors such as poor diet, exposure to environmental chemicals, and taking antibiotics can disrupt the microbiome. However, it's important to mention that microbial colonization begins at birth, which plays a role in determining the health of the gut microbiota. For example, the method of delivery (vaginal birth vs. cesarean section), as well as whether you were breastfed or given formula as a baby played a role in your gut microbiota. While you can't go back in time and change these factors, you can take action now to improve the health of your gut, which I'll discuss in detail in section four of this book.

Chapter Highlights:

- A leaky gut involves damage to the intestinal barrier, which allows proteins and other larger molecules to pass into the bloodstream, which, in turn, causes an immune system response.
- Dr. Alessio Fasano concluded that a genetic predisposition, miscommunication between innate and adaptive immunity, exposure to environmental triggers, and loss of intestinal barrier function secondary to dysfunction of intercellular tight junctions all seem to be key components in the pathogenesis of autoimmune diseases.
- It's important to understand that the lack of gastrointestinal symptoms doesn't rule out a leaky gut.
- The research shows that an increase in intestinal permeability occurs after gluten exposure in all individuals.
- Other factors that can cause a leaky gut include infections, stress, and certain medications.
- Two methods of testing for a leaky gut include the lactulose-mannitol test, and the Intestinal Antigenic Permeability Screen by Cyrex Labs.
- Many natural healthcare professionals don't do any leaky gut testing and assume that everyone with Hashimoto's has a leaky gut.
- In order to heal a leaky gut, you must remove those factors that caused the leaky gut in the first place.
- The gut microbiota play a role in the development Th1, Th2, and Th17 cells, along with regulatory T cells.
- Having an unhealthy microbiome can lead to a loss of immune tolerance, which can set the stage for a condition such as Hashimoto's.

CHAPTER 4

HASHIMOTO'S AND THE HYGIENE HYPOTHESIS

I WAS DEBATING WHETHER TO include this chapter in this section, or in the triggers section. I decided on the former because the hygiene hypothesis doesn't relate directly to environmental triggers, or to "leaky gut" triggers. The basis behind the hygiene hypothesis is that we're not being exposed to as many microorganisms, which weakens or suppresses our immune system. This, in turn, can make us more susceptible to developing infections, allergies, and autoimmune conditions such as Hashimoto's.

The *New England Journal of Medicine* published an interesting article entitled "Eat Dirt—The Hygiene Hypothesis and Allergic Diseases".[54] This article begins by pointing out that there has been an epidemic of both autoimmune and allergic diseases, which are more common in Western, industrialized countries. It goes on to discuss how this increase in the prevalence of autoimmune and allergic diseases results from a decrease in the exposure to both good and bad microorganisms. In other words, according to the hygiene hypothesis, a decreased prevalence of childhood infections can actually be a factor in the increases in autoimmunity.

This might seem to be counterintuitive to some people, as many believe that it is wise to avoid all potentially pathogenic microorganisms. This is one of the reasons why many vaccines are given during childhood these days, and why many people receive an annual flu shot. I'm not suggesting that it's beneficial for adults to get the flu, or for children to get serious illnesses such as polio or tetanus. However, we are going to extremes to avoid exposure to all of these microorganisms, and, according to the hygiene hypothesis, there can be negative consequences for those who take this approach.

Why Are We Not Being Exposed to as Many Microorganisms?

1. We spend too much time indoors. As a child, I didn't have access to all of the electronics that are available these days, so I frequently went outside to play with my friends. These days, many children spend too much time on electronic devices and not enough time exploring the environment. But it's not just children who don't spend enough time outdoors. On average, adults are spending more and more time indoors as well.

2. We are becoming too sanitary. Widespread access to clean water, soap, and chemicals to aid in cleaning dates back to the end of the 19th century;[55] thus, this is unlikely to be a big factor in the development of autoimmunity. However, one thing that has changed greatly is the use of hand sanitizers. When I was a child, there wasn't the widespread use of hand sanitizers as there is today. While soap was available, chemicals such as Triclosan weren't in all of the soaps like they are these days. Triclosan is a chemical commonly used in soaps and hand sanitizers, and I'm going to discuss it in greater detail shortly.

3. The birth process. Most births take place in a hospital setting, and, frequently, the baby is bathed too soon. Babies are born covered in a white substance called vernix, which is a protective material that helps to prevent common infections. While this chapter focuses on how we should be exposed to a greater number of microorganisms, in this situation, you want to delay bathing a newborn due to the antimicrobial properties of the vernix.[56] This is why some hospitals enforce "delayed bathing."

If the hygiene hypothesis is true, then the increase in cesarean deliveries can also play a role in the development of autoimmunity related to the hygiene hypothesis[57] because being born via a C-section can potentially lead to a change in long-term colonization of the developing intestinal tract, which, in turn, can alter the development of the immune system.[57] Approximately one third of births in the United States are through cesarean delivery. While some of these are necessary, many others are due to maternal request.

4. Vaccines. I've dedicated a separate chapter in section two that focuses on vaccinations (Chapter 19). However, I will say here that many more vaccines are given these days than in the past, which further reduces the chances of children and teenagers getting infections. I realize that some of these infections can be life threatening, and everything comes down to risks vs. benefits. While it's understandable for parents to be concerned about their children developing certain infections, they should also be concerned about the risks associated with vaccines as well, not only as they relate to the hygiene hypothesis, but also the additives included in them. According to the Centers for Disease Control (which is in favor of vaccines), some of the common substances found in vaccines include aluminum, antibiotics, formaldehyde, monosodium glutamine (MSG), and thimerosal.[58]

More About Triclosan

Since many people use hand sanitizers, I'd like to spend a little more time discussing triclosan, and why you should avoid this as much possible. Triclosan has broad-spectrum antimicrobial activity against most gram-negative and gram-positive bacteria.[59] Because of this, one of the most common uses of triclosan is in hand sanitizer products. Millions of people use hand sanitizer to kill the germs they're exposed to, but most don't realize the potential risks of using products with triclosan.

In addition to commonly being found in hand sanitizer, triclosan is also commonly found in antibacterial soap, as well as in some toothpastes. Researchers have detected triclosan in breast milk, urine, and plasma, with levels of triclosan in the blood correlating with consumer use patterns of the antimicrobial.[60] So let's look at some of the potential health risks of using triclosan:

1. Using hand sanitizers consisting of triclosan can lead to antimicrobial resistance. Many bacterial strains have become resistant to oral antibiotics. This, of course, is a big problem because, while antibiotics are overused, they can save lives in certain situations. However, many people take them unnecessarily, and because some don't take the antibiotics for the recommended duration, this has contributed to the development of bacteria that are resistant to these antibiotics.

The concept is similar with triclosan, as, these days, you see hand sanitizer dispensers almost everywhere you go. I can understand wanting to practice good hygiene, but what happened to using regular soap and water? Evidence shows that the overuse of triclosan has been linked to antimicrobial resistance to E. Coli, Salmonella, and Staphylococcus aureus.[61,62]

2. Triclosan is an endocrine disruptor. Having endocrine disrupting properties is a concern with everyone, but it is arguably an even greater cause for concern with those who have Hashimoto's. Current laboratory studies in various species provide strong evidence for triclosan's disrupting effects on the endocrine system, especially reproductive hormones.[63] Evidence exists that triclosan directly affects thyroid hormone, as one study showed that thyroid hormone levels were suppressed by triclosan,[64] while another study mentioned that triclosan impairs thyroid homeostasis.[65] One study did show that triclosan toothpaste had no detectable effect on thyroid function.[66] However, while research shows that triclosan-based toothpastes provide a more effective level of plaque control and gingival health,[67] I still would be cautious about using a toothpaste that includes this chemical.

3. Evidence indicates that triclosan can cause cancer or enhance cancer progression. One study showed that the progression of breast cancer cells was enhanced by triclosan, as well as another chemical called octylphenol.[68] This isn't suggesting that triclosan will cause breast cancer, but it may promote the progression of breast cancer that is already present. Another study showed that prostate cancer cells are promoted by triclosan.[69] Yet another study showed that triclosan is a promoter of liver tumors.[70]

To be fair, these studies were conducted on rats, which don't always translate to humans. However, we also can't assume that triclosan is safe just because there is a lack of human studies. In fact, I would take the opposite approach with this and other chemicals, as I would assume something isn't safe unless human studies prove otherwise.

4. Triclosan causes mitochondrial dysfunction. Mitochondria are organelles that play a critical role in the generation of energy derived from the breakdown of carbohydrates and fatty acids. A 2017 journal article revealed that triclosan, at low micromolar concentrations, causes mitochondrial dysfunction in many cell types, although the mechanisms are not fully understood.[71]

What Can You Do?

Most people reading this book already have Hashimoto's. If you are one of them, preventing the development of this autoimmune thyroid condition doesn't apply to you. However, this doesn't mean that you should ignore the information in this chapter. If the hygiene hypothesis is one of the factors responsible for the increase in autoimmunity over the last few decades, then following some of the advice given in this chapter can still help benefit your immune system health. In addition, if you have children or grandchildren or plan on having children in the future, then this information can greatly benefit them.

Accordingly, here are some things you should consider doing:

1. Spend more time outdoors. This admittedly is something I need to do more of, as, without a doubt, I spend too much time indoors.

2. Use more natural soaps and avoid soaps and hand sanitizers with triclosan. If you frequently use antimicrobial soaps and hand sanitizers, then I would encourage you to switch to more natural products. There are plenty of natural options for soaps and hand sanitizers, including essential oils. The essential oils thyme, mint, cinnamon, salvia, clove, and tea tree oil all have antimicrobial properties. One review study discussed how essential oils could potentially combat bacterial antibiotic resistance.[72] Another study compared the effects of tea tree oil versus triclosan, and found that regarding the antimicrobial efficacy, there was no difference between the soap with triclosan and the soap with the tea tree oil.[73]

3. You want to be cautious about taking antibiotics, and educate yourself about vaccines. While antibiotics are necessary at times, without question, they are overused. This not only can lead to antimicrobial resistance, but antibiotics can also cause a leaky gut. With regards to vaccines, I recommend educating yourself about them, especially if you have young children, grandchildren, or are planning on having children. If you are still in favor of vaccinations, consider spacing them out. Many adults receive vaccinations as well, including the flu shot, which I discuss in Chapter 19.

4. Get a cat and/or a dog. Numerous studies have demonstrated that early-life exposure to pets offers protection against allergic disease.[74,75] I have two cats and two dogs, and my life wouldn't be the same without them!

The Relationship Between Helminths and The Hygiene Hypothesis

Evidence shows an inverse relationship between certain parasitic infections and autoimmune conditions. In other words, certain parasites can modulate the immune system by increasing regulatory T cells (Tregs) and immune tolerance,[76] thus preventing autoimmunity from developing and/or benefiting those who currently have autoimmune conditions. In Chapter 9, I discuss parasites such as Blastocystis hominis as being a potential trigger of Hashimoto's; thus, the theory that parasites can be beneficial might seem contradictory.

However, it's important to understand that while some parasites can promote autoimmunity, others can potentially be beneficial to the human host. Although I considered discussing helminth therapy in a different section, I decided to bring it up here because it relates to the hygiene hypothesis. While more than 25% of the world's populations are infected with helminth parasites,[77] many years ago, most humans carried these types of parasites, and as a result, it is thought that our immune system has "co-evolved" with these organisms.[78]

What Are Helminths?

Helminths are eukaryotic parasitic worms. These parasites are divided into two phyla: Platyhelminthes (flatworms), including both trematodes and cestodes (tapeworms), and Nemathelminthes, which are nematodes (roundworms).[79] Helminths usually live in the gastrointestinal tract, although they can also colonize other organs. As I mentioned earlier, helminths are thought to suppress autoimmunity by increasing Tregs, along with inhibiting Th1 and Th17 cells.

In addition to its effects on the immune system, helminths might also have a positive effect on the microbiome by increasing the diversity of the microbiota.[80] In other words, helminth therapy might help promote the growth of "good" bacteria in the gut.

How Can Helminth Therapy Benefit Those With Hashimoto's?

Since Hashimoto's thyroiditis is a considered to be a Th1 dominant condition that is also characterized by increased Th17 cells, based on what I said earlier, it would make sense for helminths to be a potential therapy. The truth is that there is currently no evidence in the research demonstrating that helminth therapy can help people with Hashimoto's get into remission. There have been a few clinical trials involving the helminths

Trichuris suis and Necator americanus parasites to see if they can help with conditions such as Crohn's disease,[81] celiac disease,[82] and multiple sclerosis.[83]

Although these studies were promising, they still didn't provide clear evidence that helminth therapy can benefit autoimmunity. However, since numerous studies show that helminths can increase Tregs while decreasing Th1 and Th17 cells, it would make sense that this type of therapy can benefit people with Hashimoto's, as well as other autoimmune conditions. Without question more research is needed, and if you want to learn more about how helminths can potentially benefit your Hashimoto's condition I would recommend reading the book *An Epidemic of Absence: A New Way of Understanding Allergies and Autoimmune Diseases,* by Moises Velasquez-Manoff.

Chapter Highlights:

- The basis behind the hygiene hypothesis is that we're not being exposed to as many microorganisms, which essentially weakens or suppresses our immune system.
- We aren't being exposed to as many microorganisms because 1) we spend too much time indoors, 2) we are becoming too sanitary, 3) the birth process, and 4) vaccines.
- Millions of people use hand sanitizer to kill the germs they're exposed to, but most don't realize that there are some potential risks of using products with triclosan, which is also an endocrine disruptor.
- In addition to commonly being found in hand sanitizer, triclosan is also commonly found in antibacterial soap, as well as in some toothpastes.
- Some things that can be done to prevent autoimmunity from developing is to 1) spend more time outdoors, 2) avoid soaps and hand sanitizers with Triclosan, 3) exercise caution with antibiotics and vaccines, 4) get a cat or dog.
- Certain parasites (helminths) can potentially modulate the immune system by increasing regulatory T cells and immune tolerance.

SECTION TWO

THE TRIGGERS OF HASHIMOTO'S

IN THIS SECTION, I'LL discuss the different triggers of Hashimoto's thyroiditis. In section one, I briefly mentioned how the triad of autoimmunity will determine whether someone will develop an autoimmune condition such as Hashimoto's. The triad includes 1) a genetic predisposition, 2) an environmental trigger, and 3) an increase in intestinal permeability (a leaky gut). Although you can't reverse the genetic predisposition, you can detect and remove the environmental trigger and heal the gut, which can help the person with Hashimoto's achieve a state of remission.

In Chapter 3, I discussed the difference between "direct" environmental triggers and "leaky gut" triggers. A leaky gut trigger is an example of an "indirect" trigger. However, I explained that in some cases the direct environmental trigger and the leaky gut trigger are the same, while in other cases these triggers can be different.

For example, Chapter 16 is dedicated to postpartum thyroiditis, which some consider to be a "direct" trigger of thyroid autoimmunity. However, as I'll explain in the upcoming chapter, in most cases, a woman with postpartum thyroiditis will have elevated thyroid antibodies before the postpartum period. Thus, postpartum thyroiditis is considered an "indirect" trigger.

Another example involves small intestinal bacterial overgrowth, also known as SIBO. Currently, this hasn't been proven to be a direct trigger of Hashimoto's, but because SIBO can cause an increase in intestinal permeability, it can be labeled as a "leaky gut" trigger. If someone has SIBO and is exposed to a "direct" environmental trigger, then not only does the direct environmental trigger need to be removed but SIBO also needs to be addressed in order to heal the gut.

Let's look at one more example. Gluten can be a direct trigger of autoimmunity through a molecular mimicry action; however, it can also be an "indirect" trigger, as it can cause a leaky gut, which is a factor in autoimmunity. Thus, it also can be referred to as a "leaky gut" trigger.

So just to clear up any confusion you might have, here are the two main types of triggers:

- Direct environmental triggers
- Indirect triggers (these include leaky gut triggers but can also include other types of triggers)

Remember that some triggers, such as gluten and infections, can act either as a "direct" environmental trigger or as an indirect trigger (e.g., a leaky gut trigger).

Can You Have More Than One "Direct" Environmental Trigger?

By now, you should understand that it is possible to have a separate "direct" trigger and "leaky gut" trigger. It is also possible to have multiple direct environmental triggers, as well as multiple leaky gut triggers. For example, on a stool panel, someone might test positive for H. pylori and Blastocystis hominis, and they also choose to do the Chemical Immune Reactivity Screen from Cyrex Labs (discussed in Chapter 25) and test positive for mercury. All three of these can be direct triggers of Hashimoto's.

Of course, it's possible that only one of these was the primary trigger. For example, perhaps this person had mercury amalgams for many years and this was the main autoimmune trigger, but then months or years later, they contracted these infections. With someone like this, it would be very challenging or, in many cases, impossible to know which one of these factors was the primary trigger. In any case, the goal in this situation should be to remove all three of these "direct" triggers.

Similarly, it's possible for someone to have more than one "leaky gut" trigger. For example, someone can have SIBO and they might be eating gluten regularly. Both of these factors can cause a leaky gut; thus, both should be addressed.

How Do You Detect and Remove Your Triggers?

Although you might be able to get a good idea about which triggers you have after reading this section, in the third section, I'll discuss how to find these triggers. In the fourth section, I'll discuss what you can do to remove your triggers, balance other compromised areas of your body, and achieve an optimal state of health.

CHAPTER 5

GLUTEN: THE PRIMARY FOOD TRIGGER OF HASHIMOTO'S

MANY NATURAL HEALTHCARE PROFESSIONALS agree that people with Hashimoto's should avoid gluten. Many will suggest that people with any autoimmune condition should not only avoid gluten while trying to restore their health, but should do so permanently. While this might make sense for those who have obvious symptoms when consuming gluten, why should this apply to those who apparently have no problems upon being exposed to gluten? Also, if someone with Hashimoto's goes on a gluten-free trial and doesn't experience an improvement in their symptoms and/or a decrease in their thyroid antibodies, then what's the benefit of continuing to avoid gluten?

What Exactly Is Gluten?

Before discussing why it's a good idea to avoid gluten, I'd like to briefly explain what gluten is. Gluten is a mixture of prolamin proteins present mostly in wheat, but is also found in barley, rye, and oats. Gliadin is the most problematic protein found in gluten, specifically wheat, with glutenin being another protein found in wheat that is responsible for the elastic properties of dough. There are other proteins as well, including hordeins (found in barley), secalins (found in rye), and avenins (found in oats). Speaking of oats, even though they are technically gluten-free, oats are commonly cross-contaminated with gluten.

Five Reasons to Avoid Gluten While Trying to Restore Your Health

Now that you have a basic understanding of what gluten is, let's discuss some of the main reasons why those people with Hashimoto's should completely avoid gluten while trying to restore their health.

Reason #1: Gluten is a common allergen. Many people are sensitive to gluten. When I say sensitive, I don't just mean having celiac disease, which is an autoimmune condition involving gluten. Many people have a non-celiac gluten sensitivity, and I'll discuss this in this chapter. As for why many people have food sensitivities to begin with, certain sequences of amino acids are more likely to cause the production of antibody formation, which is one reason why certain foods such as gluten and dairy are more likely to result in food allergies and sensitivities.

Reason #2: Gluten cannot be completely digested. If you don't have an allergy or sensitivity to gluten, and if you don't experience an improvement in your symptoms and/or a decrease in thyroid antibodies when avoiding gluten, is it okay to eat foods with gluten? Well, even if you don't have a gluten sensitivity and you don't experience any symptoms when consuming it, the gluten proteins of wheat, rye, and barley can't be completely broken down by human digestive enzymes. The reason for this has to do with the high proline content of gluten molecules.[1] One of the consequences of not being able to fully degrade these prolines is that there are large proline-rich gluten fragments, which can cause an increase in proinflammatory cytokines.[1]

Reason #3: Gluten causes a leaky gut in EVERYONE. You are reading this correctly, as the research shows that eating gluten causes an increase in intestinal permeability (a leaky gut) in every single person,[2] even those who don't have a sensitivity to gluten. I mentioned this in Chapter 3, but it's worth repeating again. Since having a leaky gut is a component of the triad of autoimmunity I discussed in section one, eating gluten can be a major roadblock for someone who has Hashimoto's thyroiditis and is trying to get into remission.

Reason #4: Gluten is a potential trigger of Hashimoto's thyroiditis. As I just mentioned, gluten causes an increase in intestinal permeability, which is a factor in autoimmunity. In addition, gluten also can lead to a loss of oral tolerance, which is characterized by a decrease in regulatory T cells.[3, 4]

In addition, some believe that gliadin has an amino acid sequence that resembles that of the thyroid gland. Although I was unable to come across any research demonstrating this, some experts feel strongly about this similarity in amino acid sequence resulting in a molecular mimicry mechanism between the immune response to gluten and some of the proteins that are involved in thyroid function, such as thyroid peroxidase.

Assuming this molecular mimicry theory is correct, if your body develops antibodies to gliadin, the immune system can also mistakenly attack the cells of the thyroid gland. This might explain why so many people with Hashimoto's feel significantly better upon avoiding gluten, and it would also explain why many people experience a decrease in their thyroid antibodies when going on a gluten-free diet.

You might wonder why everyone who eats gluten doesn't develop an autoimmune condition. First, you need to remember the two other components of the triad of autoimmunity. In addition to having a leaky gut, you also need to have a genetic predisposition for Hashimoto's and be exposed to an environmental trigger. I also discussed how you need to have a loss of oral tolerance, which can take years to develop. This is why someone can consume gluten for many years without a problem, but, later in life, develop autoimmunity. Also, we need to keep in mind that gluten isn't always a factor in the development of Hashimoto's, but it is a big factor for many people.

Reason #5: You should focus on eating whole foods. When trying to restore your health, you want to focus on eating whole, healthy foods. No good reason exists to eat bread, pasta, cookies, etc. This is true even if you eat gluten-free versions of these foods, as just because a food is gluten-free doesn't mean that it's healthy for you. I'm not suggesting that you need to eat 100% whole foods permanently, but you should strive to do this while trying to get into remission.

Is Eating a Small Amount of Gluten Every Now and Then Okay?

Even after reading this, I'm sure that some people think that eating a small amount of gluten every now and then isn't a big deal. For some people, it might not be, but if someone has Hashimoto's, or any other autoimmune condition, eating even a small amount of gluten might prevent them from getting into remission. This is true, even if you don't experience any symptoms when eating gluten.

Gluten causes a leaky gut in everyone, and, in order to have a healthy immune system, you need to have a healthy gut. Thus, for this reason alone, I would try to avoid eating gluten while restoring your health.

But what if you have been tested for a gluten sensitivity and it came back negative? Although the third section of this book focuses on all of the different types of testing, I will further discuss testing for gluten in this chapter. However, I'll say the following here: most people who test for gluten antibodies don't obtain comprehensive testing. For example, many people only get the alpha gliadin antibodies tested, and I have had other patients who only were tested for tissue transglutaminase IgA and nothing else. These are individual components of a celiac panel.

In addition, if someone gets a complete celiac panel (I'll describe the components later in this chapter) and it comes back negative, this doesn't rule out a non-celiac gluten sensitivity. Even if the person obtained more comprehensive testing for gluten that came back negative, eating gluten will still increase the permeability of the gut, regardless of whether or not someone is sensitive to it. Thus, it's important to understand that even if you don't have a gluten allergy or sensitivity, avoiding it is still important in order to heal the gut.

Is It Safe to Eat Gluten After Getting Into Remission?

If someone has celiac disease, then, without question, they need to strictly avoid gluten permanently. Eating even a small amount can cause inflammation and an increase in autoantibodies. If someone has a non-celiac gluten sensitivity, then it also is a good idea to continuously avoid gluten. I realize it's not easy to completely avoid gluten, and what makes it even more challenging is that there are many hidden sources of gluten. If you visit **www.naturalendocrinesolutions.com/resources** you can see some of the common sources. Even if you purchase a packaged food that is gluten-free, it still might have traces of gluten in it.

According to the U.S. Food and Drug Administration, one of the criteria proposed is that foods bearing the claim "gluten-free" cannot contain 20 parts per million (ppm) or more gluten.[5] The problem is that some people with celiac disease or a non-celiac gluten sensitivity problem might react to trace amounts of gluten. Also, if you are trying to avoid gluten and plan on purchasing packaged gluten-free foods, you ideally want to make sure that the food is "certified gluten-free," which means that there is a third-party confirming that the food, drink, or nutritional supplement or herb meets the standards for being labeled as gluten-free.

So far, we have established that you should avoid gluten if you have celiac disease, and if you have a non-celiac gluten sensitivity. I'll also add that many healthcare professionals recommend that everyone with any autoimmune condition permanently avoid gluten, whether or not they have celiac disease or a non-celiac gluten sensitivity problem. While I can't say I have always agreed with this, when you do the research, it makes sense, as gluten can be an environmental trigger in many people, and it causes a leaky gut in everyone. Thus, if you want to be on the safe side, then after you get into remission, you should ideally avoid gluten permanently.

Is the Problem Really With Glyphosate?

In Chapter 20, I'll discuss how this chemical can be a factor in why so many people have problems with gluten. In other words, there is the possibility that some people don't have a problem with gluten, but instead have a problem with the glyphosate that's sprayed on wheat and other grains. Others suggest that the hybridization of wheat is the main culprit.

In his book, *Eat Wheat: A Scientific and Clinically-Proven Approach to Safely Bringing Wheat and Dairy Back Into Your Diet,* Dr. John Douillard discusses how the problem with gluten and dairy relates to congested lymphatic vessels in the brain and central nervous system. According to Dr. Douillard, this congestion can lead to food sensitivities, including those related to gluten and dairy. While he isn't necessarily encouraging everyone to eat gluten, he does say that improving upper digestion and having a healthy intestinal tract can help decongest the lymphatic system, which, in turn, will allow many people to tolerate gluten.

He adds that if you have weak digestion or a congested lymphatic system, then eliminating wheat and dairy won't do anything to address the root cause of the issue. Not surprisingly, the quality of the food you eat can make a big difference. For example, concerning grains, he discusses sourdough bread and ancient wheat such as einkorn.

My goal isn't to confuse you by presenting different sides to the story, and I'm not encouraging you or anyone else with Hashimoto's to eat gluten, but I want to teach you to keep an open mind. Avoiding gluten forever probably is the best option for everyone who has Hashimoto's.

However, I realize that some will choose to reintroduce gluten in the future, regardless of what the research shows.

You might wonder what my opinion is on this subject. I think that those with celiac disease or a non-celiac gluten sensitivity should completely avoid gluten permanently. Every now and then, I'll be asked if it's okay for someone who has celiac disease to eat sourdough bread. This question is based on a few small studies that showed sourdough wheat baked goods degrading the gluten and thus being supposedly safe for those with celiac disease.[6,7] However, a more recent study shows that this is not considered to be safe for those with celiac disease.[8]

As for whether someone with Hashimoto's who doesn't have celiac disease or a non-celiac gluten sensitivity can safely reintroduce healthier forms of wheat or other forms of gluten (i.e., rye, barley) upon improving their digestion and lymphatic system, this remains controversial. Some people who get into remission might be able to occasionally tolerate small amounts of gluten without relapsing, but the problem is that there is no way to know for certain if you are one of these people, which is why many healthcare professionals recommend avoiding gluten permanently. In fact, many healthcare professionals recommend to avoid ALL grains, even after achieving a state of remission.

What's the Difference Between a Food Allergy and Sensitivity?

In Chapter 23, I'll discuss the differences between a food allergy, sensitivity, and intolerance. Many people use these terms interchangeably, and I'm guilty of doing this at times. But there are differences between an allergy, sensitivity, and an intolerance.

Celiac Disease vs. Non-Celiac Gluten Sensitivity

What I'd like to do next is discuss the difference between celiac disease and having a non-celiac gluten sensitivity. Celiac disease is an autoimmune condition that is triggered by gluten. This condition affects both adults and children. While people with this condition can experience gastrointestinal symptoms such as bloating, gas, stomach pain, diarrhea, or constipation, it's common to experience other types of symptoms. Some of these signs and symptoms include anemia, osteoporosis, weight loss, infertility, neurological problems, skin conditions, and other health issues.

To better understand the mechanisms behind celiac disease, I will briefly discuss some of the common proteins and enzymatic structures associated with this condition. The reason why I feel this is important to discuss is because there is a much higher prevalence of celiac disease in people with autoimmune thyroid conditions such as Hashimoto's.[9,10,11,12]

By the way, many children also have celiac disease, and a few studies have shown a higher prevalence of thyroid autoimmunity in children with this condition.[13,14] This is very important, since a child with celiac disease, even if they aren't experiencing any thyroid symptoms, should probably be screened for the presence of thyroid antibodies, especially anti-thyroglobulin antibodies and anti-thyroid peroxidase antibodies.

Therefore, let's look at some of the common proteins and enzymatic structures associated with celiac disease:

Gliadin. I briefly mentioned gliadin earlier, as this is a protein of gluten. Gliadin antibodies are produced by your body against one of the gluten proteins. It's possible for someone to have celiac disease yet test negative for the gliadin antibodies. The reverse is true as well, as it's possible to have positive gliadin antibodies yet not have celiac disease. I'll elaborate on this shortly.

Transglutaminase. This is a calcium-dependent enzyme that forms a complex with ingested gliadin and causes specific deamidation of gliadin,[15] which means that it modifies the protein structure of gliadin. It's a complex process, but what's important to understand is that the presence of transglutaminase-2 autoantibodies confirms that someone has celiac disease, and thus will need to avoid gluten permanently. If you only have positive gliadin antibodies, then this isn't considered to be an autoimmune process, since gliadin is a protein of gluten and not a structure located in your body. However, transglutaminase is an enzyme produced by your body; thus, when there are transglutaminase autoantibodies, then this confirms the presence of autoimmunity.

Endomysium. The endomysium wraps around the muscle fibers, and if you have positive anti-endomysial antibodies, then this also confirms that you have an autoimmune component and will need to avoid gluten permanently. In fact, it has been consistently demonstrated that the IgA endomysial antibody has superior sensitivity and specificity than the antigliadin antibodies.[16] However, if someone has an immunoglobulin A (IgA) deficiency, then one can't rely on this test. For this reason, most celiac panels will test for IgA.

Why Do Some People Develop Celiac Disease?

Just as is the case with Hashimoto's, celiac disease is triggered by a combination of genetic and lifestyle factors. Concerning the genetics of celiac disease, more than 95% of patients with celiac disease share the major histocompatibility complex II class human leukocyte antigen (HLA) DQ2 or DQ8 haplotype.[17] Thus, if someone tests negative for these markers then there is a very good chance they don't have celiac disease, although not having these markers doesn't completely rule this condition out, and there is the possibility that the person will have a non-celiac gluten sensitivity issue.

Thus, without making this too difficult to understand, what happens in someone who has celiac disease is that they consume gluten, and the HLA-DQ2 and HLA-DQ8 antigen presenting cells present the gluten peptides to the T cells of our immune system. This results in immune system activation. In a case of "mistaken identity," the body will begin to produce antibodies against tissue transglutaminase, and anti-endomysium antibodies might also be present.

When tissue transglutaminase-2 antibodies are present, this will result in damage to the cells of the small intestine by the immune system, and can lead to digestive symptoms, malabsorption, anemia, and some of the other problems previously discussed. Tissue transglutaminase-3 antibodies primarily relate to damage caused to the epidermis (the skin), whereas elevated tissue transglutaminase-6 means that the immune system is attacking the tissues of the nervous system.

A small percentage of people with celiac disease have what's referred to as "silent celiac disease".[18,19] This means that they have celiac disease but no digestive symptoms. This is yet another reason why you can't always rely on symptoms.

What Is Non-Celiac Gluten Sensitivity?

Non-celiac gluten sensitivity is defined as a condition in which symptoms are triggered by gluten ingestion, in the absence of celiac-specific antibodies and of classical celiac villous atrophy, with variable Human Leukocyte Antigen (HLA) status and variable presence of first generation anti-gliadin antibodies.[20] What this is saying is that this condition doesn't necessarily cause damage to the villi of the small intestine, and there are no transglutaminase-2 autoantibodies or anti-endomysial antibodies present. However, in some cases, there are elevated gliadin antibodies.

Many people with a non-celiac gluten sensitivity will experience symptoms upon ingesting gluten. As I discussed earlier, they might experience gastrointestinal symptoms, or they might experience extraintestinal symptoms, such as fatigue, brain fog, dermatitis, anemia, or muscle and joint pain. The pathophysiology of non-celiac gluten sensitivity is still unclear.

Additional Testing for Celiac Disease

In addition to testing for the genetic markers of celiac disease, one can also obtain a celiac panel. Although a negative celiac panel doesn't always rule out celiac disease, obtaining such a panel is usually a good place to start if someone suspects a problem with gluten. Some people get the gliadin antibodies tested, but it's possible for these to be negative even if someone has celiac disease.

If a problem with gluten is suspected, you want to not only test the gliadin antibodies but also the antibodies to tissue transglutaminase, along with the anti-endomysial antibodies. It's also a good idea to test both immunoglobulin A (IgA) and immunoglobulin G (IgG) because if one of these immunoglobulins happens to be depressed, it can result in a false negative result.

Cyrex Labs has a comprehensive test for gluten called the Wheat/ Gluten Proteome Reactivity and Autoimmunity Panel. This test measures the antibody production against eight wheat proteins and peptides, three essential structure enzymes, and the gliadin-transglutaminase complex. Although it's a great test, very rarely do I order it, as I usually just advise my patients to avoid gluten. However, if someone wants to find out if they react to gluten then this is a test to consider obtaining, as this is a more comprehensive test than a celiac panel.

In addition, whereas a celiac panel will only measure transglutaminase-2 antibodies, the Cyrex Labs panel will also test for the antibodies against transglutaminase-3 and transglutaminase-6. This is important, as is it possible to test negative for the transglutaminase-2 antibodies, yet be positive for either the transglutaminase-3 or transglutaminase-6 antibodies.

As mentioned earlier, the transglutaminase-2 antibodies are associated with celiac disease,[21] whereas elevated transglutaminase-3 antibodies are associated with the skin,[22] and transglutaminase-6 antibodies are associated with the nervous system.[23] In other words, someone with elevated transglutaminase-6 antibodies who is exposed to gluten might not experience the digestive symptoms commonly associated with celiac disease, but instead might experience neurological symptoms.

Read This Before You Do Any Testing for Gluten...

When doing a celiac panel, or any other test involving gluten, you need to be consuming gluten or have recently eaten gluten-containing foods in order for the test to be accurate because these tests are measuring antibody production, and you won't be producing antibodies unless you are eating the food you're testing for. Thus, if you have been on a gluten-free diet for a few months or longer, then it would be a waste of money to test for a gluten sensitivity.

Even if you decided to reintroduce gluten to get an accurate test, you would still need to wait at least a few weeks before the antibodies develop. The same concept applies to other foods. For example, if you wanted to test for a casein sensitivity but have been dairy-free for a few months, then the test probably will come back negative, even if you have a sensitivity to casein.

By the way, since celiac disease can affect the absorption of some of the nutrients and can cause anemia, some other tests are important to obtain if one tests positive for this condition. This includes a complete blood count, a comprehensive metabolic panel, an iron panel, as well as checking the vitamin B12 and vitamin D levels. Bone density can also be affected, so obtaining a bone density scan might be a good idea in some cases.

Steps to Take After Being Diagnosed With Celiac Disease or a Non-Celiac Gluten Sensitivity

1. Avoid gluten...permanently. If someone has celiac disease, eating a small amount of gluten can result in the production of autoantibodies. If you have been diagnosed with celiac disease, you need to avoid eating gluten permanently. And if you have a non-celiac gluten sensitivity, it also is a good idea to permanently avoid gluten.

2. Be cautious about eating other foods that cross-react with gluten. When someone has celiac disease, or a non-celiac sensitivity, they might not feel better after avoiding gluten for a few reasons. One reason is because they are still being exposed to gluten, which frequently happens through cross contamination. However, one also needs to consider that other foods can cross-react with gluten.

What is cross-reactivity? With cross-reactivity, certain antibodies that form against gluten can also cross-react with other foods that share similar amino acid sequences. As a result of this, your body not only produces gluten antibodies against gluten, but they also produce gluten antibodies against other proteins that have a similar amino acid sequence.

Some of the foods that cross-react with gluten include cow's milk, whey, oats, millet, rice, and corn. For example, if someone completely eliminates gluten from their diet, but consumes dairy, then besides the possibility that they are sensitive to the proteins of dairy, there is also the chance they can produce gliadin antibodies, since dairy cross-reacts with gluten.

Avoiding all of the cross-reactive foods isn't always necessary, although one does need to consider that eating these cross-reactive foods can cause problems in people with celiac disease, as well as those with a non-celiac gluten sensitivity. So once again, if someone with celiac disease or a non-celiac gluten sensitivity completely eliminates gluten from their diet but still has overt symptoms, then they might be reacting to a different type of food that cross-reacts with gluten. It's also important to understand that not everyone experiences overt symptoms when eating cross-reactive foods, which is when a test such as the Gluten-Associated Cross-Reactive Foods and Foods Sensitivity Test from Cyrex Labs can come in handy.

3. Conduct tests for anemia, nutrient deficiencies, and bone density. Because celiac disease results in the malabsorption of many nutrients, it is a good idea to do some additional testing. For example, everyone with celiac disease should receive a complete blood count and an iron panel. Testing for vitamin B12, RBC folate, and RBC magnesium also would be wise. Although the blood isn't the best method of evaluating mild to moderate deficiencies of many nutrients, if someone has a severe nutrient deficiency, this frequently will show up on blood testing.

Since widespread nutrient deficiencies are common, most people with celiac disease should be on a high potency multivitamin with minerals. Due to the malabsorption of nutrients, many people with celiac disease also have a decrease in bone density. The good news is that completely avoiding gluten and correcting nutrient deficiencies will almost always help increase the bone density.

4. Consider testing for a leaky gut. If someone has celiac disease and has been consuming gluten, then they might want to consider doing a leaky gut test, or, in this situation, they can just assume that they have a leaky gut and then take measures to help restore the health of the gut, which I discuss in Chapter 28.

5. Eat whole, healthy foods. This might seem obvious, but it is possible to be 100% gluten-free but still eat an unhealthy diet. Many people with celiac disease avoid gluten but eat many "gluten-free processed foods." This includes gluten-free cookies, cakes, potato chips, cereal, pasta, pizza, etc. I'm not suggesting that you can never eat these foods, but you, of course, want to eat mostly whole foods, and minimize the consumption of processed foods, even if they are gluten-free. This is especially true while you are trying to restore your health, but even after you achieve a state of remission, it's also important to eat well to help maintain a state of wellness.

Gluten-Free Diet vs. Low FODMAP Diet

Although gluten is undoubtedly problematic for many people, grains such as wheat, rye, and barley are high in FODMAPs, which can also be a problem. A low FODMAP diet will be discussed in Chapter 21. FODMAP stands for fermentable oligosaccharides, disaccharides, monosaccharides, and polyols. If someone has SIBO, they very well might have problems with grains not because of the gluten, but because of the indigestible oligosaccharides, fructans, and galacto-oligosaccharides, which, in turn, can result in increased gas production and other digestive symptoms.

So how can you distinguish between having problems with gluten or high FODMAP foods? This admittedly can be challenging at times, and some people will have problems with both gluten and high FODMAP foods. An example would be a person who has celiac disease and SIBO. Without question, if someone is diagnosed with celiac disease or a non-celiac gluten sensitivity then gluten should be avoided. However, if someone experiences gas and other digestive symptoms even when eating gluten-free grains and/ or other high FODMAP foods (e.g., fermented vegetables, beans, starchy vegetables) then this would suggest a problem with FODMAPs.

A Gluten Sensitivity Case Study

Although many people who work with me are fine giving up gluten, Samantha was initially resistant to do so, as she felt fine when eating wheat bread, pasta, and other foods that contained gluten. It's also important to mention that she had tested for celiac disease in the past and this came back negative. I explained to Samantha that it's possible to have a non-celiac gluten sensitivity, and the absence of symptoms when consuming gluten doesn't always rule out a gluten sensitivity, so she agreed to avoid gluten. In addition to avoiding gluten and other foods as part of an AIP diet, she did some testing, and upon following my recommendations she noticed a gradual improvement in her symptoms, blood test results, etc. Eventually her thyroid panel and antibodies normalized. Although I explained the risks of reintroducing gluten after getting into remission, Samantha decided to add gluten back into her diet. She told me that she would minimize the amount of gluten-containing foods she ate initially. Unfortunately the next test revealed elevated thyroid peroxidase antibodies, and the only major change she made was reintroducing gluten. Based on these findings Samantha decided to give up gluten permanently. I provided this case study to demonstrate that not everyone with a gluten sensitivity will experience overt symptoms upon consuming gluten, and testing also isn't perfect, which is why reintroducing gluten after getting into remission is a risk.

Chapter Highlights:

- Here are five reasons why gluten should be avoided: 1) gluten is a common allergen, 2) gluten is a common trigger of Hashimoto's, 3) gluten cannot be digested, 4) gluten causes a leaky gut in everyone, 5) you should focus on eating whole healthy foods.
- For someone with Hashimoto's, eating even a small amount of gluten can cause inflammation and increase the permeability of the gut.
- Celiac disease is an autoimmune condition that is triggered by gluten, and is triggered by a combination of genetic and lifestyle factors.
- Non-celiac gluten sensitivity doesn't cause damage to the villi of the small intestine or the elevation of autoantibodies.
- Cyrex Labs has a comprehensive test for gluten called the Wheat/Gluten Proteome Reactivity and Autoimmunity Panel.
- When doing a celiac panel, or any other test involving gluten, you need to be consuming gluten or have recently eaten gluten-containing foods for the test to be accurate.
- It's possible that some people don't have a problem with gluten, but instead have a problem with the glyphosate that's sprayed on wheat and other grains.
- With cross-reactivity, certain antibodies that form against gluten can also cross-react with other foods that share similar amino acid sequences.
- In addition to the problems with gluten, grains such as wheat, rye, and barley are high in FODMAPs, which can also be problematic.

CHAPTER 6

DAIRY AND OTHER FOOD TRIGGERS OF HASHIMOTO'S

T **HE PREVIOUS CHAPTER FOCUSED** on gluten, which is the main food allergen that can be problematic for those with Hashimoto's. Other foods can also be potential triggers. Of course, this doesn't mean that these foods will be a trigger for everyone, but the problem is that it is difficult, if not impossible, to know who will do fine when eating these foods and who won't. While it's probably safe to say that those who experience overt symptoms to dairy, corn, or other allergens should avoid these foods, the lack of symptoms doesn't rule out a food sensitivity. This can make it even more challenging to know what foods to avoid.

Should Dairy Be Avoided in Those With Hashimoto's?

Many people don't do well when consuming dairy, which is also true for a lot of people with Hashimoto's. During my childhood and teenage years, I drank plenty of cow's milk, which many people perceive as being healthy. Although drinking cow's milk is very healthy for baby cows, it's not necessarily healthy for humans.

That being said, dairy has some potential health benefits. In addition, some people do well when consuming raw dairy, while others do fine consuming dairy from a goat or a sheep. However, I recommend for my patients with Hashimoto's to avoid all types of dairy while trying to get into remission. While some people do fine with raw dairy or other forms of dairy such as ghee, everyone is different, and some people do react to these healthier forms of dairy products. I'm not asking you to give up dairy forever (although some people will need to do this), but try to avoid it while restoring your health.

Why Is It Important to Avoid Drinking "Conventional" Cow's Milk?

Many people still think of cow's milk as being healthy and drink it regularly. Some people with Hashimoto's have been told to avoid dairy; thus, they no longer drink any milk and might avoid other forms of dairy such as yogurt, whey, and cheese. Why is commercial cow's milk bad for you? Here are four reasons:

1. The hormones. In addition to growth hormone that is commonly added, cow's milk also contains estrogens, which, in some people, could stimulate the growth of hormone-sensitive tumors.[24] While drinking organic cow's milk would be a healthier choice, it's important to understand that organic milk might not have growth hormones added but may have estrogens because it's common for the milk to be collected from cows while they are lactating. Due to these and other factors I'm about to discuss, avoiding cow's milk altogether is probably best, regardless of whether it's organic or non-organic.

2. The Pasteurization Process. The pasteurization process, developed by Louis Pasteur in 1864, involves heating the milk to a specific temperature in order to kill harmful bacteria. When you think about pasteurization this might sound like a wonderful idea. However, heating the milk decreases many of the nutrients such as vitamin B1, B2, folate, B12, vitamin C, and vitamin E.[25]

In addition, the pasteurization process will modify the proteins of dairy, and can potentially lead to a greater increase in food allergies, although some argue that the opposite occurs, as by denaturing the proteins this might make someone less susceptible to a dairy allergy. You might wonder if the pasteurization process will inactivate estrogens, but the research shows that pasteurized organic and conventional dairy products do not have substantially different concentrations of estrogens.[26]

3. The Homogenization Process. Why is commercial milk homogenized? The process of homogenization helps to give milk its white color and smooth texture, and might help with the digestibility of milk.[27] Homogenization changes the physical structure of milk fat and, because of this, might alter the health properties of milk. A review of studies shows an increased risk of cardiovascular disease and type 2 diabetes in those who drink homogenized milk.[28] To be fair, most of these were observational studies, and it's difficult to use these to prove a direct correlation between milk consumption and these diseases.

4. The mTORC1 pathway. There is something called the mammalian TOR complex 1 (mTORC1) and this signaling pathway plays a big role in the development and progression of a number of different health conditions. This includes conditions such as acne,[29,30] as well as chronic conditions such as obesity,[31,32] type 2 diabetes,[33] and cancer.[34,35,36]

Does this mean that drinking commercial milk will always lead to a condition such as obesity, type 2 diabetes, or cancer? While some people do fine drinking milk, others don't. As with gluten, it's unnecessary to drink cow's milk, although I admit that unlike gluten, dairy has certain health benefits, and it is also very tasty.

Many people are aware of the glycemic index, and milk has a low glycemic index. However, cow's milk, along with other types of dairy, has a high insulin index, which means that it causes a high insulin response. You might wonder if it's healthier to drink other types of milk such as from a goat or sheep. There hasn't been as much research on these types of milk, although it appears that the insulin index is similar to cow's milk.

Another Problem With Cow's Milk: Beta Casein A1

Cow's milk consists of both casein and whey protein with approximately 80% of it consisting of casein. Although many people are lactose intolerant, it's also common to be sensitive to casein. Other dairy products include casein, such as yogurt and cheese. There are different types of casein in dairy cows. The most common forms of beta-casein in dairy cattle breeds are A1 and A2.

It is thought that beta-casein variant A1 yields the bioactive peptide beta-casomorphin-7 (BCM-7). This may play a role in the development of certain human diseases, such as diabetes mellitus and ischemic heart disease. There also might be a relationship of BCM-7 to sudden infant death syndrome.[37]

Some people react to beta-casein A1, but do perfectly fine when consuming beta-casein A2. The challenge is finding out where the dairy you purchase is coming from, and, unfortunately, most of the milk in the United States comes from "A1 cows." I'll discuss raw milk shortly, as this is a better option than conventional milk. However, from what I understand, not all raw milk is made from "A2 cows," which might explain why some people don't do well when drinking raw milk.

What's the best way to get milk that has beta-casein A2? You might need to go directly to the source, which means contacting some of the local farmers to find out whether they have "A1 cows" or "A2 cows." I have seen "A2 milk" sold at my local Whole Foods store, although it is pasteurized. Goat or sheep milk doesn't have BCM-7, which is probably why many people do better when drinking these types of milk.

What About Other Types of Dairy?

Most of this information focuses on the risks associated with drinking cow's milk, but is it okay for people with Hashimoto's to consume other types of dairy? I recommend that my patients with Hashimoto's avoid all forms of dairy while trying to restore their health. This includes not only milk, but yogurt, cheese, kefir, and whey, because some people are sensitive to these other forms as well.

Since butter is low in casein, some feel that it is fine to consume. This might be true in some cases, but if someone has a known or suspected casein allergy or sensitivity, then I would still recommend they avoid it. They also need to consider the type of casein they're consuming. It admittedly can be challenging at times to know exactly what a person should and shouldn't eat, but when someone is trying to restore their health back to normal, I would rather play it safe and have them avoid all types of dairy while they are restoring their health.

Although some healthcare professionals think that everyone with Hashimoto's should avoid both gluten and dairy permanently, some people can eventually reintroduce dairy into their diet once they get into a state of remission. After all, not everyone has problems with dairy, and consuming certain types of dairy has some health benefits.

However, it does depend on the person, as some people might need to avoid dairy permanently. There admittedly are risks of reintroducing dairy, especially if someone has a sensitivity to dairy proteins such as casein or whey. Thus, some people choose to avoid dairy permanently, while others choose to reintroduce healthier forms of dairy (i.e., raw dairy) in the future.

Yet Another Problem With Dairy: Cross-Reactivity

While someone can have a direct sensitivity to dairy, it also is possible for one or more of the dairy proteins to cross-react with gluten. This is one of the main reasons why many natural healthcare professionals recommend that their patients with autoimmune conditions such as Hashimoto's avoid dairy permanently.

If you insist on eating dairy, then, in this situation, you might want to consider ordering a test such as the Gluten-Associated Cross-Reactive Foods & Foods Sensitivity by Cyrex Labs (Array #4). This tests for cow's milk, along with the following individual proteins of dairy: alpha-casein and beta-casein, casomorphin, milk butyrophilin, whey protein, and milk chocolate. If you test positive for any of these, then Cyrex Labs recommends avoiding dairy permanently. However, some other foods on this panel can be reintroduced once the gut has been healed.

Where Will You Get Your Calcium From?

Many people are concerned about getting enough calcium if they are avoiding dairy. Although dairy is the primary source of calcium for many people, other foods are high in calcium. Kale is high in calcium, so you can eat steamed kale and/or add kale to a smoothie. You might be concerned that kale is goitrogenic, along with other cruciferous vegetables, and can potentially disrupt the production of thyroid hormone.

The truth is that most people with Hashimoto's do fine eating a few servings of cruciferous vegetables each day, and cooking kale will reduce the goitrogenic properties. I'll discuss goitrogens in Chapter 26.

Chinese cabbage is also an excellent source of calcium.[38] Collard greens, broccoli, almonds, and blackstrap molasses can also provide a sufficient amount of calcium. Sardines are also a good source of calcium. Thus, there are plenty of non-dairy sources of calcium to choose from.

Additional Food Allergens to Avoid

Although gluten and dairy are the two most problematic allergens, several others should be avoided while trying to restore your health:

Corn. This is yet another common allergen, and one that cross-reacts with gluten. Research has shown that the proteins from corn can cause a celiac-like immune response due to similar or alternative pathogenic mechanisms to the proteins found in wheat.[39] In other words, eating corn can cause a similar response as gluten.

Anyone who eats processed foods regularly most likely is being exposed to corn. This is especially true if you are eating gluten-free processed foods such as gluten-free cookies, crackers, cereals, etc. If you are trying to avoid corn then obviously you will want to avoid ingredients such as corn starch, corn syrup, etc. However, many other ingredients contain corn, including the following: ascorbic acid, caramel, confectioners' sugar, hydrolyzed vegetable protein, corn-based maltodextrin, modified food starch, and xanthan gum. Keep in mind that this is just a small sample of ingredients that may include corn.

In addition to corn being a common allergen, most corn in the United States is genetically modified. So if you do choose to eat corn, or a product that includes corn, make sure that it is either certified organic or labeled as being non-GMO. Just keep in mind that many people are sensitive to corn, even when it's not genetically modified. Thus, when trying to restore your health, do everything you can to avoid corn.

Soy. Like corn, most soy is genetically modified. Thus, if you choose to eat soy, you also want to make sure that it's either certified organic or non-GMO. However, many people are sensitive to soy, even when it is not genetically modified. While it should be obvious to avoid foods such as soy milk, soy yogurt, soy burgers, etc., many packaged foods include soy ingredients.

A few studies have shown that soy has goitrogenic properties.[40,41,42] One of these studies demonstrated that the effect on the thyroid hormones was minimal, although the study involved short-term soy consumption, lasting only seven consecutive days. Another study involving soy supplementation for eight weeks in those with subclinical hypothyroidism showed that there is a threefold increased risk of developing overt hypothyroidism, although soy did demonstrate some health benefits, as it helped to decrease insulin resistance, inflammation, and blood pressure.[43]

One more reason to avoid soy is the phytates. Phytic acid is an antinutrient that is found in grains, nuts, seeds, and legumes, including soybeans. Studies show that the phytates in soy can lead to a decrease in iron and calcium absorption.[44,45] However, soaking and fermenting soy can significantly decrease the levels of phytic acid.

Some people wonder whether eating some organic fermented soy such as miso, tempeh, and natto is okay. Some people do fine eating a small amount of fermented soy. Fermented soy does have health benefits, and soaking and fermenting soy can significantly decrease the levels of phytic acid. However, if someone has a soy allergy or sensitivity, then even organic fermented soy should be avoided. Another thing to keep in mind is that fermenting soy doesn't make it less goitrogenic.

Other Food Allergens. Eliminating gluten, dairy, corn, and soy will greatly benefit the health of most people with Hashimoto's. These are four of the most problematic foods, and sometimes just eliminating these alone will greatly improve one's symptoms and test results, although I would also add refined sugars to this list. However, some people, upon eliminating these allergens, won't notice any improvement in their symptoms or tests, but this doesn't mean that they should freely eat these. Even if these foods aren't the main trigger, they still can cause inflammation and prevent their gut from healing.

Of course, other food allergens can cause problems. Eggs and peanuts are two common allergenic foods, and while I think it's a good idea for people with Hashimoto's to avoid eating peanuts and other legumes while restoring their health, some people do fine when eating eggs, especially egg yolks. Since eggs are nutrient dense, I'm usually fine with someone reintroducing eggs if they are struggling to follow a strict autoimmune Paleo (AIP) diet.

Some people find they don't tolerate eggs well upon reintroducing them, while others do fine and can continue to eat them. Just keep in mind that even if you don't have an egg allergy or sensitivity, eggs have compounds that can increase the permeability of the gut. This is why they are excluded from an autoimmune Paleo diet. I'll further discuss eggs in Chapter 26.

A Brief Overview of the Autoimmune Paleo Diet

I will go into greater detail about the AIP diet in Chapter 26, but I did want to briefly discuss it here. Many people with Hashimoto's are told to follow an AIP diet, which is similar to a standard Paleo diet. A standard Paleo diet allows vegetables, fruits, meat and fish, eggs, nuts and seeds, and unrefined oils. It excludes refined and processed foods, dairy, grains, and legumes. An AIP diet excludes some additional foods, including eggs, nuts, and seeds, along with the nightshade vegetables such as tomatoes, eggplant, and white potatoes.

Although I commonly recommend for my patients with Hashimoto's to follow an AIP diet initially, this doesn't mean that everyone needs to follow this diet strictly until they achieve a state of remission. Everyone is different, and while some people thrive on an AIP diet, it's a major struggle for others, and some people do better following a standard Paleo diet.

Can Red Meat Be an Autoimmune Trigger?

Neu5Gc is a compound found in beef, pork, lamb, and dairy products.[46] Some have expressed a concern that we produce antibodies against Neu5Gc, which can cause inflammation and other health conditions in those who eat red meat.[47] Thus, when we eat red meat, Neu5Gc might become incorporated into human tissues. If someone has anti-Neu5Gc antibodies, this can cause inflammation.

The problem is that the evidence is far from conclusive, and people have been eating red meat for a very long time without developing all of the chronic health conditions we see today. Thus, even if some people do have anti-Neu5Gc antibodies, can we conclude that these develop due to eating all types of red meat? More research is definitely needed in this area.

One study I came across did show increased anti-Neu5Gc antibodies in patients with hypothyroidism and Hashimoto's.[48] The authors concluded that the correlation of anti-TPO antibodies with increased anti-Neu5Gc antibodies means that there might be an association between anti-Neu5Gc antibodies and autoimmune hypothyroidism.[48] Does this mean that the consumption of animal products can cause or exacerbate the autoimmune component of Hashimoto's due to the development of anti-Neu5Gc antibodies?

Perhaps, but keep in mind that the incidence of Hashimoto's has skyrocketed over the last few decades, yet humans have been consuming animal products for a very long time. It's also worth mentioning that the same study showed that rheumatoid arthritis does not involve elevated anti-Neu5Gc antibodies; therefore, the authors concluded that increased anti-Neu5Gc antibodies are not a common characteristic of all autoimmune diseases.

Some might also be concerned about red meat being inflammatory. However, what's important to understand is that not all red meat is created equal. Many people reading this are aware of the differences between grass-fed beef and grain-fed beef. Studies clearly show that grass-fed beef has a greater amount of omega 3 fatty acids and a decreased amount of omega 6 fatty acids when compared to grain fed beef.[49,50,51,52]

However, it's important to make sure the cow was 100% grass fed, as many are fed grass initially, but for the last few weeks of their lives, they are fed grains, which will affect the fatty acid ratio. Thus, when you purchase red meat, you want to make sure it says 100% grass fed.

Can Sugar and Salt Trigger Hashimoto's?

Although sugar doesn't directly trigger autoimmunity, eating a lot of sugar frequently can cause blood sugar imbalances, including insulin resistance, which can be a factor in the development of Hashimoto's. I have dedicated Chapter 17 to blood sugar imbalances. I will say here that you should avoid refined sugars while restoring your health, and once in remission, you still should minimize your consumption of these.

Another thing to keep in mind is that eating a lot of sugar can be a factor in the overgrowth of Candida. I'll discuss Candida albicans in Chapter 9, and how it can be a factor in the development of some cases of Hashimoto's.

For those who may think that artificial sweeteners are a better option, evidence shows that certain non-caloric artificial sweeteners can cause glucose intolerance by altering the intestinal microbiota.[53,54,55] In other words, consuming artificial sweeteners such as aspartame, saccharin, sucralose, and acesulfame-K may lead to imbalances in the gut flora and metabolic abnormalities. Thus, while many people eat foods and drink beverages with artificial sweeteners in order to lose weight, some of these studies suggest that they might actually increase the risk of obesity.

What about salt? Much evidence shows that a high salt diet increases Th17 cells, which are associated with autoimmunity. One study showed that increasing sodium chloride consumption might increase the risk of developing autoimmunity by activating Th17 cells.[56] Another study looked at the effect of a high salt diet on intestinal immunity and the risk of inflammatory diseases, and confirmed that a high salt diet stimulates the Th17 cells of the intestine, while inhibiting regulatory T cells.[57]

Does this mean that everyone with Hashimoto's should avoid salt? The key here is moderation, as the studies that demonstrate a correlation between salt and autoimmunity specifically show that "excess" sodium chloride consumption can have a negative effect on the immune system, with one of these studies discussing the salt content in processed foods (i.e., fast food).[58] Thus, if someone is eating many packaged and processed foods, there is a good chance that they are consuming high amounts of sodium chloride. However, if someone eats mostly whole foods and adds some high quality sea salt to their food, this shouldn't trigger autoimmunity or exacerbate the autoimmune response in someone who has Hashimoto's.

Can Caffeine Trigger Hashimoto's?

The good news is that caffeine has been reported to decrease the production of both Th1 and Th2 cytokines.[59] Since Th1 cytokines are associated with most cases of Hashimoto's, this would suggest that people with this autoimmune thyroid condition might actually benefit from consuming caffeine in the form of coffee, tea, and dark chocolate. However, the reason why I recommend that my Hashimoto's patients avoid caffeine while restoring their health, especially in the form of coffee, is because most people with this condition have adrenal problems, and caffeine can have a negative effect on adrenal health.

If you're a coffee drinker, this might sound discouraging, but I find that most people with Hashimoto's are eventually able to reintroduce coffee. However, if you happen to be a slow metabolizer of caffeine (break down and excrete caffeine slowly), then it is a good idea to minimize your consumption of caffeine permanently.

According to the research, slow metabolizers of caffeine have an increased risk of having a heart attack[60] and impaired fasting glucose.[61] This doesn't mean that slow metabolizers can never drink coffee again, but it probably would be wise to limit their consumption if this is the case and ideally drink only a good quality organic coffee.

How can you tell if you are a slow or fast metabolizer of caffeine? Well, most people will have a good idea without doing any testing, as those who are "wired" after drinking coffee are probably slow metabolizers, while those who can drink plenty of coffee without a problem are most likely fast metabolizers. However, genetic testing can also be done to confirm how you metabolize caffeine. Caffeine is metabolized by the cytochrome P450 1A2 (CYP1A2) enzyme, and If someone is homozygous for the CYP1A2*1A allele then this means they are a fast metabolizer of caffeine.[62]

On a genetic test this usually will show up as an A/A genotype. Either the A/C or C/C genotype means that the person is a slow metabolizer.

How Can You Determine if You Have an Allergy, Sensitivity, or Intolerance?

In Chapter 23, I'll discuss the difference between a food allergy, food sensitivity, and food intolerance. However, I'll also give a brief summary here:

Food allergy. This usually involves an immediate reaction to a food, and is considered to be IgE-mediated. This is the type of testing that most conventional allergists will conduct.

Food sensitivity. This usually involves a delayed reaction. Thus, it frequently will take a few hours and, sometimes, a few days before someone will have a negative reaction to a food. While most food sensitivity panels involve Immunoglobulin G (IgG), other types of panels are used, including the ALCAT and Mediator Release Testing (MRT).

Food intolerance. This is usually the result of an enzymatic defect, and a good example of this is having a lactose intolerance. Having a histamine intolerance can be due to a defect in the enzyme diamine oxidase (DAO), although there can be other causes of this type of intolerance as well.

What's the Best Method of Managing Food Allergies and Sensitivities?

If someone tests positive for an IgE-mediated food allergy, then the person will need to avoid that food, sometimes permanently. Conventional treatment methods are looking at a number of different strategies for IgE allergies, including sublingual/oral immunotherapy, injection of anti-IgE antibodies, and cytokine/anticytokine therapies.[63] Of course, one does need to be aware of the potential side effects of certain conventional treatment methods.

When someone has a food sensitivity, then they still want to avoid the food while trying to get into remission. For example, if someone follows an elimination diet and they have a negative reaction to a few foods, then they should avoid these foods while trying to restore their health. Similarly, if you are relying on serum IgG testing for food sensitivities, then you will want to avoid those foods that show up as positive until the gut has healed.

How do you know when the gut has been healed? Well, perhaps the best way to know for certain is through testing. Tests are available that can detect an increase in intestinal permeability. The lactulose-mannitol test is the classic test for intestinal permeability, and I have used an intestinal permeability test from Cyrex Labs on my patients. Keep in mind that most of my patients don't do leaky gut testing, as many will rely on the improvement of their symptoms and other tests (i.e., blood tests, adrenal testing). However, some people will obtain a baseline intestinal permeability test, and if it is positive, they might do another test three to six months later to see if their gut has healed.

Chapter Highlights:

- Like gluten, dairy should also be avoided in those with Hashimoto's, as it is a common allergen, and casein cross-reacts with gluten.
- This includes not only milk but also yogurt, cheese, kefir, and whey.
- Four reasons to avoid conventional cow's milk are 1) the hormones, 2) the pasteurization process, 3) the homogenization process, and 4) the mTORC1 pathway.
- Dairy can cross-react with gluten and cause someone to produce gliadin antibodies.
- Corn and soy are two other common allergens that should be avoided by those with Hashimoto's thyroiditis.
- There are other common allergens, and an autoimmune Paleo diet will exclude these, along with other foods that can increase the permeability of the gut.
- Sugar can indirectly lead to autoimmunity through blood sugar imbalances, while high salt intake can directly lead to conditions such as Hashimoto's by increasing Th17 cells.
- While caffeine has been reported to decrease the production of both Th1 and Th2 cytokines, caffeine can also have a negative effect on adrenal health.

CHAPTER 7

THE IMPACT OF STRESS ON HASHIMOTO'S

CHRONIC STRESS IS A TRIGGER that is overlooked by many people. This poses a problem, since most people deal with chronic stress daily. But how does stress specifically lead to Hashimoto's thyroiditis? In this chapter, I'm going to discuss the relationship between stress and autoimmunity, and I have to warn you upfront that some of the information presented in this chapter will be somewhat advanced, although I'll try my best to make it easy for you to understand.

During an acute stress situation, the adrenal glands secrete the hormone cortisol, along with epinephrine and norepinephrine. Epinephrine and norepinephrine are part of the sympathetic nervous system, which is associated with the fight-or-flight response. The release of epinephrine and norepinephrine causes an increase in heart rate, increased contraction of the heart, dilation of the pupils, increased ventilation, the release of glucose from the liver, and has many other functions.

Cortisol is a glucocorticoid, and like epinephrine and norepinephrine, is also involved in the fight or flight reaction, as it is important for the production of glucose during a process called gluconeogenesis. Glucose is used as an energy source. Cortisol also is involved in the breakdown of fatty acids for energy. If the stressor is acute, then once it has been removed, the hormone levels will usually go back to normal.

What happens when the stressor isn't removed? This describes a chronic stress situation, and when this happens, the body will continue to secrete cortisol, and eventually it does so at the expense of DHEA, which is another adrenal hormone. The DHEA will eventually become depressed, while cortisol remains elevated. Over a prolonged time, the person can no longer adapt to the stress, and, as a result, the cortisol levels will also become depressed.

This is what's commonly referred to as adrenal fatigue (when both the DHEA and cortisol levels are depressed). However, the adrenals aren't truly in a state of fatigue when both cortisol and DHEA are low. In addition, this process involves more than just the adrenals, as it also involves dysregulation of the hypothalamic-pituitary-adrenal (HPA) axis.

Why Are Prolonged Elevated Cortisol Levels Harmful to Your Health?

Before I discuss the problems associated with prolonged elevations in cortisol, it's important to understand that cortisol has many essential roles. It is necessary to help control swelling and inflammation, it helps to balance the blood sugar levels, it's important for the utilization of carbohydrates and fats, and it even plays a role in gastrointestinal health. So healthy cortisol levels are important to maintain healthy blood sugar levels, maintain normal blood pressure, help with immunity and inflammation, and regulate metabolism of fat, protein, and carbohydrates.

Hopefully, you understand that cortisol isn't inherently bad. It's when cortisol becomes chronically elevated that we need to become concerned. Prolonged elevation of cortisol can decrease immune system function,[64] lower bone density,[65] cause insulin resistance,[66] and cause an increase in weight gain and blood pressure,[67] thus increasing the risk of cardiovascular disease. Having high cortisol levels is one reason why many people with Hashimoto's have difficulty losing weight. Elevated cortisol levels can also inhibit the conversion of T4 to T3.[68]

How Does Elevated Cortisol Affect the Immune System?

Stress suppresses the immune system, and, therefore, can make someone more susceptible to infections and even conditions such as cancer. Stress can also exacerbate the autoimmune response. So, how can stress suppress the immune system, yet exacerbate autoimmunity? Well, chronic or long-term stress can suppress immunity by decreasing immune cell numbers and function and/or increasing immunosuppressive mechanisms, such as regulatory T cells.[69]

However, chronic stress can also dysregulate immune function by increasing the production of both type-1 and type-2 cytokines.[69] In addition, the timing of the stress exposure can play a role, as an increased immune system response is observed when acute stress is experienced at early stages of immune activation, while suppression of the immune system may be observed at later stages of the immune response.[69]

Chronic stress can also affect immunity by decreasing secretory immuno-globulin A (SIgA).[70,71] SIgA plays a role in immune system defense at muco-sal surfaces, including the gastrointestinal tract. As a result, decreasing SIgA can increase one's susceptibility to an infection.[72] This infection, in turn, can directly cause an autoimmune thyroid condition such as Hashimoto's through a molecular mimicry mechanism (which I'll discuss in Chapter 9), or indirectly by causing an increase in intestinal permeability (a leaky gut). This is why I recommend testing the SIgA levels when ordering an adrenal saliva test, and some comprehensive stool panels also test for this.

Chronic Stress and Thyroid Autoimmunity

Although this book focuses on Hashimoto's, in my practice, I also work with people who have Graves' disease, which is another type of autoim-mune thyroid condition. And many of the patients I have worked with who have Graves' disease have mentioned stress as being a potential factor in the development of their condition. In other words, months or years before they were diagnosed with Graves' disease they were dealing with a great amount of stress.

I'm pretty sure that chronic stress was a big factor in the development of my Graves' disease condition. I'm not suggesting that stress was the only factor, but, at the very least, it contributed to the development of my condition. Also, the literature shows a strong correlation between chronic stress and Graves' disease.[73,74,75]

Is there a correlation between chronic stress and Hashimoto's? Over the years, I have consulted with many people with Hashimoto's who felt stress was a big factor in the development of their condition. However, according to the research, stress seems to be a more common trigger in those people with Graves' disease. Why is this the case? Well, it has to do with the way stress affects the immune system.

In a properly functioning immune system, you ideally want to have a healthy balance between T-helper 1 (Th1) and T-helper 2 (Th2) activity. But certain factors can affect these pathways and make someone Th1 or Th2 dominant. This, in turn, can increase the chances of the person developing an autoimmune condition such Hashimoto's.

In most cases, Graves' disease is considered to be a Th2 dominant condition. Stress may influence the expression of thyroid autoimmunity in susceptible individuals by shifting the Th1-Th2 balance away from Th1 and toward Th2.[76] In other words, chronic stress seems to make someone more Th2 dominant and less Th1 dominant. Since most cases of Hashimoto's are thought to be Th1 dominant, this would explain why stress wouldn't be as likely to trigger this condition. This doesn't mean that stress can't be a trigger in those with Hashimoto's, which is why I would still recommend working on improving your stress coping skills.

After all, while chronic stress might not directly trigger autoimmunity in most cases of Hashimoto's thyroiditis, it does cause a decrease in regulatory T cells (Tregs) along with an increase in proinflammatory cytokines. This decrease in Tregs will make someone more susceptible to developing an autoimmune condition such as Hashimoto's. And Hashimoto's is also characterized by an increase in proinflammatory cytokines.

Let's not forget about the relationship between stress and SIgA. I commonly see depressed SIgA levels in my patients with Hashimoto's, and along with having a decrease in Tregs, this increases the likelihood of getting an infection,[77] and it can also cause an increase in intestinal permeability,[78] which is a factor in autoimmunity. In addition, a journal article that discussed the relationship between stress and thyroid autoimmunity suggested that one reason why there have been few reports concerning the possible relationship between stress and Hashimoto's might be because the onset and course of the condition is more gradual when compared to Graves' disease, and, therefore, the effect of stress might be overlooked.[79]

I discussed this in section one when I discussed the autoimmunity timeline, and how people with Hashimoto's will typically develop thyroid autoantibodies many years prior to experiencing symptoms and being diagnosed with Hashimoto's. Thus, even if stress were a trigger of someone's Hashimoto's condition, many people won't be able to make this connection. Even if they were able to make a correlation, it's unlikely that they would be able to prove with certainty that stress was the main trigger, as it's possible that the chronic stress set the stage for another trigger.

It's the Perception of Stress That Causes Problems

The way one perceives the stressor can play a huge role in determining whether or not someone develops a health condition. The good news is that it is possible to change your perception of stress. Although you might not be able to make this transition overnight, if you put your mind to it, you can modify the way you perceive common stressors. I'm not suggesting that you will get to the point where you are never stressed, as this is highly unlikely, but if you make a sincere effort to change the way you perceive the stress in your life, you can accomplish this within a reasonable amount of time. Making this change will have a huge impact on your overall health.

How Can You Modify Your Perception of Stress?

What can you do to modify your perception of stress? Is it just a matter of telling yourself that you're not going to let stress bother you? Well, this definitely is a step in the right direction. However, it probably is a good idea to incorporate one or more mind-body medicine (MBM) techniques such as meditation, yoga, or biofeedback.

I'll further discuss this in Chapter 27, but one of the keys is to set aside time each day to incorporate one or more of these techniques. Many people who practice yoga, meditation, or other MBM techniques don't do so daily. However, you want to practice some type of MBM every day if you want to successfully modify your perception of stress.

I realize this is easier said than done for many people, including myself. I personally set aside approximately 15 minutes every day to focus on stress management. Sure, it would be better if I spent more time daily on MBM, but the reason I brought this up is because I have a never-ending to-do-list, and I also enjoy spending time with my wife and two daughters.

While I realize that you also might not have a lot of time to focus on MBM, it all comes down to setting priorities, and the key is to get into the routine of doing this. Even if you can only set aside five minutes initially to do some deep breathing daily this will still be beneficial. Then, once you get into the routine, you may eventually increase the amount of time you spend each day improving your stress-management skills.

The Role of the Hypothalamic-Pituitary-Adrenal (HPA) Axis

Many natural healthcare professionals who do adrenal testing will focus on improving the health of the patient's adrenal glands, even though the problem is frequently with the HPA axis. With regards to adrenal health, the hypothalamus secretes hormones called corticotropin-releasing hormone (CRH) and vasopressin, which, in turn, stimulates the pituitary to release adrenocorticotropic hormone (ACTH), and this hormone acts on the adrenal cortex to produce glucocorticoids.

Cortisol is the main hormone produced by the adrenal cortex. Just as is the case with thyroid hormone, through negative feedback, cortisol will inhibit the hypothalamus and pituitary gland, which, in turn, will decrease the secretion of CRH, vasopressin, and, ultimately, cortisol. Epinephrine and norepinephrine are produced by the adrenal medulla.

In order to improve the communication between the hypothalamus and pituitary gland, it's important to understand some of the common factors that can cause dysregulation in the first place.

1. Chronic stress. I have already discussed the role of stress, and chronic stress is probably the biggest factor that causes dysregulation of the HPA axis. Obviously the adrenals are greatly affected with regards to stress, but chronic stress affects both the HPA axis and the hypothalamic-pituitary-thyroid (HPT) axis.[80,81] And the activation of the HPA axis will also inhibit the hypothalamic-pituitary-gonadal (HPG) axis. [82,83]

What is the consequence of this? Well, one big consequence is that chronic stress can have a negative effect on fertility. The pregnenolone steal is a condition in which the body prioritizes the production of cortisol at the expense of the sex hormones. This make sense, since for someone in a stressed state, reproducing usually isn't a priority. This is why if someone has low sex hormones (e.g., estrogen, progesterone, or testosterone) it is necessary to first focus on improving the health of the adrenals.

2. Inflammation. Cytokines regulate inflammation and play a role in the communication between the hypothalamus and the pituitary gland, as they normally stimulate the HPA axis, while suppressing the HPT axis and HPG axis.[84,85,86] However, autoimmune thyroid conditions such as Hashimoto's usually involve an increase in proinflammatory cytokines, which, in turn, can cause miscommunication between the hypothalamus and pituitary gland,[87,88] which, in turn, can affect the adrenals, thyroid, and/or gonads.

3. Neurotransmitter imbalances. Some of the neurotransmitters can modulate the HPA Axis. Numerous studies show that serotonin activates the HPA axis.[89,90] Dysregulation of the HPA axis seems to be a factor in depression,[91] and serotonin is the primary neurotransmitter implicated in the pathophysiology of depression. It also appears that dopamine plays a role in modulating the HPA axis.[92,93] The neurotransmitter gamma-aminobutyric acid (GABA) can also influence the HPA axis.[94]

4. Medications. Certain medications can cause problems as well. For example, evidence shows that inhaled corticosteroids, such as those used in asthma, can result in HPA axis suppression, and thus lead to adrenal insufficiency.[95,96] Corticosteroids can also inhibit the HPT axis, and thus lead to hypothyroidism.[97,98] Statins are another drug that can potentially affect the hypothalamus and pituitary gland, as I came across a study showing that statins can potentially lower testosterone levels by affecting the HPG axis.[99]

Can Physical and Emotional Trauma Trigger Hashimoto's?

Research indicates that both physical and emotional traumas can be a factor in autoimmunity. Although I wasn't able to find any studies that related directly to Hashimoto's, I did come across a study showing that severe tissue trauma can result in a profound proinflammatory response that can trigger autoimmunity in those with a susceptibility to systemic lupus erythematosus.[100] Thus, I suppose it is possible that if someone had severe trauma to the thyroid gland then this might result in autoimmunity, assuming other factors I have discussed in this book were also present (e.g., a genetic predisposition or a leaky gut).

As for emotional trauma, based on what I have discussed in this chapter, it probably isn't surprising that there is evidence that posttraumatic stress disorder (PSTD) can increase the risk of developing autoimmunity,[101,102] perhaps by exhibiting a different type of regulatory T cell that might be less suppressive.[103] I also came across a study showing that childhood traumatic stress can increase the chances of being hospitalized with a diagnosed autoimmune condition decades into adulthood.[104] Another study showed that childhood maltreatment is associated with an increased risk of subclinical hypothyroidism in pregnancy.[105]

How Can You Test for Adrenal Problems and HPA Axis Dysregulation?

I'll discuss testing for adrenal imbalances in section three. However, I did want to mention here that most endocrinologists don't do any adrenal testing unless they suspect a severe case of adrenal insufficiency such as Addison's Disease. Otherwise, they usually will dismiss adrenal problems as having any relationship to conditions such as Hashimoto's, despite the evidence I have discussed in this chapter. I'm not suggesting that everyone who has Hashimoto's has adrenal problems and/or HPA axis dysregulation, but these imbalances are very common, and, in my opinion, it is foolish to dismiss them as not being a potential cause or contributing factor.

Chapter Highlights:

- With chronic stress, the adrenals continue to secrete cortisol, and, while this might initially result in elevated cortisol levels, over a prolonged period this can result in depressed cortisol levels, along with a depressed DHEA.
- Healthy cortisol levels are important to maintain healthy blood sugar levels, maintain a normal blood pressure, help with immunity and inflammation, and regulate metabolism of fat, protein, and carbohydrates.
- Chronic stress can dysregulate immune function by increasing the production of proinflammatory and type-2 cytokines.
- Chronic stress can affect immunity by decreasing secretory IgA.
- The perception of the stressor is more important than the actual stressor itself, and the good news is that you can change your perception of stress.
- One way to modify your perception of stress is by incorporating one or more mind-body medicine techniques such as meditation, yoga, or biofeedback.
- Chronic stress is probably the biggest factor that causes dysregulation of the hypothalamic-pituitary-adrenal (HPA) axis.
- Other factors that can cause dysregulation of the HPA axis include inflammation, neurotransmitter imbalances, and certain medications.
- Evidence shows that both physical and emotional traumas can be a factor in autoimmunity

CHAPTER 8

ENVIRONMENTAL TOXINS

WE LIVE IN A TOXIC world with tens of thousands of chemicals in our environment, and we're exposed to many of these daily. Unfortunately many toxins are considered to be safe until proven otherwise, when the opposite should be true. It is impossible to completely avoid these toxic chemicals, thus the next best thing would be to minimize your exposure to environmental toxins while, at the same time, detoxifying these chemicals from your body regularly.

I can easily write an entire book on environmental toxins, and perhaps one day I'll do so! But for now, I will dedicate two chapters to environmental toxins. This chapter will focus on some of the common environmental toxins that can potentially trigger an autoimmune condition such as Hashimoto's. Then, in the fourth section, Chapter 29 will discuss how to reduce your toxic load and support your detoxification pathways. I'll also discuss some of the different options available for testing environmental toxins in the third section.

The Problem With Most Research Studies on Environmental Toxins

The research regarding environmental toxins and thyroid autoimmunity is incomplete. Tens of thousands of chemicals are in our environmental, but most of the long-term side effects of these environmental toxins are unknown. In addition, most of the research studies that have been conducted involve testing these chemicals in isolation. This is problematic because the combination of certain chemicals can be even more toxic to our health.

A good example of this involves glyphosate, which is the active ingredient in the herbicide Roundup, to which I've dedicated Chapter 20. But I'll say here that most studies involving glyphosate have been conducted in isolation. Most pesticide and herbicide formulations also contain something called adjuvants, which are labeled as being inert by most manufacturers. Roundup contains glyphosate in combination with ethoxylated adjuvants, which makes the formulation even more toxic than if it only included glyphosate alone.[106]

While I'll discuss some of the research of individual environmental toxins that can potentially trigger Hashimoto's, the truth is that we have no idea what the cumulative effects of these toxins have on our body. Another thing to keep in mind is that being exposed to many chemicals over time can lead to a glutathione deficiency, which is a factor in experiencing a loss of chemical tolerance, also known as toxicant-induced loss of tolerance (TILT). This can lead to "multiple chemical sensitivity syndrome," and eventually Hashimoto's thyroiditis.

What's the Difference Between Toxins and Toxicants?

Although I use the word "toxins" throughout this book, most chemicals we're exposed to are actually "toxicants." "Toxin" refers to a substance produced by living cells or organisms, whereas a "toxicant" refers to a synthetic substance. For example, snake venom would be an example of a "toxin," while bisphenol A (BPA) would be an example of a "toxicant." Thus, when I discuss "environmental toxins," in most cases, I am actually referring to "environmental toxicants."

What Outdoor Air Pollutants Are We Most Commonly Exposed to?

When going through my masters in nutrition degree, I took a biotransformation and detoxification course taught by Dr. Walter Crinnion, a naturopathic doctor for over 30 years who focuses on environmental pollution and detoxification. I learned from Dr. Crinnion that the following are some of the top sources of outdoor air pollution:

- Transportation: cars, buses, trucks
- Fuel consumption in stationary sources
- Industrial processes

- Solid waste disposal
- Chemical dumps
- Aerial spraying of farms
- Forest fires

Some of the most common pollutants include volatile organic compounds (VOCs), which are solvents and include benzene and xylene. Other environmental toxins we're commonly exposed to include Polycyclic aromatic hydrocarbons (PAH), carbon monoxide, ozone, heavy metals, pesticides, and herbicides.

The Effect of Outdoor Air Pollution on Thyroid Health

An interesting study revealed the impact of certain chemicals on thyroid peroxidase (TPO) activity.[107] Thyroid peroxidase is an enzyme that plays an important role in thyroid hormone production. The study showed that benzophenones, PAHs, and persistent organic pollutants altered TPO activity at low doses.

Some of the chemicals in this study decreased TPO activity, while others increased TPO activity. So when looking to restore the health of someone with Hashimoto's, one can't overlook the impact of these environmental toxins. Another study showed that certain benzene-related compounds could lead to thyroid dysfunction.[108]

Another study showed that perflurocarbons from common household products such as food containers; stain-resistant protection for clothing, furniture, and carpets; and paints are associated with thyroid disease in women.[109] Some studies have shown that certain solvents such as benzene have a negative effect on thyroid function.[110] Regarding the products we use, one study showed that parabens could affect thyroid hormone levels, especially in women.[111]

Pesticides Can Directly Affect Thyroid Health and Thyroid Autoimmunity

One study examined the association between the use of organochlorines and risk of hypothyroidism and hyperthyroidism.[112] They found that the use of chlordane, the fungicides benomyl and maneb/mancozeb, and the herbicide paraquat were significantly associated with hypothyroidism. The data in the study showed that there was a role of organochlorines and fungicides in the etiology of thyroid disease.

Another study assessed the burden of organochlorine pesticides and their influence on thyroid function in women.[113] Out of the analyzed pesticides, the concentration of p,p'-DDT and its metabolites was higher in all subjects, but dieldrin was found to be significantly high in the hypothyroid women.

Yet another study evaluated the pesticide effects on reproductive and thyroid hormones of cotton farmers.[114] The study concluded that pesticide exposure is associated with thyroid and reproductive hormone level disturbance. Other studies show that pesticides and other environmental factors can be a factor in thyroid autoimmunity.[115,116] We also can't ignore the harmful effects these chemicals have on babies and children. One study showed that prenatal exposure to organochlorines could lead to an increased prevalence of thyroid antibodies, along with other health issues, in those born to highly exposed mothers.[117]

Please don't overlook the importance of the previous sentence, as this is probably one of the reasons why we see more and more children and teenagers with Hashimoto's. Regarding chemical exposure during pregnancy, one study mentioned that the major sources of exposure for six classes of concern include phthalates, phenols, perfluorinated compounds, flame retardants, polychlorinated biphenyls, and organochlorine pesticides.[118] For this reason, before trying to conceive, it is a very good idea to take at least a few months to reduce your toxic load, as doing this might help to reduce the incidence of autoimmune conditions such as Hashimoto's.

Can Bisphenol A Trigger Hashimoto's?

Bisphenol A (BPA) is a chemical commonly found in plastic water bottles and many other sources, including food packaging, dental materials, healthcare equipment, thermal paper (i.e., receipts), as well as toys and articles for children and infants.[119] A few studies show a relationship between BPA and thyroid autoimmunity. One study showed a relationship between BPA and thyroid peroxidase antibodies.[120] The study discussed how BPA might enhance autoimmunity through a few different mechanisms.

Dr. Datis Kharrazian is the author of *Why Do I Still Have Thyroid Symptoms When My Lab Tests Are Normal?* In a journal article, he mentions that a potential mechanism for the role of BPA in autoimmunity may be structural molecular mimicry.[121] He suggests that there might be a structural similarity between BPA and triiodothyronine (T3), which leads to a potential cross-reactivity. In a more recent study, Dr. Kharrazian mentions many other immunological mechanisms for BPA to induce autoimmunity, including the following:[122]

- Altered hepatic biotransformation
- Pituitary lactotrophic cell activation to synthesize prolactin
- Estrogen receptor endocrine disruption
- Altered cytokine expression
- Lipopolysaccharide-induced nitric oxide promotion
- Altered antigen-presenting cell reactivity
- Altered immunoglobulin activity
- Th17 aryl hydrocarbon receptor activation

What Are Polychlorinated Biphenyls?

Polychlorinated biphenyls (PCBs) are synthetic organochlorine chemicals that were useful industrial products in the past, but their production was ended because they persist in both the environment and in living organisms.[123] Even though they are no longer manufactured, they persist in our environment and can be a factor in many health conditions, including Hashimoto's. One study involving 2,046 adults from Slovakia found that exposure to PCBs was associated with hypothyroidism and an increase in thyroid autoantibodies.[124] Another study showed an increase in thyroid peroxidase antibodies in those exposed to persistent organic pollutants, including PCBs.[125]

Can Ionizing Radiation Trigger Hashimoto's?

Ionizing radiation is a known cause of thyroid cancer.[126] Can it trigger Hashimoto's? While primary hypothyroidism is the most common radiation-induced thyroid dysfunction,[127] evidence also shows that external radiation increases the risk of autoimmune thyroiditis, especially with regards to radiation treatment for cancers of the neck region.[128,129]

Evidence also shows an increased prevalence of thyroid autoimmunity in Chernobyl-contaminated regions. One study demonstrated findings of autoimmune thyroid disease at markedly increased frequency in a population of children with poor iodine status.[130] Another study found a dose-response relationship between I131 doses and thyroid peroxidase antibodies[131] in that a higher dose of ionizing radiation was associated with a greater prevalence of thyroid peroxidase antibodies.

Common Sources of Indoor Pollutants

I discussed volatile organic compounds (VOCs) earlier, and while these are factors in outdoor air pollution, according to the Environmental Protection Agency (EPA), there is actually greater exposure to VOCs from the air inside our homes. Some examples of the solvents found in breath samples include chloroform, trichloroethane, and benzene.

Here are some of the sources of these solvents that are commonly found indoors:

- Mothballs and deodorants (have paradichlorobenzene)
- Plastics, foam rubber, and insulation (styrene)
- Dry cleaning (tetrachloroethylene)
- Paints (styrene and xylene)
- Tap water (chloroform)

If someone in the house is a smoker then the people living there will be exposed to a greater amount of these chemicals. Benzene is a known carcinogen that is present in tobacco smoke, along with many other chemicals.

While I did come across one study that suggested that cigarette smoking may increase the risk of hypothyroidism in people with Hashimoto's,[132] many more studies show a correlation between smoking and Graves' disease.[133,134] Regardless of what the research shows, those with Hashimoto's should avoid smoking cigarettes and try to minimize their exposure to second-hand smoke.

Are the Chemicals From Your Carpet Making You Sick?

Carpets are also a big source of chemicals, as they can contain VOCs, formaldehyde, dust mites, and other environmental toxins. One study showed that carpets of different type (wool, synthetic) emitted benzene, toluene, xylenes, styrene, 4-phenylcyclohexane, 2, 2-butoxyethoxy-ethanol, along with acetone and formaldehyde.[135] Although some of these were emitted in low concentrations, these chemicals still can have a negative impact on your health.

Hardwoods also aren't free from chemicals. Compounds such as methanol, acetaldehyde, and acetic acid are commonly released from hardwoods.[136] Thus, if you get hardwoods installed you want to choose those that are low VOC.

There is also a concern when it comes to flame retardants, also known as polybrominated diphenyl ethers (PBDEs). These are found in mattresses, couches, and other furniture. An article in USA Today focused on this. It discussed a study led by Duke University, which showed that out of 102 couches tested, 85% were treated with some kind of untested or potentially toxic flame retardant. The same study discussed how these flame retardants "are linked to hormone disruption, cancer, and neurological toxicity in hundreds of animal studies and several human ones".[137]

Flame retardants are included not only in products such as furniture but also in clothing. The next time you are visiting a retail store, look at some of the children's pajamas. They come with a large warning tag stating that they are treated to be fire-resistant, and if you have children or grandchildren, you want to avoid buying clothes with these tags.

Another study found a high prevalence of primary hypothyroidism (11%) in workers from a factory that produced polybrominated biphenyls.[138,139] The hypothyroidism was frequently associated with an elevation of thyroid peroxidase antibodies, and less frequently, anti-thyroglobulin antibodies.[139] It was suggested that the bromine might be a factor in the thyroid dysfunction, although they didn't elaborate as to whether this also was responsible for the elevated thyroid autoantibodies. Another study showed that PBDE exposure was associated with increased thyroglobulin antibodies.[140]

Can PBDEs Cause the Extinction of Giant Pandas?

While conducting my research on PBDEs, I came across a 2017 journal article that discussed how these chemicals pose a risk to captive giant pandas.[141] Although the focus of this book is on Hashimoto's, I admit that I have a soft spot for animals, especially those that are endangered. According to the journal article, the Qinling subspecies of giant panda are highly endangered, as fewer than 350 that inhabit the Qinling Mountains.

The blood and feces of captive and wild pandas were tested to find 13 types of PBDEs and a total PBDE concentration that was 255% higher than in wild pandas. Nine types of PBDEs were found in the blood samples, and the PBDEs in the blood were significantly higher in the captive pandas than in the wild pandas. The study concluded that these chemicals could be threatening the panda's health.

While I'm guessing that most people reading this don't have a pet panda, many do have other types of pets that are being affected by harmful chemicals. If you're not an animal lover, then I'm hoping that reading this information will make you realize the impact these chemicals can have on the health of you and your family.

Switch to Natural Household Cleaners, Air Fresheners, Cosmetics, etc.

When I discuss environmental toxins in my articles, webinars, or directly with my patients, I commonly recommend making the switch to natural products. Now, I'm making this recommendation to you in this book. The chemicals from these products can, without question, have a harmful effect on your thyroid and immune system health. Fortunately, natural substitutes exist for just about every household product.

It would be great if you can switch to all natural and organic products, but I realize that doing this can be expensive. However, in the long run, it will be less costly when you consider the impact these chemicals have on your health. Nevertheless, I realize that many people still won't change their products, so if you can't afford to buy everything natural, then you need to prioritize.

I would begin with any sprays or air fresheners you use, as these will have a big impact on your respiratory tract and immune system. Put aside the harsh brand name cleaning chemicals and purchase some natural household cleaners, or simply use vinegar, baking soda, and/or an essential oil such as Melaleuca alternifolia (tea tree oil) as a cleaning agent.

Regarding cosmetics, use a natural deodorant that is free of aluminum, and if you use body creams or lotions you want these to be free of any chemicals since you're rubbing them into your body. If you don't want to buy natural soaps and shampoos, at least try to purchase products without artificial fragrances. This topic deserves its own chapter, as there's so much I can discuss about natural products and cosmetics.

Check Out the Skin Deep Website

When choosing skincare products you might want to consider visiting the Environmental Working Group's Skin Deep website. This consists of a database of over 70,000 products, including soaps, shampoos, deodorants, sunscreen, makeup, toothpaste, and many other products. The information regarding the ingredients from the personal care products listed on their website is from the published scientific literature, and the ratings given indicate the level of concern due to the ingredients in the product.

For example, if you visit **www.ewg.org/skindeep** and search for Acure Organics Night Cream, you'll see that the overall hazard is low, the risk of developing cancer is low, and the risks of allergies and immunotoxicity is low. This doesn't mean that there is absolutely no risk from using this product, but it is on the low side. If you look at the overall rating of the Acure Organics brand, you'll see that the overall hazard is low, the risk of cancer is low, the risk of developmental and reproductive toxicity is low, but the risk of allergies and immunotoxicity is moderate.

Let's Not Forget About the Chemicals Found in Foods

Not surprisingly, the chemicals found in certain foods can have a negative impact on your health. This is why you want to try to eat as many organic foods as possible. While organic food won't be free of environmental toxins, in most cases, they will have significantly less chemicals than non-organic food. Pesticides are found in many fruits and vegetables.

According to a recent review of certain studies comparing the health effects of organic and conventional foods,[142] two studies reported significantly lower urinary pesticide levels among children consuming organic versus conventional diets. Even though there are still risks of pesticide exposure when consuming organic food, if you minimize your exposure to pesticides but don't completely eliminate them, it would still be worth eating organic in my opinion.

Since the discovery of DDT in 1939, numerous pesticides (organo-chlorides, organophosphates, carbamates) have been developed and used extensively worldwide with few guidelines or restrictions.[143] In 1992, the World Health Organization (WHO) reported that roughly three million pesticide poisonings occurred annually, resulting in 220,000 deaths worldwide. Over the last few decades since this was reported, things have only gotten worse.

Farmers seem to be at high risk for being affected by endocrine disrupting chemicals, as they are exposed to a greater amount of pesticides than the general public. Some studies have shown that the incidence of hormone-related organ cancers, or hormonal cancers, is elevated among farmers.[144] Pesticides have been classified as carcinogens in humans by the International Agency for Research on Cancer.[145]

Among the organochlorine pesticides tested, toxaphene, dieldrin, and endosulfan had estrogenic properties comparable to those of DDT and chlordecone.[146] Several environmental chemicals are capable of binding to the androgen receptor and interfering with its normal function, includ-ing the organophosphate pesticide fenitrothion.[147]

Can Botox Injections Trigger Hashimoto's?

Botox injections use various forms of botulinum toxin to temporarily paralyze muscle activity. It works by blocking the release of the neurotrans-mitter acetylcholine, which leads to inactivity of the muscles or glands innervated.[148] Botox injections are commonly used to reduce the appear-ance of facial wrinkles, although they can also treat other problems including neck spasms, an overactive bladder, and lazy eye. One case study showed a possible link between Botox injections and Hashimoto's thyroiditis.[149] It involved a woman who experienced elevations of TSH after Botox injections in her eyelids, and the authors suggested that there might be a link between the Botox injections and the TSH elevations through a molecular mimicry mechanism, as they found that Botox and thyroid autoantigens shared a similar amino acid sequence.

The Relationship Between Toxic Metals and Hashimoto's

Just as is the case with other environmental toxins, nobody is going to eliminate all of the toxic metals from their body. Everyone has mercury, cadmium, arsenic, and other heavy metals stored in their tissues. Some people have small amounts of these toxic metals, while other people have larger amounts. Either way, the goal is to minimize your exposure to toxic metals, while trying to take measures that will help eliminate these (and other environmental chemicals) from your body.

Mercury. Many factors can trigger Hashimoto's, and a few studies have shown evidence of a link between mercury exposure and thyroid autoim-munity, along with other autoimmune conditions.[150,151] Some of the sources of mercury exposure include dental amalgams, fish, vaccines, and indus-trial use. Also, many babies are being born with high levels of mercury passed on from the mother. This is the case with other heavy metals as well.

One study looked at the total mercury concentrations in the liver, kidney, and cerebral cortex of 108 children aged 1 day to 5 years, and the mercury levels of 46 fetuses were determined.[152] The study found that the mercury in the fetuses and older infants correlated significantly with the number of dental amalgam fillings of the mother. Evidence also shows that methylmercury from fish can affect the fetus.

Even though mercury can potentially trigger autoimmunity, the organ most affected by this heavy metal is the brain. Evidence indicates that mercury from dental amalgam fillings may contribute to the body burden of mercury in the brain.[153] Thus, for those people with Hashimoto's who are suffering from the symptoms of brain fog, if you have mercury amalgams, then this can be one potential cause.

To help reduce your exposure to mercury, you want to avoid eating larger fish, consider replacing mercury amalgams, and try to avoid vaccines. However, you need to be very cautious when getting dental amalgams removed, and if you choose to get this done, I would recommend working with a biological dentist. A good resource for finding one is by going online and visiting the website for the International Academy of Oral Medicine and Toxicology. Their website is **www.IAOMT.org**. The International Academy of Biological Dentistry & Medicine is another resource, and their website is **www.iabdm.org**.

Aluminum. Some of the common sources of aluminum include pots and pans, aluminum cans, deodorant, aluminum foil, and some vaccines. Aluminum is another environmental toxin that can be found in tap water. Evidence suggests that high levels of aluminum can be a factor in the development of Alzheimer's Disease.[154,155]

Although I didn't find any research that showed a link between aluminum exposure and Hashimoto's, keep in mind that aluminum is a demonstrated neurotoxin and a strong immune stimulator.[156] This is why aluminum is commonly added to vaccines as an adjuvant.

An adjuvant is a substance that is added to a vaccine to increase the body's immune response to the vaccine. Experimental evidence shows that simultaneous administration of as little as two to three immune adjuvants can overcome genetic resistance to autoimmunity.[157] In other words, even if you have a genetic resistance to developing autoimmune conditions such as Hashimoto's, there is the possibility this condition can be triggered by exposure to multiple adjuvants.

Exposure to multiple adjuvants happens quite frequently in children through the routine administration of vaccinations. In some countries, by the time children are four to six years old, they will have received a total of 126 antigenic compounds along with high amounts of aluminum adjuvants through routine vaccinations.[158] Perhaps this is another factor behind the higher incidence of Hashimoto's in children and teenagers. I'll further discuss adjuvants in Chapter 19.

Arsenic. Some of the sources of arsenic include pesticides, herbicides, chicken, and brown rice. Exposure to arsenic in drinking water is common in many countries.[159] Inorganic arsenic is considered to be toxic. The highest levels of these arsenics in groundwater occur in the West, Midwest, and Northeast regions of the United States.

A recent journal article discussed how high concentrations of inorganic arsenic are found in some rice-based foods and drinks widely used in infants and young children.[160] Thus, while adults need to be cautious about consuming large amounts of inorganic arsenic, if you have children, then you want to make sure that they aren't eating large amounts of these foods. Poultry and seafood are the primary sources of organic arsenics, which are considered to have very low toxicity.

The health consequences of chronic arsenic exposure include increased risk for various forms of cancer and many noncancer effects, including diabetes, skin diseases, chronic cough, and toxic effects on the liver, kidney, cardiovascular system, and peripheral and central nervous systems. While I couldn't find any research that shows a relationship between arsenic exposure and Hashimoto's, evidence indicates that exposure to arsenic can directly affect thyroid health,[161] possibly by affecting the thyroid hormone receptors.[162]

Cadmium. Some of the sources of cadmium include cigarette smoke, tap water, coffee, shellfish, refined foods, and marijuana. Studies suggest that cadmium is associated with several clinical complications, such as renal dysfunction and bone disease, but also some cancers.[163] A few studies have shown that cadmium exposure can cause thyroid dysfunction.[164,165] Just as mercury can potentially trigger autoimmunity, the same might be true of cadmium.[166]

Lead. Some of the common sources of lead exposure include cigarette smoke, colored inks, lead-based paints, ceramic glazes, and congenital causes. Diets deficient in calcium, magnesium, and/or iron can make someone more susceptible to a lead toxicity problem. Evidence indicates lead exposure can lead to depressed thyroid hormone levels.[167,168] However, other studies show no relationship between lead exposure and thyroid health. It is possible that the amount of lead can play a role on how it affects thyroid health. While lead might play a role in autoimmunity,[169] I wasn't able to find any correlation in the research between lead and Hashimoto's.

Electronic Pollution

We are surrounded by electromagnetic fields, also known as EMFs. Every electronic device emits EMFs. This includes televisions, computers, refrigerators, cell phones, vacuum cleaners, and fluorescent lights. Much controversy surrounds the effects of EMFs on the cells and tissues of the body. The safe limit of EMF exposure seems to be 2.5 milligauss, according to the Environmental Protection Agency.

How do EMFs affect thyroid health? Studies in rats have found that exposure to both 50 Hz and 900 MHz EMFs decrease the production of thyroid hormone.[170] Cell phones emit about 900 MHz.

However, does this translate to humans? One study on the correlation between cell phone use and thyroid health showed a higher than normal TSH and lower thyroid hormone levels in those who used their cell phones more frequently.[171] The study concluded that there are possible harmful effects of mobile microwaves on the hypothalamic-pituitary-thyroid axis.

As for whether electromagnetic fields can cause Hashimoto's, I did come across a journal article that looked at the relationship between electromagnetic fields and autoimmunity.[172] The authors mentioned how exposure to electromagnetic fields may induce a stress-like situation, which can be a factor in autoimmunity. Of course, this doesn't confirm a direct relationship between EMFs and autoimmune conditions such as Hashimoto's.

Another study conducted on rats showed that there were no adverse effects of long-term EMF exposure on T cell populations, including Th17 cells, regulatory T cells, or the Th1/Th2 balance.[173] More studies are needed in this area.

Even if EMFs weren't a direct trigger of Hashimoto's, I still would recommend trying your best to minimize your exposure to them. Evidence suggests that EMFs can potentially cause infertility[174] and cancer,[175] although more research is needed.

Chapter Highlights:

- Some of the top sources of outdoor air pollution include transportation, fuel consumption in stationary sources, industrial processes, solid waste disposal, chemical dumps, aerial spraying of farms, and forest fires.
- Some of the common environmental pollutants we're exposed to include VOCs such as benzene and xylene, polycyclic aromatic hydrocarbons, carbon monoxide, ozone, heavy metals, pesticides, and herbicides.
- Common sources of volatile organic compounds include mothballs and deodorants, plastics, foam rubber, dry cleaning, paints, and tap water.
- Tobacco smoke includes benzene and other harmful chemicals.
- Carpets can contain VOCs, formaldehyde, dust mites, and other environmental toxins.
- Compounds such as methanol, acetaldehyde, and acetic acid are commonly released from hardwoods.
- Flame retardants, also known as polybrominated diphenyl ethers (PBDEs), are found in mattresses, couches, and other furniture.
- Fortunately, natural alternatives to household cleaners, air fresheners, and cosmetics exist.
- A few studies have shown evidence of a link between mercury exposure and thyroid autoimmunity.
- Although I wasn't able to find studies that showed a direct relationship between other heavy metals and Hashimoto's, they can potentially trigger autoimmunity.
- Much controversy still surrounds the effects of EMFs on the cells and tissues of the body, but I recommend doing everything to minimize your exposure to them.

CHAPTER 9

THE ROLE OF INFECTIONS IN HASHIMOTO'S

C ERTAIN INFECTIONS CAN CAUSE autoimmunity, including bacteria, viruses, parasites, and fungal infections. In this chapter, I will start out by explaining how an infection can potentially lead to an autoimmune condition such as Hashimoto's. Then I'll discuss some of the common infections that can be potential triggers. In section three, I'll discuss what you can do to test for common infections, and in section four, I'll discuss the different treatment options for infections that you test positive for.

In order to better understand the relationship between infections and Hashimoto's, I'd like to start out by discussing dendritic cells and toll-like receptors, and then I'll discuss some of the different mechanisms in which an infection can lead to autoimmunity. If you don't want to understand how an infection can lead to an autoimmune condition such as Hashimoto's, you can always skip ahead and start reading about the different types of infections.

What Are Dendritic Cells?

Dendritic cells are part of your immune system and play a role in antigen presentation. An antigen is a foreign molecule such as a pathogenic bacteria. If someone has a bacterial infection, the dendritic cell will bind to the bacteria (antigen) and then present it to the immune system, which will do everything it can to destroy the bacteria.

In addition to dendritic cells, other antigen presenting cells include macrophages and B lymphocytes. Different antigen-presenting cells cause responses in different T cell populations.[176] Dendritic cells will cause responses in different T cells than macrophages, which will cause responses in different T cells than B lymphocytes.

What Is a Major Histocompatibility Complex?

A major histocompatability complex (MHC) aids in allowing the immune system to recognize these antigens. For example, if pathogenic bacteria invade the body, the MHC molecules are what actually bind to the proteins of these pathogens. After doing this, it displays them on the surface of the antigen presenting cell so that the appropriate T cells can recognize them, and these T cells then attempt to eradicate the bacteria.

What happens after the T cells recognize the antigens? Eventually, the T cells will attempt to destroy the pathogen, but before this happens, the T cell that binds to the MHC class II molecule is called a "naive" helper T cell. This naive helper T cell will become either a Th1 cell, a Th2 cell, a Th17 cell, or a regulatory T cell.[177] In a healthy immune system, you want a balance of Th1 and Th2 cells, a large amount of regulatory T cells (Tregs), and a low number of Th17 cells. But with autoimmunity, you commonly get an imbalance of the Th1 and Th2 pathways, along with an increase in Th17 cells and a decrease in Tregs.

What Are Toll-Like Receptors?

Toll-like receptors play an essential role in the development of autoimmune conditions such as Hashimoto's thyroiditis.[178,179] Toll-like receptors are a type of pattern recognition receptor, and these, in turn, recognize a wide range of something called pathogen-associated molecular patterns, also known as PAMPS.[180] PAMPs are found in pathogens such as viruses and bacteria.

An example of a PAMP is a lipopolysaccharide, which are large molecules found in gram-negative bacteria. These PAMPs are not normally found in the body of humans; thus they are immediately identified as being a foreign substance by the immune system. There is also something called DAMPs, which stands for "damage-associated molecular patterns." Unlike PAMPs, which are associated with infections, DAMPs are usually associated with trauma. Both PAMPs and DAMPs are involved in the inflammatory response.

Three Mechanisms of Autoimmunity

What I'd like to do now is discuss three possible mechanisms by which infections can trigger an autoimmune response and lead to the development of a condition such as Hashimoto's:

1. Molecular mimicry is one of the primary mechanisms, as this is where a foreign antigen (i.e., bacteria) shares a sequence or structural similarities with self-antigens.[181] Perhaps the best way to think of this is that certain pathogens (i.e., bacteria) have amino acid sequences that are similar to the amino acid sequences in our body. Thus, what happens is that the immune system essentially gets confused, and it not only attacks the proteins of the pathogen, but because their proteins are similar to our proteins, the immune system will also end up attacking our proteins as well.

2. Epitope spreading can also be a possible mechanism or contributing factor to autoimmunity. An epitope is the part of an antigen that is recognized by the immune system, and it's what the antibody binds to. With epitope spreading, the immune response to an infection causes damage to the tissues.[182,183]

3. Bystander activation describes an indirect or non-specific activation of autoimmune cells caused by the inflammatory environment present during an infection.[184,185] For example, if someone has a lot of inflammation due to gut dysbiosis, this can lead to the activation of immune system cells; thus, it can result in dysregulation of the immune system and potentially be a factor in autoimmunity.

Natural vs. Conventional Treatment Methods for Pathogens

One dilemma someone with an infection faces is whether to use conventional treatment methods, such as prescription drugs, or take a natural treatment approach. I will briefly discuss this here but will go into greater detail about treating infections in the fourth section. With an infection such as H pylori, triple therapy, consisting of a proton pump inhibitor (PPI), amoxicillin, and clarithromycin, was once commonly used, although more and more doctors are using quadruple therapy on H. pylori, which consists of a PPI plus three antimicrobials (clarithromycin, metronidazole/tinidazole and amoxicillin), or a PPI plus a bismuth plus tetracycline and metronidazole[186,187] because antibiotic-resistant strains of H. pylori are more prevalent.[188,189]

One of the downsides of using these drugs is that they have a negative effect on the health of the gut. Antibiotics can eradicate not only pathogenic bacteria but also good bacteria. They also can cause a leaky gut. Using PPIs also comes with some risks, which I discuss in Chapter 28.

What about natural treatment methods? Taking a natural treatment approach can be effective, and although I usually recommend natural treatment methods over prescription drugs, one of the downsides of using nutritional supplements and herbs is that they will almost always take longer to eradicate an infection such as H. pylori. Also, while natural antimicrobials usually won't be as harsh on the good bacteria, some herbs are more potent than others, and the good bacteria can be impacted to some extent even when taking a natural approach. Thus, you still need to be cautious when using natural antimicrobials.

Thus, one has to weigh both the benefits and risks of using conventional and natural treatment methods when eradicating infections. In most cases, taking prescription drugs will be a quicker process, but they also are harsher on the gut flora and are associated with greater side effects. However, it frequently will take longer to eradicate an infection using natural antimicrobials. Regardless of whether you take prescription drugs or natural antimicrobials, you want to take measures to improve the health of the gut environment, which I'll discuss in section four.

Different Types of Infections Associated With Hashimoto's

I will now discuss some of the pathogens that are commonly associated with Hashimoto's. Please keep in mind that this list isn't necessarily all-inclusive, and I'm sure future studies will demonstrate that other infections are linked to the development of Hashimoto's.

Epstein-Barr. Epstein-Barr virus (EBV) is one of the most common viruses in humans. EBV is usually spread through bodily fluids, primarily through the saliva.[190] Although many people with EBV are asymptomatic, some of the symptoms associated with an EBV infection include fatigue, fever, sore throat, swollen lymph nodes in the neck, a rash, and an enlarged spleen.[190]

Numerous studies have associated EBV with autoimmunity, including systemic lupus erythematosus (SLE), rheumatoid arthritis, and Sjögren's syndrome.[191] Also, evidence shows that Epstein-Barr can be a trigger for autoimmune thyroid conditions, including Hashimoto's. One study suggested that the high prevalence of EBV infection in cases of Hashimoto's (and Graves' disease) imply a potential role of EBV in triggering thyroid autoimmunity.[192] Another small study showed that EBV antibodies are more common in those with autoimmune thyroiditis.[193]

Can Epstein-Barr Be Responsible for All Thyroid Conditions?

As I was making the final changes to this book, a new book entitled *Medical Medium Thyroid Healing* was released by Anthony Williams. This book mentions that most thyroid and autoimmune thyroid conditions are due to the Epstein-Barr virus. This includes hypothyroidism and Hashimoto's thyroiditis, along with hyperthyroidism and Graves' disease, and even thyroid nodules and cysts. According to the author, the EBV attacks the thyroid gland, and the immune system attacks the virus, which is responsible for all of the different thyroid conditions. In other words, he doesn't consider EBV to be one of many different triggers of Hashimoto's, but labels it as being the sole cause behind this condition. He discusses how many other health conditions are related to EBV, including other autoimmune conditions, Lyme disease, and some types of cancers, including breast and prostate cancer.

While I don't agree that EBV is the sole factor behind most cases of Hashimoto's and other chronic health conditions, I must admit that I found this book to be very interesting, and I commend the author for trying to improve the health of others. While I'm thrilled that you are reading my book on Hashimoto's Triggers, I recommend reading other books on Hashimoto's as well. This way, you can come to your own conclusions based on the information presented.

I'll add that one of the keys to addressing viral infections is to improve the overall health of the immune system, thus even if EBV isn't the main cause behind your Hashimoto's condition, it can only benefit your health to eat well, improve your stress-management skills, and to do other things to improve your immune system health. I'll further discuss treating EBV and other infections in Chapter 31.

Herpes Simplex Virus. Genital herpes is a sexually transmitted disease caused by two types of viruses. The viruses are herpes simplex type 1 and herpes simplex type 2.[194] This usually results in mild symptoms, and genital herpes sores usually appear as one or more blisters on or around the genitals, rectum, or mouth.[194] Other areas that can be infected include the liver, lung, eye, and central nervous system.[195] Research suggests that herpes simplex virus infections are involved in a variety of autoimmune conditions, which may include the development of Hashimoto's.[196]

Hepatitis C. Hepatitis C virus is the most common chronic blood-borne infection in the United States.[197] Most people who become infected with this virus do so by sharing needles or other equipment to inject drugs, as well as the inadequate sterilization of medical equipment.[198,199] Although the infection can be mild in some people, in others, it can lead to liver cirrhosis or even liver cancer.

A relationship exists between hepatitis C and Hashimoto's. One study showed that the prevalence of hepatitis C virus is slightly increased in those with Hashimoto's.[200] This was confirmed in another study that showed that chronic hepatitis C infection could be associated with autoimmune thyroid conditions and hypothyroidism.[201] Another study showed that hepatitis C had a higher incidence in those with Graves' disease but not in patients with Hashimoto's.[202]

Parvovirus B19. The most common illness as a result of this virus is Fifth disease.[203] This is a mild rash illness, and some of the initial symptoms people present with include fever, runny nose, and headaches.[203] Parvovirus B19 can also lead to rashes, along with painful or swollen joints. The virus spreads through respiratory secretions such as saliva, sputum, or nasal mucus.[204] Parvovirus B19 has been associated with a few different autoimmune conditions, and strong evidence shows it also being involved in the development of some cases of Hashimoto's.[205]

HTLV-I. Human T-lymphotropic virus (HTLV-I) is estimated to infect 10 to 20 million people worldwide.[206] One study showed a high prevalence of thyroid peroxidase and thyroglobulin antibodies in HTLV-1 carriers.[207] Another study showed that HTLV-1 had a role in the development of both Hashimoto's and Graves' disease.[208]

Yersinia enterocolitica. Studies show evidence of a relationship between Yersinia enterocolitica and Hashimoto's. One study involving 71 patients showed that the prevalence of Yersinia enterocolitica plasmid-encoded outer proteins was 14-fold higher than those in the control groups.[209]

Helicobacter pylori. While an H. pylori infection is more commonly associated with Graves' disease, it can also be a potential trigger for Hashimoto's.[210,211,212] Although H. pylori can cause gastric and duodenal ulcers over a prolonged time, people infected with this bacteria are frequently asymptomatic. H. pylori infection can cause a deficiency of vitamin C, vitamin A, vitamin E, vitamin B12, folic acid, and essential minerals such as iron.[213]

Lyme disease. Borrelia burgdorferi is the pathogen associated with Lyme disease, and it is a potential trigger of Hashimoto's thyroiditis through molecular mimicry mechanisms.[214] I have dedicated Chapter 10 to Lyme disease and Hashimoto's.

Blastocystis hominis. Blastocystis hominis is a parasite that can inhabit the gastrointestinal tract of humans, as well as many animals. Some researchers question whether this parasite is beneficial to the host, or if it is pathogenic. The more recent research seems to point towards Blastocystis hominis as being a pathogenic parasite that should be eradicated. Some evidence indicates that it can be a potential trigger for Hashimoto's.

The most frequent symptoms associated with Blastocystis hominis include abdominal pain and diarrhea. Other symptoms include anorexia, fever, anal itching, and nausea.[215] However, not everyone with Blastocystis hominis experiences symptoms. Another thing to keep in mind is that other types of parasites can cause similar symptoms.

Blastocystis hominis is usually tested for through a stool panel. I'll discuss this type of testing in Chapter 25.

More About Blastocystis Hominis and Hashimoto's

I'd like to discuss specifically how Blastocystis hominis affects the immune system. Blastocystis appears to increase proinflammatory cytokines, including interleukin 1β (IL-1β), IL-6, and tumor necrosis factor alpha.[216] These proinflammatory cytokines are linked to autoimmune diseases, including Hashimoto's thyroiditis. In addition, Blastocystis hominis can increase intestinal permeability.[217,218] In other words, it can cause a leaky gut, which as you now know is also a factor in most, if not all autoimmune conditions.

One case report involving a 49-year old man with chronic urticaria and Hashimoto's showed that treating Blastocystis hominis with the drug metronidazole got rid of the urticaria, and normalized the thyroid hormones while decreasing the thyroid antibodies.[219] This is just a single case study, although I have worked with a few Hashimoto's patients who tested positive for Blastocystis hominis and went into remission upon eradication. Other healthcare professionals I know also have seen this with some of their patients.

Research also shows an increased risk of infection with Blastocystis hominis when stress is present[220] because Blastocystis hominis is opportunistic in immunocompromised patients, and stress can suppress the immune system and make someone more susceptible to such an infection.

Can Candida Albicans Trigger Hashimoto's?

People with Hashimoto's thyroiditis commonly have an overgrowth of Candida. As for whether a Candida overgrowth can be a trigger of autoimmunity, I think it's safe to say that in most cases having a Candida overgrowth isn't going to be a direct trigger of thyroid autoimmunity. However, evidence shows that a Candida overgrowth can result in an increase in proinflammatory cytokines,[221] which are a factor in autoimmune conditions such as Hashimoto's. In addition, a few studies show evidence of Candida causing an increase in autoantibodies,[222,223] although these don't involve thyroid peroxidase or thyroglobulin antibodies. However, a study by Dr. Aristo Vojdani did show immunological cross-reactivity between Candida albicans and human tissue, including the thyroid gland.[224]

In his book *Nutritional Medicine,* Dr. Alan Gaby mentions a possible mechanism of Candida-induced autoimmunity, as he discusses how the acetaldehyde produced by Candida can bind to serum proteins to form acetaldehyde-haptenated proteins. Dr. Gaby goes on to state that "haptenization of proteins could result in loss of functional activity and may induce antibody formation, potentially leading to the development of autoimmune disease".[225]

A hapten is an antigenic compound, and haptenization involves the reaction of this antigenic compound with a carrier protein. This, in turn, causes an immune system response. Thus, according to Dr. Gaby, the acetaldehyde produced by the Candida will bind with proteins in the blood, which, in turn, can trigger an autoimmune response. Even if having a Candida overgrowth doesn't directly trigger autoimmunity, there is evidence that it can disrupt the intestinal barrier.[226,227] Thus, a Candida overgrowth can potentially cause a leaky gut, which, in turn, is a factor in autoimmunity.

A Couple of Things to Keep in Mind...

Now that you are familiar with some of the more common pathogens that have been linked with Hashimoto's, a few other things are important to understand. First, not everyone with one or more of these infections will develop Hashimoto's. Even if someone has a genetic predisposition for Hashimoto's and is exposed to one of these pathogens, it won't always trigger an autoimmune response.

Second, this list of pathogens isn't all-inclusive, as I'm sure other pathogens can potentially cause thyroid autoimmunity and lead to a condition such as Hashimoto's. While we currently know much about certain infections and the role they play in autoimmunity, there is also a lot we don't know.

How Can You Determine if You Have One or More of These Infections?

I discuss testing for infections in the third section of this book, but I will briefly mention that different types of panels can determine if someone has one or more of these infections. For example, a comprehensive stool panel can be used to detect certain pathogenic bacteria, yeast overgrowth, and parasites. However, it's important to keep in mind that false negatives are possible, especially with yeast and parasites.

Concerning yeast overgrowth, I find an organic acids test to be the best method of determining if someone has a yeast overgrowth. This is a urine test and also tests for metabolites of bacterial overgrowth. While it would be great to have everyone order both a comprehensive stool panel and an organic acids test, these tests are expensive, and not everyone can afford to obtain both tests. Thus, if you suspect a yeast overgrowth or a pathogenic infection, then many times you have to try to determine which test would be most beneficial to obtain.

Blood tests are necessary for detecting some pathogenic infections. This includes testing for Borrelia burgdorferi (the bacteria associated with Lyme disease) and many of the co-infections. I'll discuss Lyme disease and the related co-infections in Chapter 10. Viruses are also usually best detected through the blood. Thus, if one suspects multiple infections then they might need to order a few different tests. Another option is to test for all of the pathogens I discussed that can potentially lead to Hashimoto's.

Chapter Highlights:

- Certain bacteria, viruses, parasites, and yeast/fungi can potentially trigger autoimmunity.
- If pathogenic bacteria invade the body, the MHC molecules actually bind to the proteins of these pathogens.
- Toll-like receptors are a type of pattern recognition receptor, and these, in turn, recognize a wide range of something called pathogen-associated molecular patterns (PAMPS),which are found in pathogens such as viruses and bacteria.
- Three ways in which infections can trigger an autoimmune response include 1) molecular mimicry, 2) epitope spreading, and 3) bystander activation.
- Some controversy exists over whether certain microbes should be eradicated, including H. pylori and Blastocystis hominis
- Some of the different pathogens associated with Hashimoto's thyroiditis include Epstein-Barr, herpes simplex virus, hepatitis C, Parvovirus B19, HTLV-1, Yersinia enterocolitica, Helicobacter pylori, Lyme disease, and Blastocystis hominis.
- One dilemma someone with an infection faces is whether to use conventional treatment methods such as prescription drugs or a natural treatment approach.
- It's very common for people with Hashimoto's to have an overgrowth of Candida.
- A Candida overgrowth is common in those with Hashimoto's, but whether it's a direct trigger of autoimmunity is controversial.

CHAPTER 10

LYME DISEASE AND OTHER TICK-BORNE COINFECTIONS

A S I DISCUSSED IN the previous chapter, infections such as H. pylori, Epstein-Barr, and Yersinia enterocolitica can trigger Hashimoto's. While these and other types of infections can be challenging to treat, Lyme disease and other tick-borne infections can be some of the most difficult infections to overcome. It's challenging enough to restore one's health when dealing with a condition such as Hashimoto's, but it's obviously even more challenging when someone has an autoimmune thyroid condition plus an infection such as Lyme disease.

Lyme disease is the most common tick-borne disease in the United States, as approximately 30,000 cases of Lyme disease are reported annually to the CDC.[228] However, many cases of Lyme disease aren't reported; thus the actual number is much higher than this. The disease is transmitted to humans through the bite of the Ixodes tick, and, in most cases, the tick must feed for at least 36 hours for transmission of the spirochete Borrelia burgdorferi to occur.[228] In some cases mosquitoes can also transmit B. burgdorferi,[229] but it's much more commonly transmitted through ticks. Treatment with antibiotics for two to four weeks will frequently help to resolve the problem, although some people end up with chronic Lyme disease.

Certain co-infections can also be transmitted along with B. burgdorferi, which can lead to a worsening of the symptoms. Having one or more of these co-infections can make Lyme disease even more challenging to treat. Here are some of the more common co-infections:[230]

- Bartonella species
- Yersinia enterocolitica
- Chlamydophila pneumonia
- Chlamydia trachomatis
- Mycoplasma pneumonia
- Babesia

Why Is Lyme Disease so Challenging to Treat?

One reason why Lyme disease is so difficult to treat is because it can invade other areas of the body, such as the nervous system. A second reason is due to the co-infections that are commonly transmitted along with Lyme disease. Most doctors don't test for these co-infections.

Lyme disease occurs in three stages, and, those in the later stages are more difficult to treat. Let's look at the different stages:

Stage #1. The symptoms of this stage will usually appear a few days or weeks after infection, and they commonly resemble the flu. Erythema migrans, also known as a "bull's-eye rash," is the most common manifestation of early Lyme disease.[231] Most doctors are trained to look for this "classic" rash, although certain variations are common.[231] However, it's important to understand that not everyone with Lyme disease has a rash, and a misdiagnosis of erythema migrans does occur, which can result in severe health consequences when left untreated. In most cases, administration of antibiotics for 2 to 4 weeks during this stage will eradicate the infection.

Stage #2. This stage of Lyme disease involves spreading of the disease. Although it is still possible to eradicate the infection during this stage, it is usually much more challenging, and a longer administration of antibiotics is recommended by most Lyme disease specialists. Cardiac manifestations such as heart block and muscle dysfunction are common during the second stage.[232] Spreading to the central nervous system can also occur within the first few weeks after skin infection,[233] yet Lyme disease may have a latency period of months to years before symptoms of late infection emerge.[234] This is yet another reason why early treatment can be very important.

Stage #3. The third stage is known as late stage Lyme disease, or chronic Lyme disease. Although Stage 2 Lyme disease involves spreading of the pathogen and can begin affecting the organ systems, in the third stage these symptoms can become more pronounced. The person might experience arthritis, neurological symptoms such as numbness in the extremities, or memory loss. The person might also develop a multitude of nonspecific CNS manifestations that can be confused with conditions such as multiple sclerosis, brain tumor, and psychiatric derangements.[234]

Some refer to chronic Lyme disease as "post-Lyme disease syndrome," which is defined as continuing or relapsing non-specific symptoms (e.g., fatigue, musculoskeletal pain, or cognitive complaints) in a patient previously treated for Lyme disease.[235] Although some healthcare professionals feel that these symptoms are caused by a persistent infection with B. burgdorferi, other sources suggest that these symptoms aren't due to B. burgdorferi but, instead, are caused by residual damage to tissues and the immune system that occurred during the infection.[236,237] This might explain why antibiotic therapy doesn't seem to offer any sustained benefit to patients with this condition.[235]

How Is Lyme Disease and Other Tick-Borne Infections Detected?

Here are some of the markers that can be used to determine if someone has Lyme disease:

Enzyme-Linked Immunosorbent Assay (ELISA). This is the most commonly used test. It doesn't test for the presence of Lyme disease, but measures the antibodies associated with this infection. The downside of the ELISA is that false negatives are common, especially with acute Lyme disease, as it takes at least a few weeks before someone develops these antibodies after becoming infected.

Western Blot. This is also a commonly recommended test, and the CDC requires 5 out of 10 "bands" for a test to be considered positive. Some bands are more significant than others; thus, some healthcare professionals will diagnose someone with Lyme disease, even if they have less than 5 bands. False results are possible with this test, and one study showed that 27.5% were found to have a false positive IgM immunoblot, which resulted in 78% of these patients receiving unnecessary antibiotic therapy.[238] False negatives can also occur, and according to **www.lymedisease.org**, using both the ELISA test and Western Blot together will result in failing to identify roughly 54% of patients with Lyme disease.

Culture for Borrelia burgdorferi. The probability of detecting B. burgdorferi through a culture depends on the specimen, the stage of the disease, and the expertise of the laboratory.[239]

CD57. This is a marker on natural killer cells, and since chronic Lyme disease is known to suppress the immune system, CD57 will typically be depressed.[240]

C4a. Chronic Lyme disease is associated with increased levels of C4a.[241] While this alone won't confirm that someone has Lyme disease, if someone with elevated C4a levels has been diagnosed with Lyme disease, a follow-up C4a can be used to determine if treatment for Lyme disease is successful.

C3a. Although C3a levels are usually elevated in acute Lyme disease, this marker is normal in chronic Lyme disease.

iSpot. This test helps to detect Borrelia antigen-specific effector/memory T cells.[242] In other words, it looks at the T cell response to B. burgdorferi, and some sources claim that it has a higher specificity and sensitivity when compared to the Western Blot.[242]

Specialty labs for Lyme disease, such as IGeneX, have something called a Complete Lyme Panel that includes the IFA (Immunofluorescent Assay) to screen for antibodies against B. burgdorferi, the IgG and IgM Western Blots that determine the type of B. burgdorferi antibodies, and a serum and whole blood PCR to help detect burgdorferi-specific DNAs.

IGeneX also offers testing for other tick-borne coinfections. This includes Babesia, Bartonella, Human Granulocytic Anaplasma, Rickettsia, and Chlamydophila pneumoniae. I will now discuss some of these common co-infections:

Babesiosis. Babesia is an intraerythroctyic protozoa that can lead to babesiosis, and it can cause symptoms similar to Lyme disease such as fatigue, muscle and joint pains, chills, and fever. It has a similar pathogenesis and clinical course as malaria.[243] IGeneX uses the immunofluorescent assay (IFA) to detect Babesia-specific IgG or IgM antibodies, as well as a PCR screen and something called the Fluorescent In-Situ Hybridization (FISH) assay.

Ehrlichia. Human monocytic ehrlichiosis is a tick-borne infectious disease transmitted by several tick species, especially Amblyomma species caused by Ehrlichia chaffeensis.[244] Two additional Ehrlichia species, Anaplasma phagocytophila and E. ewingii act as human pathogens.[244] IGeneX uses the Ehrlichia Indirect Immunofluorescence Assays and PCR tests to diagnose this infection.

Bartonella. Bartonella are bacteria, and many people with Lyme disease also have Bartonella infections.[245,246] Symptoms can include fatigue, headache, fever, swollen glands, along with other symptoms. IGeneX uses Immunofluorescence Assays and PCR testing to detect bartonella infections.

Rickettsia. Rickettsia species are gram-negative, obligate intracellular bacteria responsible for the spotted fever and typhus groups of diseases around the world.[247] Rickettsia rickettsii and Rickettsia conorii are transmitted by the bite of a tick, and thus can be a common co-infection associated with Lyme disease. Rocky Mountain spotted fever (RMSF), which is caused by Rickettsia rickettsii, is among the deadliest of all infectious diseases.[248] IGeneX has something called the Rickettsia species PCR test, which detects Rickettsia specific DNA.

Mycoplasma. Mycoplasma pneumonia is a common respiratory pathogen that produces diseases of varied severity ranging from a mild upper respiratory tract infection to severe atypical pneumonia.[249] This organism is also responsible for producing a wide spectrum of non-pulmonary manifestations including neurological, hepatic, cardiac diseases, hemolytic anemia, polyarthritis, and erythema multiforme.[249] The differential diagnosis between Lyme disease and Mycoplasma pneumoniae infection, or the recognition of the co-infection by Mycoplasma pneumoniae is problematic because both diseases result in similar manifestations.[250] PCR testing is commonly used to detect the presence of this infection.

Can Lyme Disease Trigger Hashimoto's?

Evidence indicates that B. burgdorferi can be a potential trigger of thyroid autoimmunity through a molecular mimicry mechanism.[251,252] In other words, thyroglobulin, thyroid peroxidase, and the proteins of B. burgdorferi can share amino acid sequences that can cause the immune system of someone with B. burgdorferi to attack these thyroid structures. Thus, there is an increased risk of developing Hashimoto's in someone who has Lyme disease.

Some of the co-infections associated with Lyme disease might also lead to Hashimoto's. For example, one case study showed that bartonella henselae could trigger autoimmune thyroiditis.[253] Mycoplasma species might also be a trigger.[254]

What Are the Treatment Options for Lyme Disease and Its Coinfections?

In Chapter 33, I'll discuss both conventional and alternative treatment options for Lyme disease. But I will say here that the conventional medical approach for both acute and chronic Lyme disease is to have the person take antibiotics. While this can be effective for many acute cases, antibiotics aren't nearly as effective for chronic cases of Lyme disease. What makes it even more challenging is that having one or more coinfections is common. Fortunately, a number of different alternative treatment options are available, although no specific natural treatment approach works in every case of chronic Lyme disease.

Chapter Highlights:

- Lyme disease is the most common tick-borne disease in the United States.
- Borrelia burgdorferi is the pathogen associated with Lyme disease.
- Some of the co-infections commonly associated with Lyme disease include Bartonella species, Babesia, Yersinia enterocolitica, Chlamydophila pneumoniae, Chlamydia trachomatis, and Mycoplasma pneumonia.
- Lyme disease has three stages with the later stages being more challenging to treat.
- Although some testing for Lyme disease and co-infections is available at conventional labs, specialty labs, such as IGeneX, offer more comprehensive testing.
- Evidence indicates that Borrelia burgdorferi can be a potential trigger of thyroid autoimmunity through a molecular mimicry mechanism.
- When Lyme disease is initially diagnosed, antibiotics are recommended by most medical doctors.
- Just as is the case with acute Lyme disease, most medical doctors will also recommend antibiotics for those with chronic Lyme disease, but they are much less effective.
- Although antibiotics might be the best option for many cases of acute Lyme disease, a natural treatment approach should be considered for chronic Lyme disease.

CHAPTER 11

TOXIC MOLD AND CHRONIC INFLAMMATORY RESPONSE SYNDROME

MOST PEOPLE DON'T CONSIDER the negative impact that mold can have on their health. But the mycotoxins produced from mold can cause many health issues and sometimes lead to debilitating symptoms. In this chapter, I'm going to discuss the negative health consequences of mycotoxins, chronic inflammatory response syndrome (CIRS), and how toxic mold can potentially lead to Hashimoto's.

Mycotoxins are frequently classified by the organ they affect. They can be hepatotoxins (affecting the liver), nephrotoxins (affecting the kidneys), neurotoxins (affecting the nervous system), immunotoxins (affecting the immune system), etc. Some mycotoxins affect multiple organs.

Over 300 types of mycotoxins are produced by molds. The concern isn't just with humans, as molds can affect livestock as well, which can indirectly affect humans. Aflatoxins are one of the most significant mycotoxins affecting livestock, although others include vomitoxin, zearalenone, fumonisin, and ochratoxin. Grains, such as corn, wheat, and barley, may be easily contaminated with mold, which is how the livestock get these mycotoxins.

How Is Mold Toxic to Your Health?

It's important to understand that not everyone has a negative reaction to mold. Genetics plays an important role with how people will react to mold. HLA is part of the immune system and is involved in antigen presentation. Certain HLA genotypes make people more susceptible to mycotoxins and cause many different symptoms. The reason why people with these genes are more likely to react to mold is because having one of these HLA genotypes will reduce the person's ability to clear the mycotoxins produced by the mold, which, in turn, is responsible for the symptoms people will experience.

Exposure to mold is well known to trigger inflammation, allergies and asthma, oxidative stress, and immune dysfunction in both human and animal studies. Mold spores, mycotoxins, and fungal fragments can be measured in buildings and in people who are exposed to these environments.

What Are the Symptoms of Toxic Mold?

There can be many symptoms associated with a mold toxicity, but the following are some of the most common ones:

- Severe fatigue
- Anxiety
- Insomnia
- Memory loss
- Migraines
- Skin rashes
- Respiratory distress
- Sinus problems
- Excessive thirst
- Neurological symptoms
- Frequent static shocks

If you happen to be dealing with many of the symptoms I just listed, then you might want to ask yourself the following questions:

- Is there a musty odor at home, at work, or in school?
- Are there any signs of water damage in these areas?
- Are there any leaks in the roof?
- Has your home (or place of work or school) ever been flooded?

How Are You Exposed to Mold?

Most people are exposed to mold through one of the following three ways:

1. Eating contaminated foods. Mycotoxins usually get into food in the field, or during storage. This is why shipping, handling, and storage practices of foods need to be considered. While most people are exposed to many mycotoxins through eating grains and other foods, such as nuts and seeds, animals consuming feeds that are contaminated with mycotoxins can produce meat and milk that contains these toxic residues.

2. Skin contact with mold. Sometimes, there is unusual growth of commensal species that is normally present on human skin or in the gut.

3. Inhalation of mycotoxins. This typically is the problem when someone is living in a water-damaged home, or if they work or go to school where there is toxic mold. If you feel worse while at home and feel better at work or school, this is a good sign of a mold problem in your home. The reverse is true as well.

If you work from home then you might notice that all of your symptoms improve when you go out of town for an extended period. And while the positive feeling of going on a vacation might play a role in you feeling better, if extreme symptoms disappear while away from your home, then you should consider hiring an indoor air inspector, which I'll discuss shortly.

Mold Toxicity vs. Chronic Inflammatory Response Syndrome

Chronic Inflammatory Response Syndrome (CIRS) occurs when genetically susceptible people are exposed to certain biotoxins. Although the focus of this chapter is on mold, CIRS can also result due to biotoxins associated with Lyme disease and its coinfections, as well as certain cyanobacteria, and a marine dinoflagellate that produces Ciguatera toxin.[255] Thus, in addition to being exposed to these biotoxins through mold, Lyme disease, and other pathogens, eating contaminated fish can also be a source.

Who is likely to develop CIRS? Well, not only does the person need to be exposed to biotoxins/mycotoxins from at least one of the sources I just mentioned, but they also need to have a genetic susceptibility. In other words, not everyone who is exposed to certain mycotoxins will develop CIRS. However, those who are exposed to certain mycotoxins (and other biotoxins) and are genetically susceptible will most likely develop CIRS. This, in turn, will lead to systemic inflammation and commonly cause vascular, neuroimmune, and endocrine imbalances.

Next I'll discuss in greater detail the testing involved, but if someone is suspicious of CIRS then they probably will want to start with genetic testing, as well as Visual Contrast Sensitivity testing. If these are positive (especially the genetics), then the person will want to proceed with some of the tests I describe next, and will also want to hire an indoor air specialist, making sure that ERMI testing is conducted.

Testing Options to Consider for Mold Toxicity/CIRS

Although I focus on the different types of testing in section three, I'll discuss the different testing options for mold toxicity in this chapter. When discussing testing for CIRS that is associated with a mold toxicity, you want to consider doing a few different things:

1. Genetic Testing for Human Leukocyte Antigens (HLAs). HLAs are found on the surfaces of cells and play a role in something called antigen presentation. Having certain HLA markers can make people susceptible to different conditions. For example, certain HLA markers can make someone more susceptible to developing an autoimmune condition such Hashimoto's.

Similarly, those who have certain HLA genetic markers will be unable to mount a proper immune response when exposed to mycotoxins, along with other types of biotoxins. Thus, they will develop a chronic inflammatory response. While the majority of people's bodies are able to get rid of mycotoxins without any intervention, this isn't the case with those who are genetically susceptible. As I'll discuss in this chapter, this chronic inflammatory process will lead to imbalances of the hormones, along with other imbalances responsible for the symptoms associated with a mold toxicity.

Testing for these markers should be considered because if a person has many of the symptoms listed earlier but test negative for all of these HLA markers, chances are they don't have a mold toxicity. However, if the person tests positive for one or more of these genetic markers then there is a much greater chance of them having a mold toxicity. You want to test for the following HLA markers:

HLA DRB1
HLA DQ

HLA DRB3
HLA DRB4
HLA DRB5

Fortunately, most local labs, including Labcorp and Quest Diagnostics, will test for these HLAs.

2. Visual Contrast Sensitivity (VCS) Test. This test can be conducted either online or in an office setting. This test determines your ability to see details at low contrast levels by presenting a series of images of decreasing contrast. Failing the test is a sign of neurological dysfunction, which can be due to the presence of neurotoxins.

While a positive finding of this test itself isn't diagnostic of a mold toxicity, in combination with some of the other tests, it can help to determine if someone has this condition. If you can't get a VCS test done in person, you can take an online VCS test, as a few different companies offer this, including **www.vcstest.com** and **survivingmold.com**.

3. Test your home for mold. With regards to testing your home for mold, you want to hire a certified indoor air testing company, preferably one that is open to ERMI testing. ERMI stands for Environmental Relative Moldiness Index. This involves DNA testing to identify the different species of molds by analyzing the dust. This test can be very helpful in identifying toxic strains of mold in the home, workplace, or schools. Keep in mind that not all air testing companies offer ERMI testing; thus, this is something you should ask when calling to schedule an appointment.

While you might not have control over testing a non-home environment such as work or school, if you feel worse while at work or school, and you don't feel as bad when you are at home, then mold very well might be an issue in these locations. If this is the case then you probably won't be able to hire an indoor air testing company to inspect the school or workplace, but you can contact the employer and/or principal about this.

4. Test the person for mycotoxins. When testing for mycotoxins, I would recommend a specialty lab that focuses on this. An example is Realtime Laboratories, as they offer a urine test that measures 15 potentially harmful mycotoxins, along with 9 macrocyclic trichothecenes. Great Plains Laboratory offers a test called the GPL-MycoTOX Profile, which also screens for mycotoxins.

Keep in mind that testing for mycotoxins isn't the same as testing for mold. For example, one well-known lab offers an IgE mold allergy test, which looks at the IgE antibodies to 15 different types of molds. I'm not suggesting that this test doesn't have any value, but when someone is dealing with CIRS, testing for mycotoxins is preferable because the mycotoxins cause the inflammatory response in those who are genetically susceptible.

5. Other tests. If you are experiencing some of the symptoms described earlier, and if one or more of the HLA genetic markers come out positive, then you probably will want to consider testing for the following markers I'm about to discuss. Fortunately, most local labs have these available.

Leptin. Leptin is an important regulator of appetite and fat storage. Sometimes, this marker is elevated in those with CIRS. What happens is that proinflammatory cytokines bind to the leptin receptor. This leads to leptin resistance, which is the main reason why many people with CIRS will put on weight. In addition, having a blocked leptin receptor will also interfere with the production of melanocyte stimulating hormone.

Melanocyte Stimulating Hormone (MSH). Because of the blocked leptin receptor, this marker is low in most patients with a mold toxicity. Low levels of MSH can lead to a widening of the tight junctions of the small intestine (a leaky gut),making someone more susceptible to developing an autoimmune condition, which is one way in which having a mold toxicity can lead to the development of Hashimoto's.

Having low levels of MSH also can cause a type of bacteria to colonize the deep nasal passages, and is known as MARCoNS. The bacteria associated with MARCoNS can create certain toxins that help perpetuate the inflammatory process.

Transforming Growth Factor (TGF) Beta-1. TGF Beta-1 can help to suppress autoimmunity, but, at the same time, it is associated with decreased function of regulatory T cells (Tregs). Because of the low number of Tregs, the person will be more susceptible to developing one or more autoimmune conditions. This is another mechanism where CIRS can lead to an autoimmune condition such Hashimoto's.

Vasoactive Intestinal Polypeptide (VIP). This marker will typically be low in those with a mold toxicity. When this is the case, the patient will frequently have shortness of breath and air hunger, especially upon exertion. Low VIP levels can also cause the upregulation of aromatase, an enzyme that converts testosterone to estradiol. As a result, having low VIP levels can lead to low testosterone and elevated estrogen levels.

C4a. This marker is associated with the complement system and plays a role in activating inflammatory responses. This is elevated in Lyme disease and is usually elevated in those with a mold toxicity.

Antidiuretic hormone (ADH). This is also known as vasopressin, and it tells the kidneys to preserve water. In those with CIRS due to a mold toxicity, ADH is usually undetectable, which means that the kidneys aren't conserving water, and, as a result, the person usually experiences dehydration and excessive thirst. In addition, this can lead to frequent static electrical shocks.

Matrix metallopeptidase 9 (MMP-9). This is a marker associated with the innate immune system, and higher levels of MMP-9 have been associated with increased tumor invasiveness, and with increased permeability in the blood brain barrier.

Vascular endothelial growth factor (VEGF). This is a marker of capillary hypoperfusion, and low levels can result in a reduced oxygenation of tissues, which, in turn, will have a negative effect on the health of the mitochondria. This commonly causes symptoms such as fatigue and muscle pain. VEGF might be elevated early in CIRS, but in the later stages, this marker is usually low. Treatment is usually accomplished by taking high dose fish oils, plus a low-amylose diet is usually followed.

NeuroQuant brain MRI. NeuroQuant is a software program that measures a few different MRI brain regions and measures the volume of each of these regions. What does this have to do with mold toxicity? Well, mold toxicity can have a negative impact on brain volume. While the NeuroQuant isn't a specific test for a mold toxicity, this test can determine if someone with a suspected or confirmed case of mold toxicity has changes in brain volume, which can cause some of the symptoms associated with mold toxicity.

How can you have this test done? Well, the first thing you'll need to do is have a brain MRI, and a special protocol is required. The results of this test can then be sent to another lab for further analysis.

How Can Mycotoxins Cause Hashimoto's?

Having a mold toxicity/CIRS can make someone more susceptible to developing Hashimoto's. I mentioned two different mechanisms earlier, as one involves low levels of melanocyte stimulating hormone causing a leaky gut, which is a factor in autoimmunity. I also discussed how increased levels of TGF Beta-1 can decrease the number of Tregs, which also will make someone more susceptible to developing Hashimoto's.

Treatment Options for Mold Toxicity/CIRS

If someone has CIRS associated with a mold toxicity, then what is the recommended treatment? I'll discuss this in Chapter 33, although I will say here that the most important factor is to eliminate the source of the mold. This might sound like common sense, but you'd be surprised as to how many people skip this step. One of the main reasons for this is because getting rid of the source isn't always easy.

If you're being exposed to mold through the food you eat, then it might not be too challenging to reduce or even completely eliminate your exposure. However, if you have mold in your home or place of work then this probably will require remediation or, in some cases, moving or quitting your job. Once again, I'll go into greater detail about the different treatment options for mold in the fourth section.

Chapter Highlights:

- Mycotoxins are frequently classified by the organ they affect, and some mycotoxins affect multiple organs.
- Not all molds produce mycotoxins, but over 300 types of mycotoxins are known to be produced by molds.
- Some of the more common symptoms associated with a mold toxicity include severe fatigue, anxiety, insomnia, memory loss, migraines, skin rashes, respiratory distress, sinus problems, and neurological symptoms.
- Three ways we're exposed to mold include 1) contaminated foods, 2) skin contact with mold, and 3) inhalation of mycotoxins.
- Some of the more common mycotoxins include aflatoxins, citrinin, ochratoxin, trichothecenes, and zearalenone.
- Chronic Inflammatory Response Syndrome (CIRS) occurs when genetically susceptible people are exposed to certain biotoxins.
- Those who have certain HLA genetic markers will be unable to mount a proper immune response when exposed to mycotoxins, along with other types of biotoxins.
- When testing your home for mold, you want to hire a certified indoor air testing company, and preferably one that is open to ERMI testing.
- Some markers that can be helpful if mold toxicity is suspected include leptin, melanocyte stimulating hormone, transforming growth factor beta, vasoactive intestinal polypeptide, C4a, antidiuretic hormone, matrix metallopeptidase 9, and vascular endothelial growth factor.
- Low levels of melanocyte stimulating hormone can cause a leaky gut, which is one way in which mycotoxins can lead to autoimmunity.

Chapter Highlights, continued:

- Increased levels of TGF Beta-1 can decrease the number of regulatory T cells, which can make someone more susceptible to developing Hashimoto's.
- When treating a mold toxicity, the most important factor is to eliminate the source of the mold.

CHAPTER 12

ESTROGEN DOMINANCE

S O FAR, YOU HAVE learned that many factors can trigger an autoimmune response, leading to a condition such as Hashimoto's. Some of
the different triggers we have covered so far include stress, gluten, environmental toxins, and infections. Can imbalances in the sex hormones
play a role? In this chapter, I'm going to discuss the role of estrogen
dominance and estrogen metabolism in the development of Hashimoto's.

Although I have worked with male patients who have Hashimoto's,
most of the people who have this condition are women. In fact, most
autoimmune disorders are more prevalent in women. According to the
research, at least 85% of thyroiditis, systemic sclerosis, systemic lupus
erythematosus, and Sjögren disease patients are female.[256] Why is this
the case? Although many factors can lead to autoimmunity, the biggest
differentiating factor between men and women are the sex hormones.
Women have higher levels of the hormones estrogen and progesterone,
while men have higher levels of androgens, such as testosterone.

Keep in mind that there might be other reasons why women are more
likely to develop an autoimmune condition than men. While one needs
to consider the impact of the sex hormones, genetics can be a factor.
Females have two X chromosomes, while males have an X and a Y chro-
mosome, which chromosomal difference may play a role in why females
more commonly developing autoimmune conditions than men.[257]

The immune system also differs to some extent between men and women. Research seems to show that women produce a more vigorous immune response,[258] and, when combined with other factors, this might make women more susceptible to developing an autoimmune condition such as Hashimoto's. While some studies show that estrogen significantly increases pro-inflammatory cytokine production,[258,259] other studies suggest that estrogen can increase regulatory T cells[260] that can suppress autoimmunity.

Healthy Levels of Estrogen vs. Estrogen Dominance

While estrogen seems to get a "bad rap" at times, the truth is that healthy levels of estrogen can be anti-inflammatory, which can help to prevent autoimmunity from developing. However, a condition such as estrogen dominance can serve as an autoimmune trigger. It's important to understand that estrogen dominance isn't only considered to be a state of excess of estrogen but can also be caused by a progesterone deficiency.

Thus, you also want to pay attention to the ratio between estrogen and progesterone. If someone has a progesterone deficiency with normal estrogen levels then this is considered a form of estrogen dominance. Progesterone can help to increase regulatory T cells (Tregs) while decreasing proinflammatory cytokines and Th17 cells,[261,262,263,264] which can help to suppress autoimmunity.

How Can You Test for Estrogen Dominance?

Testing is the best method to determine if someone has an imbalance between estrogen and progesterone. I'll discuss the different methods of testing the sex hormones in the third section of this book. Much confusion surrounds hormone testing. You need to consider the different types of testing (i.e., blood, saliva, urine) and whether the person taking the test is male or female. For females, different options are available depending on whether someone is cycling, perimenopausal, or in postmenopause. Of course, if someone is taking bioidentical hormones, this can affect the results of such testing.

What Are Some Common Causes of Estrogen Dominance?

How does someone develop estrogen dominance? Here are a few of the different ways:

1. Hormone replacement therapy. No evidence I'm aware of shows a correlation between taking exogenous forms of estrogen and developing

Hashimoto's. However, studies show that hormone replacement therapy can exacerbate the autoimmune condition systemic lupus erythematosus.[265] Other studies show that hormone replacement therapy can be beneficial with multiple sclerosis.[266]

If you choose to take estrogen, I would recommend bioidentical estrogen, and not conjugated forms such as Premarin. Of course, the dosage you take is very important, as hormones are very powerful. It's common to see high estradiol levels in patients who are taking bioidentical estrogen. This is especially true with saliva testing, which measures the free form of the hormone.

2. Oral contraceptives. Not all oral contraceptives include estrogen, as some only include progestin. Others include a combination of estrogen and progestin, and these can affect estrogen metabolism. I haven't seen any studies demonstrating a link between oral contraceptives and autoimmunity, although a few studies show the use of certain oral contraceptives is associated with a slight increase in breast cancer risk.[267,268] However, this depends on the formulation. Also, evidence suggests that oral contraceptives can potentially reduce the risk of developing ovarian cancer.[269]

While oral contraceptives might not directly cause autoimmunity, they can lead to nutrient deficiencies including folic acid, vitamins B2, B6, B12, vitamin C and E, magnesium, selenium, and zinc.[270] As I discuss in Chapter 13, certain nutrient deficiencies can play a role in autoimmunity.

3. Xenoestrogens. Many studies show that xenoestrogens can have a negative effect on estrogen metabolism. I discussed this in Chapter 8. I also gave examples of how certain xenoestrogens can be a factor in thyroid autoimmunity.

The xenoestrogen I focused on the most was bisphenol A (BPA), as this is one of the xenoestrogens we're commonly exposed to, which is a known endocrine disruptor.[271,272,273] Drinking out of BPA-free plastic bottles doesn't necessary mean you aren't being exposed to endocrine-disrupting chemicals, as bisphenol S (BPS) and bisphenol F (BPF) are two commonly used BPA substitutes which also have endocrine-disrupting properties.[274,275] While many people realize that plastic water bottles are a big source of BPA, many aren't aware that thermal paper receipts are a major source as well.[276] Phthalates are another common xenoestrogen, and these can also affect estrogen metabolism.[277,278]

4. Pregnenolone steal. The pregnenolone steal is what happens when someone deals with prolonged chronic stress. The body prioritizes the production of cortisol, and if someone is in a stressed state, cortisol will be produced at the expense of the sex hormones. This can cause estrogen dominance by resulting in low progesterone levels, and healthy progesterone levels are important for preventing the development of autoimmunity by increasing Tregs and decreasing proinflammatory cytokines.

5. Problems with the HPA and/or HPG Axis. The hypothalamic-pituitary-gonadal (HPG)axis regulates the secretion of the sex hormones. The hypothalamus communicates with the pituitary gland, and the pituitary hormones follicle stimulating hormone (FSH) and luteinizing hormone (LH) are responsible for signaling the release of estrogen and progesterone from the gonads. Plus, dysregulation of the HPA axis can affect the adrenals, which can affect the sex hormones.

Another Factor in Estrogen Dominance: The Clearance of Estrogen from the Body

It's not just the levels of estrogen that can be problematic; we also need to consider how efficient or inefficient the body is at clearing estrogen from the body. If someone has problems with their detoxification pathways, or if they have certain genetic polymorphisms, then this can affect the clearance of estrogen from the body. Let's take a look at four pathways that play an important role in the detoxification of estrogen:

1. Glucuronidation. A process called glucuronidation is involved in the detoxification of estrogen. Estrone and estradiol undergo glucuronidation by enzymes called glucuronosyltransferases (UGTs). These in turn catalyze the conjugation of something called UDP-glucuronic acid to steroid hormones, including estrogen. This conjugation process can vary from person to person, and can be one reason why someone can do a better job of detoxifying estrogen when compared to another person.

Another factor involves an enzyme called beta-glucuronidase, which can prevent the excretion of estrogen and allow it to re-enter the circulation. Thus, you ideally want to have low levels of this enzyme. Elevated beta-glucuronidase is associated with an increased risk of certain types of cancers.

Some comprehensive stool panels test for this enzyme because having imbalances in the gut flora can lead to elevated levels of beta-glucuronidase.

When this is the case, you will want to inhibit this enzyme. Supporting the gut flora can help, and some of the nutrients and herbs that can inhibit this enzyme include broccoli, Brussels sprouts, apricots, watercress, calcium d-glucarate, milk thistle, and licorice.

2. Sulfation. Sulfation is the main pathway for estrogen metabolism, although some prescription drugs can also be biotransformed through this pathway. Estrone and estradiol, along with their metabolites, undergo sulfation by enzymes called sulfotransferases (SULTs). Nutrients that activate these enzymes include genistein, vitamins A and E, selenium, and phenethyl isothiocyanate, which is found in cruciferous vegetables such as watercress and cabbage.

What's important to understand is that sulfation is important for the inactivation of estrogens. Polymorphisms of the SULT enzymes can affect the detoxification of estrogen. Sulfite oxidase in an enzyme that catalyzes the transformation of sulfite to sulfate, and two important cofactors to this enzymatic reaction are vitamin B6 and molybdenum.

3. Glutathione. Research shows that catechol estrogen quinones produce free radicals that can cause DNA mutations, which, in turn, can lead to certain types of cancer.[279] Although this doesn't directly relate to being a trigger of Hashimoto's, I thought it was important to discuss how these quinones can be conjugated with glutathione, which, in turn, will prevent damage to the DNA.[280] You can support glutathione through diet by eating sulfur-rich foods such as cruciferous vegetables and garlic. Supplementing with N-acetylcysteine, or a liposomal or an acetylated form of glutathione are also options.

4. Methylation. The enzyme catechol-o-methyltransferase (COMT) is involved in the detoxification and excretion of estrogens. Thus, supporting detoxification/methylation can help with the elimination of estrogens. Not surprisingly, if someone has a genetic polymorphism of the COMT gene, then this can affect the methylation of estrogens. In addition, certain cofactors are necessary to support the methylation of estrogen, including S-adenosylmethionine (SAMe) and magnesium. Certain precursors present in the diet are necessary for the formation of SAMe, including methionine, folate, choline, betaine, and vitamins B2, B6, and B12.[281] Thus, not only can a genetic defect involving the COMT gene affect the clearance of estrogens but being deficient in one or more of the nutrients mentioned can also be a factor.

I realize that this chapter was probably somewhat advanced for some people, but the takeaway is that estrogen dominance and problems with estrogen metabolism can be factors in the development of Hashimoto's. I'll further discuss balancing the sex hormones and how to support estrogen metabolism in Chapter 27.

Chapter Highlights:

- Women are more likely to develop Hashimoto's than men, and having problems with estrogen metabolism can be a factor, although there can be other factors as well.
- The research seems to show that women produce a more vigorous immune response, which, in turn, can make them more susceptible to developing an autoimmune condition such as Hashimoto's.
- Healthy levels of estrogen can be anti-inflammatory, while a condition such as estrogen dominance can cause an increase in proinflammatory cytokines.
- Some of the common causes of estrogen dominance include hormone replacement therapy, oral contraceptives, xenoestrogens, the pregnenolone steal, and problems with the HPA and/or HPG axis.
- Progesterone can help to prevent autoimmunity from developing by increasing regulatory T cells and decreasing proinflammatory cytokines.
- Increased beta-glucuronidase levels can prevent the excretion of estrogen and allow it to re-enter the circulation.
- Sulfation is important for the inactivation of estrogens, and polymorphisms of the sulfotransferases can affect the detoxification of estrogen.
- The enzyme catechol-o-methyltransferase (COMT) is involved in the detoxification and excretion of estrogens; thus, if someone has a genetic polymorphism of the COMT gene, then this can affect the methylation of estrogens.

CHAPTER 13

NUTRIENT DEFICIENCIES

HAVING CERTAIN NUTRIENT DEFICIENCIES can make someone more susceptible to developing Hashimoto's, which is why I have included this chapter in the triggers section. Although being deficient in any nutrient will have a negative effect on one's health, I'm not going to discuss all of the different nutrients in this chapter, but instead will focus on some of the ones more relevant to immune system health.

Before discussing some of the different nutrients, you might be wondering how having one or more nutrient deficiencies can make someone more susceptible to developing an autoimmune condition such as Hashimoto's. First of all, being deficient in certain nutrients can lead to a decrease in regulatory T cells (Tregs), which play a role in preventing autoimmunity from developing. Two of the more important nutrients that have a positive effect on Tregs are vitamin A and selenium, among others. Healthy vitamin D levels are also important for optimal immune system health.

It's not just the health of the immune system that's important when discussing the different nutrients. Some nutrients, such as zinc, play an important role in gut health, which, in turn, is important for optimal immune system health. Other nutrients are required to support the detoxification pathways. Thus, having certain nutrient deficiencies can make you more susceptible to the negative impact of environmental toxins, and certain environmental toxins can be a trigger of Hashimoto's.

I will focus on seven nutrient deficiencies that can make someone more susceptible to developing a condition such as Hashimoto's. This doesn't mean that other nutrients aren't important, as, of course, ALL nutrients are essential in helping someone achieve and maintain a state of optimal health. It is difficult to prioritize the importance of certain nutrients, but I'll try my best.

NUTRIENT DEFICIENCY #1: SELENIUM

Although selenium has many roles in the body, the predominant bio-chemical action of this mineral in both animals and man is to serve as an antioxidant via the selenium-dependent enzyme, glutathione peroxidase, and, thus, protect cellular membranes and organelles from oxidative damage.[282] If someone is deficient in selenium, they will also be low in glutathione, and this is a concern because glutathione helps to protect the cells from the damaging effects of free radicals. While taking precursors such as N-acetylcysteine (NAC) can increase glutathione levels, you also need to have healthy selenium levels.

Signs and Symptoms of a Selenium Deficiency

A severe selenium deficiency is characterized by cardiomyopathy (disease of the heart muscle), while a moderate deficiency usually results in symptoms such as muscular weakness and pain,[283] along with dry skin.[284] Since selenium is important for the conversion of T4 to T3, having a moderate to severe selenium deficiency can lead to symptoms of hypothyroidism.

Signs and Symptoms of a Selenium Toxicity

Although supplementing with selenium can be beneficial in some cases, you do want to be careful about supplementing with high doses of selenium supplements, as doing this can result in a selenium toxicity. A few years ago, 201 people were affected by an error in a liquid dietary supplement that contained 200 times the labeled concentration of selenium.[285] Fortunately, only one person was hospitalized. The symptoms associated with the selenium toxicity include diarrhea (78%), fatigue (75%), hair loss (72%), joint pain (70%), nail discoloration or brittleness (61%), and nausea.[285]

How Does Selenium Relate To Hashimoto's?

Selenium can be beneficial for people with Hashimoto's in a few different ways. I'm going to discuss two of them here.

1. Selenium plays a role in the conversion of T4 to T3. Certain deiodinase enzymes play a role in the conversion of T4 into T3. And a few studies show that having a selenium deficiency can result in a decrease in this conversion.[286,287] On a blood test, a person with a conversion problem will usually have normal levels of T4 and low or depressed levels of T3. Keep in mind that other factors can affect the conversion process, and, in most cases, a selenium deficiency isn't the primary reason for a conversion problem, as liver and gut problems are even greater factors.

2. Selenium can help to decrease thyroid peroxidase (TPO) antibodies. A few studies have demonstrated that supplementing with 200 mcg of selenium per day can result in a decrease in TPO antibodies.[288,289] Why is this the case? Hydrogen peroxide is a necessary substrate for TPO activity. If someone has low levels of antioxidants then the hydrogen peroxide that is generated can cause excessive oxidative stress, which, in turn, can increase TPO antibodies.

Earlier, I mentioned that selenium is a cofactor of glutathione; thus, having sufficient selenium levels can increase glutathione levels, which, in turn, will reduce the hydrogen peroxide levels. This can help to reduce TPO antibodies. However, if someone has a selenium deficiency, then this can cause excessive amounts of hydrogen peroxide, which, in turn, will lead to oxidative stress and can be a factor in the pathogenesis of an autoimmune condition such as Hashimoto's.[290]

Food Sources vs. Supplements

Food Sources: Seafood and organ meats are considered to be the richest food sources of selenium.[291] Brazil nuts are also a good source of selenium, and one study showed that the consumption of two Brazil nuts is as effective for increasing selenium status and enhancing glutathione peroxidase activity as 100 mcg of selenomethionine.[292] However, the amount of selenium in a Brazil nut is dependent on the amount of selenium in the soil, along with other factors, including soil pH.

For example, according to the U.S. Department of Agriculture Food Composition Database, Brazil nuts have 544 mcg of selenium per ounce, but values from other analyses vary widely.[291] One study showed that selenium concentrations in individual Brazil nuts can vary between 8 and 83 mcg,[293] which, of course, is a huge difference. This is why one can't assume that they are getting plenty of selenium by eating a few Brazil nuts, as this isn't always the case. In addition, those following a strict autoimmune Paleo (AIP) diet are not allowed to eat Brazil nuts, as nuts and seeds are excluded from this diet.

Supplements: Some of the different types of selenium include selenomethionine, selenocysteine, sodium selenite, and selenium-enriched yeast. I personally prefer either selenomethione or selenium-enriched yeast, although the other forms I mentioned can also correct a selenium deficiency.

NUTRIENT DEFICIENCY #2: VITAMIN A
Vitamin A is yet another nutrient whose deficiency can make someone more susceptible to developing a condition such as Hashimoto's.

Signs and Symptoms of a Vitamin A Deficiency
Although a mild vitamin A deficiency will frequently present with no symptoms, two of the more common symptoms caused by a moderate to severe vitamin A deficiency include night blindness and xerophthalmia, which is abnormal dryness of the eyes. Some of the other symptoms associated with a vitamin A deficiency include dry skin and frequent infections.

Signs and Symptoms of a Vitamin A Toxicity
Like selenium, it is possible to overdose with vitamin A. Some of the possible vitamin A toxicity symptoms include nausea and vomiting, headache, fatigue, loss of appetite, dizziness, and dry skin. While it is possible to take too much active vitamin A, high doses of beta-carotene isn't toxic, although eating many carotene-rich foods (i.e., carrots and sweet potatoes) can result in carotenemia, which results in a yellow pigmentation of the skin. In addition, not everyone is able to convert beta-carotene into active vitamin A.

How Does Vitamin A Relate to Hashimoto's?
Having sufficient vitamin A levels is important for immune tolerance, which seems to relate to vitamin A increasing Tregs.[294,295] Some sources question whether even a marginal vitamin A deficiency can have a profound effect on the health of the immune system.[296] Many people are aware that taking large doses of vitamin A can be toxic, and, while this usually isn't a problem when taking vitamin A as part of a multivitamin, you do want to be cautious if you take a separate vitamin A supplement. This is especially true if you take a supplement that consists of retinol, which is the

bioavailable form of vitamin A, whereas carotenoids (i.e., beta-carotene) need to be converted into active vitamin A.

Food Sources vs. Supplements

Food Sources: Animal products such as liver and other organ meats, eggs, cheese, and butter are some of the best sources of active vitamin A. Sweet potatoes, carrots, spinach, and kale are good sources of carotenoids.

Supplements: When taking vitamin A as a supplement the label will usually read either retinyl acetate or retinyl palmitate, which are the active forms, or beta-carotene. Some supplements will have a combination of these. Although it's fine to take beta carotene, the problem with relying on this is that not everyone can convert the carotenoids into active vitamin A.

NUTRIENT DEFICIENCY #3: ZINC

Zinc is yet another nutrient whose deficiency can make someone more susceptible to developing a condition such as Hashimoto's. Having a zinc deficiency is common due to inadequate intake, malabsorption, and impaired utilization, with inadequate dietary intake the primary cause.[297]

Signs and Symptoms of a Zinc Deficiency

A moderate to severe zinc deficiency can cause rough skin, poor appetite, mental lethargy, delayed wound healing, taste abnormalities, hypogonadism, oligospermia, and weight loss.[298]

Signs and Symptoms of a Zinc Toxicity

One of the main concerns with consuming too much zinc, usually in the form of supplements, is that it can cause an imbalance of copper.

How Does Zinc Relate To Hashimoto's?

Zinc can prevent the development of Hashimoto's in a few different ways. Zinc deficiency impairs both the innate and the adaptive immune system and can be normalized by zinc supplementation.[299] Also, a few studies show that zinc can decrease Th17 cells.[300,301,302] In addition, zinc can increase Tregs.[303] Finally, a zinc deficiency can make someone more susceptible to developing an infection,[304,305,306] which can trigger Hashimoto's.

Zinc can also improve the health of the gut, which, of course, is important for a healthy immune system. One study showed that zinc substantially alters the gut microbiota and reduces the minimum amount of antibiotics needed to eradicate pathogens such as Clostridium difficile.[307] Zinc also plays a role in the function of the epithelial barrier, which seems to be due to modifications of the tight junctions.[308] If you recall, damage to these tight junctions is a factor in a leaky gut. Another study showed that zinc carnosine could help to prevent an increase in intestinal permeability.[309]

Food Sources vs. Supplements

Food Sources: Some good food sources of zinc include beef, lamb, turkey, spinach, asparagus, pumpkin seeds, cashews, lentils, and quinoa.

Supplements: Although zinc picolinate is commonly used in studies, other good quality forms include zinc glycinate, zinc citrate, zinc gluconate, and zinc aspartate. One study I came across showed that zinc citrate absorption is comparable with zinc gluconate, and both are far superior to zinc oxide.[310] Another study compared the bioavailability of zinc glycinate to zinc sulfate, and found that the bioavailability of zinc glycinate was significantly superior.[311] Another study showed that zinc glycinate changes zinc status better than zinc gluconate,[312] and that taking higher doses of both forms (60 mg/day) over a 6-week period didn't affect copper status.[313] I also mentioned a study that showed that zinc carnosine could prevent a leaky gut from occurring.

NUTRIENT DEFICIENCY #4: IRON

Iron is one of the most commonly deficient minerals seen in people with Hashimoto's. It's surprising that many medical doctors don't recommend an iron panel to their patients. It's even more surprising when someone is experiencing symptoms such extreme fatigue or hair loss, yet an iron panel isn't ordered.

Even though I'm going to discuss iron deficiency anemia, it's important to understand that you can have an iron deficiency without having anemia, and you can have anemia without having an iron deficiency. To better understand this, let's discuss what happens when someone has anemia. Anemia results when the body doesn't produce enough red blood cells or hemoglobin.

Although many medical doctors don't perform an iron panel, most doctors routinely order a complete blood count to look at the red blood cells, hemoglobin, and hematocrit. When someone has anemia one or more of these values are depressed. Hemoglobin is an iron-rich protein that gives blood its red color; thus, when iron is low, typically, hemoglobin is low, along with the red blood cell count and hematocrit. But this isn't always the case; thus, just because all three of these are normal doesn't mean you can't have an iron deficiency.

While a complete blood count is commonly recommended by primary care physicians when someone has a routine physical examination, in my opinion, an iron panel should also be ordered. If someone has a normal iron panel but has depressed red blood cells, hemoglobin, and/or hematocrit, then other potential causes of the anemia should be investigated. However, if someone has an iron deficiency, regardless of whether or not they have anemia, the cause of the deficiency should be addressed.

Signs and Symptoms of an Iron Deficiency
Some of the common signs and symptoms of an iron deficiency include fatigue, weakness, pale skin, dizziness, shortness of breath, and chest pain.[313]

What Are Common Causes of an Iron Deficiency?
Someone can become deficient in iron for one of three main reasons. One reason is due to blood loss, which is why some doctors will refer the patient with iron deficiency anemia to a gastroenterologist in order to rule out gastrointestinal bleeding. Not surprisingly, women who have a heavy menstrual flow are more likely to have an iron deficiency than women who have a lighter menstrual flow.

A second reason for an iron deficiency is iron malabsorption. This can be caused by a number of different factors, such as having an infection, inflammatory bowel disease, celiac disease, and, in some cases, small intestinal bacterial overgrowth. Even exposure to glyphosate can lead to the chelation of minerals such as iron, thus leading to an iron deficiency.[314] Glyphosate, the active ingredient in the herbicide Roundup, is discussed in Chapter 20.

A third common reason for an iron deficiency relates to low dietary intake of iron. Iron is found in two different forms. Heme iron is found in foods such as meat, poultry, and fish. It is more absorbable than non-heme iron, which is found in plant-based foods.[315,316]

Thus, vegetarians and vegans are more likely to develop an iron deficiency than those who eat meat. It's also important to know that vitamin C and hydrochloric acid help to increase the absorption of iron; thus, having hypochlorhydria (low stomach acid) or low vitamin C levels can have a negative effect on iron absorption.

Signs and Symptoms of an Iron Toxicity

If someone has a severe iron toxicity, they may experience vomiting, diarrhea, and abdominal pain initially, and liver failure can eventually develop. However, over the years, I have had a few patients with elevated iron markers in the blood who didn't experience such symptoms. Even in these cases, it's important to get the iron levels down, as too much iron can cause oxidative stress. This is why you never want to supplement with iron unless if an iron deficiency has been confirmed. And then, even if taking an iron supplement is necessary, you want to address the cause of the problem.

I will add that there is a possible link between genetic hemochromatosis (iron overload) and Hashimoto's.[317,318] However, one of these studies involved only two people, and the other study involved only men who were homozygous for the hemochromatosis allele, as the study showed that they developed thyroid antibodies and hypothyroidism. While more research is probably needed to see if there is a connection between iron overload and autoimmunity, without question, excess iron causes an increase in oxidative stress,[319] and excessive oxidative stress is a factor in autoimmune conditions such as Hashimoto's.

How Does Iron Relate To Hashimoto's?

Many minerals are important for normal thyroid hormone metabolism. Iodine and selenium are two of the more well-known minerals involved in the formation of thyroid hormone. However, iron deficiency impairs thyroid hormone synthesis by reducing the activity of heme-dependent thyroid peroxidase.[320,321] This isn't to suggest that most cases of hypothyroidism are due to an iron deficiency, but a severe iron deficiency can be a factor. For example, if someone with Hashimoto's has depressed thyroid hormone levels, and also has iron deficiency anemia, while the damage to the thyroid gland by the immune system very well might be the primary reason for the low thyroid hormone levels, it is possible that the low iron levels are also a factor.

Although you now know that iron is important for thyroid hormone metabolism, at this point, you might be wondering how an iron deficiency can play a role in the development of Hashimoto's. Cytochrome

P450 enzymes are produced by the liver, and are found in the kidney, small intestine, lung, adrenals, and most other tissues. They are utilized in phase one detoxification. These CYP450 enzymes are heme-dependent, which means that they require iron to function properly.

I'm not going to get into detail about the detoxification pathways here, but environmental toxins are one of the potential triggers of Hashimoto's, and an iron deficiency can have a negative effect on the CYP450 enzymes that are necessary for phase one detoxification. Thus, having an iron deficiency can have a negative effect on this phase one process, causing a buildup of reactive intermediates, which, in turn, causes an increase in oxidative stress, which, once again, is a factor in the development of autoimmune conditions, including Hashimoto's.

Food Sources vs. Supplements
Food Sources: Heme iron is found in foods such as meat, poultry, and fish. Some non heme sources of iron include spinach, Swiss chard, collard greens, and asparagus.

Supplements: Ferrous sulfate is the most common form of iron supplement recommended. However, I usually recommend iron glycinate to my patients, as this has less gastrointestinal side effects when compared to ferrous sulfate and ferrous fumarate. Also, it seems to be better absorbed.

The Components of an Iron Panel
Please refer to Chapter 24, as I discuss the components of an iron panel, including the optimal reference ranges. One thing I want to say here is that for those medical doctors who do testing to determine if a patient has an iron deficiency, many will just order a serum iron test and/or ferritin. But after reading this chapter along with the one on testing, I'm hoping you will understand why it's necessary to obtain a complete iron panel.

When Is Someone Considered to Be Iron Deficient?
Most medical doctors will consider someone to be iron deficient if they fall outside of the lab reference range. For example, if a patient has a serum iron of 65 mcg/dL, a ferritin of 15 ng/ml, and an iron saturation of 18%, they would be considered to have healthy iron levels by most medical doctors. However, just as is the case with most other blood tests, there is a difference between the "lab" reference range and the "optimal" reference range.

For example, if ferritin is on the low side but still within the normal lab reference range, you need to be suspicious of an iron deficiency. This is especially true if the person also has a low iron saturation, serum iron, and/or high TIBC. I consider someone to be deficient in iron when they are outside of the "optimal" reference range, which is discussed in Chapter 24.

Can Iron Supplements Feed Pathogenic Organisms?

Although iron is an important mineral, it also is essential to pathogenic microorganisms.[322,323] Thus, many healthcare professionals recommend that their patients avoid taking iron supplements if they have a suspected or confirmed infection, as the iron can feed the pathogen, making it more difficult to eradicate. Thus, while it is important to correct an existing iron deficiency, it might be a good idea to address any infections that are present first.

One can make the argument that if someone has a mild iron deficiency, it might be best to focus on improving iron absorption prior to taking iron supplements. For example, both vitamin C and gastric acid are necessary for iron absorption; thus, those with an iron deficiency can take a whole food vitamin C supplement and either betaine HCL with pepsin, or one tablespoon of apple cider vinegar 15 minutes before each major meal. They would then want to retest the iron panel in a couple of months to see if the numbers have improved. In addition, improving the health of the gut will also help with the absorption of nutrients, including iron. I'll discuss this in section four.

NUTRIENT DEFICIENCY #5: VITAMIN D

Many people are deficient in vitamin D. Others fall within the recommended lab reference range, but have less than optimal levels. Although vitamin D is referred to as a vitamin, the active form is a prohormone. Vitamin D increases the intestinal absorption of calcium and phosphorus, which in turn promotes bone mineralization and remodeling. It is also involved in regulating serum calcium and phosphorus levels and plays a big role in immunity, which of course is important for those with Hashimoto's.

Signs and Symptoms of a Vitamin D Deficiency

While most lab reference ranges suggest that optimal levels should be above 30 ng/ml, some sources, including the vitamin D Council, suggest for these levels to be greater than 50 ng/ml. Many people who are deficient in vitamin D don't experience any noticeable symptoms. If the vitamin D deficiency is severe, then they might experience symptoms such as muscle pain or weakness. But other factors can cause such symptoms, and not everyone with depressed vitamin D levels will experience muscle pain or weakness. Thus, the best way to determine if you have a vitamin D deficiency is through testing.

Signs and Symptoms of a Vitamin D Toxicity

The main concern with elevated vitamin D levels is hypercalcemia, which is an excess of calcium in the blood. This can lead to symptoms such as nausea, vomiting, poor appetite, weakness, and, sometimes, kidney problems. But once again, you don't want to look only at the vitamin D levels, as you should also look at the serum calcium levels, which is part of a comprehensive metabolic panel.

How Does Vitamin D Relate To Hashimoto's?

Numerous studies show a correlation between vitamin D deficiency and autoimmune thyroid disease. A few studies have shown that low levels of vitamin D are associated with the presence of antithyroid antibodies and abnormal thyroid function.[324,325] Many people with Hashimoto's have low levels of vitamin D.[326,327] This doesn't mean that a vitamin D deficiency is the cause of their condition, although having such a deficiency might make someone more susceptible to developing Hashimoto's.

Having healthy vitamin D levels is also important for optimal gut health. One study showed that a vitamin D deficiency could be a factor in the development of a leaky gut and intestinal inflammation.[328] Another study looked at the effects of vitamin D supplementation on intestinal permeability (along with other markers) in people with Crohn's disease. The study found that increasing vitamin D levels through supplementation prevented a leaky gut from developing and reduced inflammation.[329]

Food Sources vs. Supplements

Food Sources: Vitamin D is very low in the food supply, as it is not found in plant materials (i.e., vegetables, fruits, or grains) and it is present in small amounts in meats and other animal food sources, except in rare cases such as fish liver oils.[330] Dairy products are commonly fortified with vitamin D, and canned salmon, sardines, and tuna can be good sources of vitamin D.[331] Overall, it is very difficult to get enough vitamin D from the diet, and it is almost impossible to correct a vitamin D deficiency through diet alone.

Regular sunlight exposure can naturally increase vitamin D levels, although keep in mind that the amount of skin that is exposed to the sun is important. For example, if someone takes a walk in the sun fully clothed, then they will produce much less vitamin D when compared to someone who is sunbathing. Other factors that can have a negative effect on vitamin D production include living in a northern latitude, having dark colored skin, air pollution, frequent use of sunscreen, having a VDR polymorphism, and being deficient in one or more cofactors, including magnesium, vitamin K2, zinc, boron, and vitamin A.

Supplements: Supplemental vitamin D comes in two primary forms. When someone purchases vitamin D in a health food store, they are usually getting cholecalciferol, also known as vitamin D3. However, when a medical doctor writes a prescription, it is for ergocalciferol, which is known as vitamin D2. Even though some sources claim that these two are equivalent, vitamin D3 is the more potent form of vitamin D.[332] In addition to vitamin D3 being more effective, vitamin D2 has diminished binding of metabolites to vitamin D binding protein in the plasma, a nonphysiological metabolism, and a shorter shelf life.[332]

NUTRIENT DEFICIENCY #6: MAGNESIUM

Magnesium is a cofactor in hundreds of enzyme reactions, and, without question, some of these enzyme reactions can play a role in preventing autoimmunity from developing. For example, magnesium plays a role in many ATP-generating reactions.[333] ATP is required for glucose utilization, the synthesis of fat, proteins, nucleic acids and coenzymes, muscle contraction, methyl group transfer and many other processes, and, as a result, interference with magnesium metabolism also influences these functions.[333]

Blood sugar imbalances also can play a role in the development of Hashimoto's, and magnesium can help to increase insulin sensitivity.[334,335,336] Also, evidence shows that chronic magnesium deficiency results in excessive production of oxygen-derived free radicals and low-grade inflammation.[337] One of the main reasons for this is because magnesium is a cofactor in the synthesis of glutathione. Thus if someone has a moderate to severe magnesium deficiency, there is a good chance they have a glutathione deficiency as well, which will increase the chances of them having oxidative stress.

Signs and Symptoms of a Magnesium Deficiency

Some of the early signs of a magnesium deficiency include loss of appetite, lethargy, nausea, vomiting, fatigue, and weakness. If someone has a moderate to severe magnesium deficiency, then this may result in tremors, muscle cramps, tetany, generalized seizures, and even cardiac arrhythmias.[338]

How Does Magnesium Relate To Hashimoto's?

Having a magnesium deficiency probably won't directly cause Hashimoto's. However, a moderate to severe magnesium deficiency can have a negative effect on the hundreds of enzyme reactions that require magnesium, which can set the stage for autoimmunity.

For example, magnesium is a cofactor in glutathione synthesis. As I mentioned earlier, low glutathione levels will lead to increases in free radicals and oxidative stress, which are factors in autoimmunity. In Chapter 17, I discuss how blood sugar imbalances could play a role in the development of Hashimoto's, and magnesium can also help in this area by decreasing insulin resistance/increasing insulin sensitivity.

Food Sources vs. Supplements

Food Sources: Green leafy vegetables are an excellent source of magnesium. Nuts, seeds, and legumes are also good sources, although these foods are excluded from an AIP diet. You can also get some magnesium through the water, although this won't be the case if you are drinking distilled or reverse osmosis water. However, a good quality spring water is a source of magnesium, along with calcium and potassium.

Supplements: I usually recommend magnesium citrate or magnesium glycinate/malate to my patients. Other forms include magnesium oxide, magnesium taurate, magnesium lactate, and magnesium orotate. All of these can be beneficial, although I would try to avoid magnesium oxide due to its low bioavailability. If you take a multivitamin, one way to find out quickly if it is of low quality is to see if it uses magnesium oxide as the form of magnesium.

NUTRIENT DEFICIENCY #7: OMEGA-3 FATTY ACIDS

It is important to have the proper ratio of omega-6 and omega-3 fatty acids. The optimal ratio of omega-6 to omega-3 fatty acids should be somewhere between 1:1 and 4:1, but most people eat somewhere in the range of 10:1 to 20:1. Since most people eat too many foods high in omega-6 fatty acids (i.e., vegetable, nut, and seed oils), it's not surprising that most people have a high ratio. Keep in mind that not all omega-6 fatty acids are bad for you. Gamma linolenic acid (GLA) is an omega-6 fatty acid, and numerous studies have shown this fatty acid to have anti-inflammatory effects.[339,340]

Signs and Symptoms of an Omega-3 Fatty Acid Deficiency

Some of the symptoms of an omega-3 fatty acid deficiency include fatigue, memory problems, dry skin, depression, and poor circulation.

Can You Consume Too Many Omega-3 Fatty Acids?

Although most people don't have a problem with consuming too many omega-3 fatty acids from food sources, there is a concern about taking too high of a dosage of fish oils. The main reason for this has to do with something called lipid peroxidation. Lipid peroxidation involves the oxidation of lipids (fats). What happens is that reactive oxygen species and free radicals attack the polyunsaturated fatty acids of the fatty acid membrane.[341]

Since lipid peroxidation is self-perpetuating, the initial oxidation of only a few lipid molecules can result in significant tissue damage.[341] Because polyunsaturated fatty acids are susceptible to oxidation, there is a concern that consuming fish oils can cause lipid peroxidation, which will lead to an increase in inflammation and tissue damage.

I agree that the consumption of rancid and/or excessive amounts of good quality fish oils can be problematic. However, much research has been done on the anti-inflammatory benefits of eicosapentaenoic acid (EPA) and docosahexaenoic acid (DHA). Although healthy people might not require higher doses of omega-3 fatty acids, many people with chronic health conditions such as Hashimoto's can benefit from higher doses of EPA and DHA. Just make sure you purchase good quality omega-3 fatty acids, and I commonly recommend between 1,000 and 2,000 mg of EPA and between 500 and 1,000 mg of DHA to my patients with Hashimoto's thyroiditis.

How Can Omega-3 Fatty Acids Benefit People With Hashimoto's?

Higher doses of EPA and DHA can help to reduce inflammation and down-regulate proinflammatory cytokines.[342,343] Also, evidence indicates that they can help reduce Th17 cells,[344] which are associated with autoimmunity.

Food Sources vs. Supplements

Food Sources: Fish is the best food source of omega-3 fatty acids, with sardines and salmon having a high omega-3 fatty acid content. Other good sources include grass-fed beef, walnuts, and flaxseeds. According to **whfoods.org**, winter squash and olive oil are good sources of omega 3 fatty acids as well.[345]

Supplements: I commonly recommend fish oil supplements to my patients with Hashimoto's because of the high amounts of EPA and DHA. I am often asked about krill oil and cod liver oil, and while these are good omega-3 fatty acid supplements to take on a wellness basis, they usually don't have enough EPA and DHA to help reduce significant amounts of inflammation.

What About the Other Nutrients?

Keep in mind that the omission of other nutrients doesn't mean that I'm dismissing their importance. For example, I'm well aware that vitamins B2, B3, B5, B6, B12, folate, vitamin C, vitamin E, vitamins K1 and K2, calcium, potassium, manganese, and chromium are all important for optimal health. In fact, all of the nutrients are important, and having a moderate to severe deficiency of any nutrient can be detrimental to your health.

As I mentioned in the beginning of this chapter, I wanted to focus on some of the nutrients whose deficiencies are more likely to be problematic in someone with Hashimoto's. Nevertheless, you could make a good argument that I should have expanded this list to include vitamin B12, vitamin C, and other nutrients.

The Relationship Between Methylation and Hashimoto's

Methylation is a process that is very important to our overall health. It is necessary when it comes to protein synthesis, detoxification, the formation of neurotransmitters, and regulation of hormones, among other functions. Before I discuss this further, I want to let you know that this is a very advanced topic, and I am only going to cover a few basics here.

What exactly is methylation? Every organic compound has something called a methyl group. This consists of one carbon atom, and three hydrogen atoms. Methylation involves the donation of a methyl group.

Why is this important? Methylation is necessary for most of the body's systems. It is involved in the repair of DNA, helps to prevent the overproduction of homocysteine, and is important when it comes to detoxification. If someone has problems with methylation, they will have a greater risk of developing certain chronic health conditions. Thus, one of the goals is to make sure you take measures to help support proper methylation.

What Is an MTHFR Polymorphism?

Although not all of my patients with Hashimoto's obtain genetic testing, for those who do, it is very common for them to have MTHFR polymorphisms. As a result, I figured I'd briefly discuss this here. Methylenetetrahydrofolate reductase (MTHFR) is an enzyme that is vital for re-methylation of homocysteine to methionine.

Although I'm sure some people reading this are familiar with genetic polymorphisms, many probably don't know what these are. A polymorphism is a common genetic defect. There are many other genetic polymorphisms one can have besides the MTHFR defect.

Concerning MTHFR and thyroid autoimmunity, one study involving 50 patients who were diagnosed with Hashimoto's found that 15 of these patients had MTHFR mutations.[346] Another study looked into the associations between factors regulating DNA methylation and the prognosis of autoimmune thyroid disease. They concluded that MTHFR +677 C/T and +1298A/C polymorphisms were not correlated with the development or prognosis of autoimmune thyroid disease.[347] Thus, having an MTHFR polymorphism apparently isn't a direct factor in the development of Hashimoto's, and it doesn't have a positive or negative effect on the prognosis of those people who already have Hashimoto's.

The Role of the Nutrients in Mitochondrial Health

Having healthy mitochondria is important for having a healthy immune system. The most well-known function of mitochondria involves the production of adenosine triphosphate, which is also known as ATP. Why is ATP important? In addition to its well-established role in cellular metabolism, extracellular ATP and its breakdown product, adenosine, have very important effects on a variety of biological processes including neurotransmission, muscle contraction, cardiac function, platelet function, vasodilatation, and liver glycogen metabolism.[348] ATP also plays an important role in DNA and RNA synthesis.[349]

Certain nutrients are important for the mitochondria to function normally. Thus, if someone eats a lot of refined foods and sugars, causing a deficiency of those nutrients important for mitochondrial function, this can result in mitochondrial decay.[350] The following are some of the main nutrients that are necessary for optimal mitochondrial health:

- CoQ10
- Lipoic acid
- Acetyl-L-carnitine
- Magnesium
- Omega-3 fatty acids
- Biotin
- Riboflavin (vitamin B2)
- Niacin (vitamin B3)
- Pyridoxine (vitamin B6)
- Resveratrol

How Can You Detect and Correct Nutritional Deficiencies?

In the third section of this book, I'll discuss some of the different tests you can perform in order to determine if you have one or more nutritional deficiencies. However, I will say that while a few comprehensive panels are available to test for many of the different nutrients, no single test can accurately measure all of the different nutrients. In the fourth section of this book, I'll discuss what you can do to correct nutritional deficiencies.

Keep in mind that while nutritional supplementation can be important, it's even more important to address the cause of the nutrient deficiency. For example, if someone has a gut infection that is affecting the absorption of nutrients, it is necessary to eradicate the infection. After this has been accomplished, it then will be necessary to take measures to heal the gut. All of this will be covered in detail in the fourth section of this book.

Chapter Highlights:

- Seven nutrient deficiencies that can make someone more susceptible to developing Hashimoto's thyroiditis include 1) selenium, 2) vitamin A, 3) zinc, 4) iron, 5) vitamin D, 6) magnesium, and 7) omega-3 fatty acids.
- Being deficient in certain nutrients can lead to a decrease in regulatory T cells.
- Certain nutrients play an important role in gut health, while others are required to support the detoxification pathways.
- A few studies have demonstrated that supplementing with 200 mcg of selenium per day can result in a decrease in TPO antibodies.
- Having sufficient vitamin A levels is important for immune tolerance, which seems to relate to vitamin A increasing regulatory T cells.
- Studies show that zinc can decrease Th17 cells and increase regulatory T cells.
- Environmental toxins are one of the potential triggers of Hashimoto's, and an iron deficiency can have a negative effect on the CYP450 enzymes that are necessary for phase one detoxification.
- A few studies have shown that low levels of vitamin D are associated with the presence of antithyroid antibodies and abnormal thyroid function.
- Having a magnesium deficiency can cause a decrease in glutathione levels and an increase in insulin resistance, both of which can be factors in the development of Hashimoto's.
- Higher doses of EPA and DHA can help to reduce inflammation and downregulate proinflammatory cytokines, and there is also evidence that they can help to reduce Th17 cells.

Chapter Highlights, continued:

- MTHFR is an enzyme that is vital for remethylation of homocysteine to methionine, and it is very common for people with Hashimoto's to have an MTHFR polymorphism.
- Having healthy mitochondria is important for having a healthy immune system.

CHAPTER 14

WHAT YOU NEED TO KNOW ABOUT IODINE AND HASHIMOTO'S

I ODINE'S ROLE IN HASHIMOTO'S thyroiditis is controversial. One can't deny that iodine is an important mineral, and since it is necessary for the formation of thyroid hormone, an iodine deficiency can lead to hypothyroidism. Iodine has many other functions as well. However, with Hashimoto's, the low or depressed thyroid hormone levels are the result of damage to the thyroid gland by the immune system, and, thus, usually isn't due to an iodine deficiency. This doesn't mean that people with Hashimoto's can't be deficient in iodine. However, there is a concern about iodine being a potential trigger of Hashimoto's, and I'll discuss this in detail in this chapter.

I will start with the basics and discuss the role of iodine in thyroid health. This will help you better understand why iodine can be beneficial in some people, but problematic in others. After reading this information, you should understand that the problem relates to the increase in oxidative stress produced when consuming excessive amounts of iodine and/or when someone has low antioxidant levels. Thus, the individual's ability to neutralize free radicals and reactive oxygen species (ROS) is the main factor that will determine who does fine when taking iodine, and who doesn't. This is one of the main reasons why some people do fine when taking higher doses of iodine, while others don't do well, even when smaller doses are taken.

The Role of Iodine in Thyroid Health

So let's briefly discuss the role of iodine in thyroid health. The thyroid follicles are cells in the thyroid gland where thyroid hormones are produced. You get iodide from the diet, which travels through the bloodstream to the thyroid follicular cells, which in turn takes up the iodide with the help of something called a sodium-iodide-symporter. Thyroid peroxidase is an enzyme that plays an important role in iodination, which involves the oxidation of iodide ions to form iodine atoms.

Thyroxine contains four iodine atoms, which is why it's referred to as "T4," and these iodine atoms attach to a tyrosine molecule. As you might have guessed, triiodothyronine contains three iodine atoms, which is why it's referred to as "T3." There is also thyroglobulin, which is synthesized by the thyroid follicular cells, which acts as a substrate for the synthesis of T3 and T4, and also stores inactive forms of thyroid hormone. What's important to understand is that iodine and tyrosine are important for the formation of thyroid hormone, and thyroid peroxidase and thyroglobulin also play important roles.

Thus, it would make sense to conclude that a deficiency in iodine can lead to a decrease in thyroid hormone production, thus resulting in a hypothyroid condition. However, too much iodine can potentially lead to an excess in thyroid hormone production, thus leading to a hyperthyroid condition. However, it would be erroneous to conclude that most hypothyroid conditions are caused by a deficiency in iodine, and similarly, that most hyperthyroid conditions are caused by an excess in iodine.

Iodine and the Autoimmune Component of Hashimoto's

This is where it begins to become somewhat controversial. With Hashimoto's, the hypothyroid condition is caused by the immune system attacking the thyroid gland, thus leading to destruction of the gland. So what's the problem with taking iodine in people with Hashimoto's? Well, the controversy seems to be centered around thyroid peroxidase (TPO) which is an enzyme that plays a role in the production of both T3 and T4.

Evidence suggests that consuming iodine can increase the TPO antibodies in some individuals. If you recall, earlier I mentioned that thyroid peroxidase is involved in iodination, which involves the oxidation of iodide ions to form iodine atoms. This process involves the formation of free radicals and ROS, including hydrogen peroxide, which I discussed in the previous chapter. If someone doesn't have sufficient antioxidants to minimize the oxidative damage, then this can cause problems, including damage to the thyroid gland.

Without question, some people with Hashimoto's don't do well when consuming iodine. However, other people with Hashimoto's not only feel better when taking iodine but also get into remission while supplementing with iodine. I'm not suggesting that the iodine was the main factor responsible for them getting into remission, although keep in mind that iodine can play a role in eradicating infections by dissolving biofilm,[351,352] in regulating estrogen metabolism,[353] and in helping with the excretion of environmental toxins such as bromine.[354] Thus, while iodine can cause problems in some people with Hashimoto's, having an iodine deficiency can also be problematic.

The Impact of Bromine, Fluorine, and Chlorine

When discussing iodine, it's important to discuss the other halogens and the impact they have on iodine metabolism, as well as our overall health. Evidence suggests that bromine might cause or exacerbate autoimmune thyroiditis.[355] Also, bromine can interfere with the metabolism of iodine (356). Since supplementing with iodine can cause the excretion of bromine, if someone has high tissue levels of bromine and takes an iodine supplement or eats foods high in iodine, then this can make the person feel worse upon supplementing with iodine due to a detox reaction because it is helping to eliminate bromine from the body.

Fluorine and chlorine are two other halogens that can also interfere with iodine metabolism, and they can have a negative effect on our health in other ways as well. This is why you want to do everything you can to avoid exposure to fluoride by drinking purified water that filters out fluoride, as well as using fluoride-free toothpaste. You also want to minimize your exposure to chlorine, which you can also do by drinking purified water, as well as having a good quality water filter on your showerhead. Some reading this will wonder if they should avoiding swimming in chlorinated pools, and I definitely would try to minimize doing this, although I will add that you also need to enjoy life and shouldn't be paranoid about completely avoiding exposure to all chemicals.

Although I discuss some of the benefits of iodine in this chapter, keep in mind that I am cautious about having my patients with Hashimoto's initially supplement with iodine. I just want you to understand that iodine isn't inherently bad, and I don't think we can completely ignore an iodine deficiency. However, in most cases, it's best to improve the person's immune system health and antioxidant status before attempting to correct an iodine deficiency.

The Role of Hydrogen Peroxide in Triggering Hashimoto's

Earlier, I discussed how an excess of oxidative stress seems to be the main issue when supplementing with iodine, and I'd like to expand on this. Hydrogen peroxide is an essential co-substrate for the thyroid peroxidase (TPO) enzyme during the oxidation of inorganic iodine for thyroid hormone synthesis.[356] In other words, during the formation of thyroid hormone, the body produces hydrogen peroxide, which is a type of ROS. Even under normal circumstances, there is a greater amount of hydrogen peroxide produced than consumed by the iodination process, which can expose the thyroid gland to excessive amounts of free radicals.[357]

What's important to understand is that it's not the iodine that actually damages the thyroid gland, but hydrogen peroxide or other ROS.[358] For example, if someone takes a 50mg potassium iodide supplement, then this will lead to higher levels of hydrogen peroxide, which can result in an increase in oxidative stress. If someone has abnormally high levels of oxidative stress and/or low amounts of antioxidants, then this, in turn, can result in damage to the thyroid gland, which can lead to an increase in thyroid antibodies, typically thyroid peroxidase antibodies.

But why then do many people do fine when taking iodine supplements? Do these people not produce higher amounts of hydrogen peroxide? Well, I mentioned the importance of antioxidants earlier, and glutathione peroxidase and thioredoxin reductase are two of the more important antioxidant enzymes that help protect cells (including cells of the thyroid gland) from oxidative damage.[359] Thus, if someone has sufficient levels of these and other antioxidants, then this will help neutralize the excess production of hydrogen peroxide.

Thus, it makes sense that people with higher levels of antioxidants can tolerate higher amounts of oxidative stress from consuming larger amounts of iodine. Unfortunately, many people have low levels of antioxidants. So how can you increase the levels of these antioxidants? Well, both of the antioxidants I just mentioned are selenium-dependent, so one of the main keys to preventing any adverse effects from iodine is to make sure you have sufficient levels of selenium. This explains why numerous studies demonstrate how taking selenium can lower thyroid antibodies by increasing glutathione peroxidase levels.[360,361] In addition, taking an acetylated or liposomal form of glutathione can also be beneficial.

Yet, if selenium can help prevent the damage to the thyroid gland caused by hydrogen peroxide by increasing selenium-dependent antioxidants, then why do some people seem to react to iodine even when they take selenium? There are a few reasons for this, such as the following:

1. They don't have an iodine deficiency. Not everyone has an iodine deficiency; therefore, not everyone needs to increase their iodine levels. The same is true with other minerals. A good example is iron. I discussed the correlation in the research between having an iron overload and Hashimoto's in Chapter 13. If someone obtains an iron panel (serum iron, ferritin, iron saturation, TIBC), and if it's determined that they have sufficient levels of iron, taking a separate iron supplement can cause oxidative stress. Thus, the problem isn't just with iodine, as taking high doses of some other minerals such as iron can also cause oxidative stress, and can potentially be a factor in thyroid autoimmunity.

2. They take excessive amounts of iodine. Although I'm a supporter of iodine testing and supplementation in those people who need it, I'm not an advocate of most people taking very high doses of iodine (i.e., 50 mg per day). Although there might be some cases when people can benefit from taking very high doses of iodine, just as is the case with everything else, one needs to weigh the risks and benefits. The problem is that it's impossible to predict how someone will respond when taking very high doses of iodine.

3. They might be reacting to selenium and not iodine. Although I'm touting the benefits of selenium, the truth is that selenium toxicity can be an issue in some people. While most people do fine taking 200 mcg of selenium per day, for some people, this is too high of a dose. Of course, some people take higher amounts of selenium. Rarely have I found problems with patients taking 200 mcg/day of selenium, although everyone is different.

4. The symptoms might be due to the detoxification of bromine. Remember that iodine and bromine compete for the same receptors, and that I mentioned earlier how supplementing with iodine, or eating iodine-rich foods can cause the excretion of bromine. Thus, if you experience certain detox symptoms such as an increase in fatigue or headaches when taking iodine, then this can be due to the excretion of bromine, and not the iodine itself. Also, selenium is a cofactor for glutathione production, so taking selenium can increase glutathione production, which, in turn, can also help with the excretion of bromine along with other toxins.

5. The symptoms might be due to the eradication of pathogens. Iodine has antimicrobial properties, and, as a result, if someone has one or more infections then they might experience die-off symptoms when taking iodine due to the pathogens being eradicated.

6. The person might have reduced glutathione peroxidase activity due to a genetic polymorphism. This would make sense in many cases, as, while this book focuses on many environmental factors that we can control, we can't dismiss the potential impact of genetics. Thus, if someone has a reduction in glutathione peroxidase activity due to a genetic polymorphism, then they won't be able to reduce the oxidative stress as efficiently as someone who doesn't have this genetic defect.

7. They are reacting to other ingredients in the iodine supplement. Some people who supplement with iodine don't do well not because of the iodine, but due to other ingredients. For example, they might be reacting to a filler in the supplement. This can be the case with any nutritional supplement you take; if you don't do well with a specific supplement or herb, then there's always the possibility that you are reacting to one of the fillers.

How Much Selenium Should You Take?

As for how much selenium you should take daily, this varies from person to person. When taking a selenium supplement, a common dose recommended by healthcare professionals is 200 mcg/day. What type of selenium supplement should you take? Although I commonly recommend selenomethionine to my patients, whole food selenium supplements are also something to consider, and evidence suggests that taking a yeast-based selenium supplement is more bioavailable than either selenomethionine[362] or selenium selenite.[363]

Are Other Antioxidants Important to Neutralize the Negative Effect of Iodine?

The focus thus far has been on how selenium can help neutralize the damaging effects of hydrogen peroxide by increasing the levels of the antioxidants I mentioned earlier. However, other antioxidants also can help minimize free radical damage. Much evidence shows that vitamin C has protective effects towards hydrogen peroxide-induced DNA strand breaks and oxidative DNA damage.[364,365,366] In addition, vitamin C might also correct the damage to the sodium iodide symporter system.[367] Thus, anyone thinking of supplementing with iodine probably will also want to supplement with high doses of vitamin C. Alpha lipoic acid can also offer protection against hydrogen peroxide-induced oxidative stress,[368] so this is also something to consider taking.

However, while I recommend nutritional supplements to my patients, we need to remember that eating well is essential. While it's fine to supplement with selenium, vitamin C, and/or other antioxidants temporarily, these aren't substitutes for eating a healthy diet. You should be getting most of your antioxidants from fruits and vegetables, and I'll discuss in greater detail about the importance of eating whole healthy foods in Chapter 26.

Why Are Some People Deficient in Iodine?

I'm not going to get into great detail about this, but according to Dr. David Brownstein, author of Iodine, Why You Need It, Why You Can't Live Without It, there are a few reasons why many people are deficient in iodine. First, due to poor farming techniques, the soils are depleted of iodine, which means the foods we eat are also deficient of this mineral. Another reason is because iodine is no longer used in bread dough conditioners, but the manufacturers replaced iodine with bromine. Bromine competes with iodine, so people who eat a lot of bread are more likely to be iodine deficient.

Yet another reason for widespread iodine deficiency is because many people are afraid of consuming too much iodized salt, which, for some people, might be the only source of iodine they get in their diet. While consuming iodized salt by itself isn't sufficient to correct an iodine deficiency, it is better to consume this minimal amount of iodine than none at all. I usually recommend that my patients avoid iodized salt and to take natural sea salt instead.

What about studies showing that increased iodine intake in certain countries correlates with an increased incidence of autoimmune thyroid disease, mainly Hashimoto's thyroiditis? Well, some suggest that these people might have been deficient in selenium. Thus, if there isn't sufficient selenium, then this can lead to a greater amount of oxidative damage due to the lack of selenium-dependent antioxidants. Also, evidence shows that increased oxidative stress is a factor in Hashimoto's.[369,370] Another explanation is that these populations might have had a greater incidence of glutathione peroxidase polymorphisms, or another genetic polymorphism, which, in turn, made them more susceptible to the damaging effects of ROS.

Should YOU Supplement With Iodine?

Based on what I have said so far, if you were to obtain a urine test that reveals low iodine levels (I discuss testing for iodine in Chapter 25), should you supplement with iodine? As I mentioned earlier, if someone with Hashimoto's has low antioxidants and consumes high amounts of iodine, this can exacerbate the autoimmune response. This is true even if they test positive for an iodine deficiency. Thus, I usually don't recommend for my patients with Hashimoto's to supplement with iodine initially, as my primary focus is to improve the health of their immune system and antioxidant status. Once this has been accomplished, I think it's important to correct an existing iodine deficiency.

Supplementation vs. Food Sources of Iodine

Although many reading this will agree that taking high doses of iodine supplements isn't a good idea, some will wonder if it's okay to eat food sources of iodine. Some natural healthcare professionals recommend that people with Hashimoto's avoid food sources of iodine as well. Eating some foods that are iodine-rich is fine for most people with Hashimoto's. Although some healthcare professionals argue that it would be best for those with Hashimoto's to avoid food sources that are very high in iodine such as seaweed and sea vegetables, other good sources of iodine that are fine for most people to eat include sardines, salmon, and eggs (for those who aren't following an AIP diet).

Is It Okay to Take a Multivitamin With Iodine?

For those with Hashimoto's who take a multivitamin, some will wonder whether they should avoid taking one that has iodine, which describes most of them, although some companies have multivitamins that are iodine-free. In most cases, I'm not concerned about the small amount of iodine that's present in a multivitamin, as this small amount usually isn't going to cause any problems, although there are exceptions. For those who are pregnant, iodine is important for the health of the developing fetus, so, in this case, I recommend taking a prenatal with iodine.

My Final Thoughts With Regards to Iodine Supplementation

So where do I stand regarding iodine supplementation in those with Hashimoto's? First, before someone supplements with iodine, they should be tested to confirm that an iodine deficiency is present. Second, even if a deficiency is confirmed, it's a good idea to work on improving the health of your immune system and antioxidant status for at least a few months before supplementing with iodine. In most cases, it's fine to wait until remission has been achieved before supplementing with iodine or eating foods very high in iodine, such as seaweed.

I realize that some people who read this book may have supplemented with iodine prior to getting into remission, and they might have felt better upon supplementing with iodine. Many years ago, when I first started working with people who have Hashimoto's, I had a lot of my patients supplement with iodine prior to improving their immune system health, and many of them did fine, but some people didn't do well. The problem with taking this approach is that it's impossible to predict who will do well when supplementing with iodine and who won't do well. Thus, I currently take a more conservative approach.

Once you have improved your immune system health, if you have an iodine deficiency and you choose to start taking iodine, I would recommend that you start with small doses while continuing to supplement with antioxidants such as selenium and vitamin C. As I mentioned earlier, you also want to eat a healthy diet consisting of plenty of vegetables. I'd also be cautious about taking massive doses of iodine, and, just to be on the safe side, it would be a good idea to work with a healthcare professional when supplementing with iodine.

Just as is the case with any nutrient deficiency, you ideally should retest after a few months to confirm that the deficiency has been corrected. Thus, if you did a urine iodine spot test that confirmed an iodine deficiency, after three or four months of iodine supplementation, do a retest.

No doubt, the iodine controversy will continue, but, hopefully, after reading this, you have a better understanding of the risks and benefits associated with iodine. If you take anything away from this chapter, I'm hoping that it will be that while iodine can be problematic for some people with Hashimoto's, iodine itself isn't inherently bad. In addition, while it's important to correct any nutrient deficiency, in the case of iodine, it probably is a good idea to first focus on improving the health of the immune system, along with other imbalances, before supplementing with iodine.

Chapter Highlights:

- Iodine is controversial in those with Hashimoto's.
- Although iodine is important for the formation of thyroid hormone, low thyroid hormone levels associated with Hashimoto's is caused by damage to the thyroid gland by the immune system.
- Iodine can help with the excretion of bromine, can help with estrogen metabolism, and can eradicate infections.
- It's not iodine that actually damages the thyroid gland, but free radicals and reactive oxygen species associated with an increase in oxidative stress.
- Selenium can help prevent the damage to the thyroid gland caused by free radicals by increasing the selenium-dependent antioxidants.
- Vitamin C also has protective effects towards the damage caused by free radicals.
- Urine testing seems to be the most accurate method of testing for an iodine deficiency.
- A reduction in glutathione peroxidase due to a genetic polymorphism can be one reason why many people don't do well with iodine supplementation.
- Even if a deficiency is confirmed, it's a good idea to work on improving the health of your immune system and antioxidant status for at least a few months before supplementing with iodine.

CHAPTER 15

CAN OVERTRAINING
TRIGGER HASHIMOTO'S?

M **OST PEOPLE UNDERSTAND THAT** regular exercise is important for optimal health. While I'm sure many people reading this are already following a regular exercise routine, other people rarely exercise. Some people with Hashimoto's live a sedentary lifestyle not because they choose to do this, but perhaps they don't have the energy to exercise, or they might experience a lot of pain and, therefore, can't exercise without the pain increasing. In this chapter, I'll discuss the types of exercise people with Hashimoto's should do, how exercise affects the immune system, and how overtraining can be a potential trigger.

What I'd first like to do is discuss some of the benefits of exercise. You probably realize that exercise benefits cardiovascular health, as it can result in a reduction in incidence of and mortality from coronary artery disease, help with weight loss, reduce stress and anxiety, can help increase bone density, and it has other health benefits as well. Physical inactivity will increase the risk of cardiovascular disease and other chronic conditions such as diabetes, obesity, hypertension, osteoporosis, depression, and even cancer.

What Type of Exercise Should You Do?

I'm going to discuss three different types of exercise and whether or not these would be suitable for those with Hashimoto's. These include high-intensity interval training, continuous aerobic exercise, and resistance exercise. Although I'm not going to discuss stretching, I think this is an important part of an exercise routine as well.

1. High-intensity interval training. More and more people are becoming familiar with the benefits of high-intensity exercise. High-intensity interval training involves repeatedly exercising at a high intensity (90–100 percent of your maximum heart rate) for 30 seconds to several minutes, separated by one to five minutes of recovery.[371] The research shows that high-intensity intermittent exercise can help with insulin resistance;[372,373] thus, it can be very effective in reducing total abdominal fat, subcutaneous fat, and abdominal visceral fat in obese women.[374] It can also help reduce oxidative stress and improve antioxidant status.[375]

As for how to incorporate high-intensity interval training, there are a few different options. You can use a treadmill, stationary bike, or a rowing machine. If you don't have access to any exercise equipment, you still can do high-intensity interval training. For example, you can go outside and do some sprints or walk up some stairs. You can do a thirty-second sprint, followed by one to two minutes of light walking, followed by another thirty-second sprint, etc. Numerous variations of high-intensity interval training routines exist, and if this is new to you, then you want to start slowly. It's also a good idea to work with a certified personal trainer for at least one or two sessions in order to make sure you do this correctly.

Should People With Hashimoto's Engage in High-Intensity Interval Training?

Although I personally use high-intensity interval training, I am very cautious about having my patients with Hashimoto's engage in this type of exercise while restoring their health. Many people with this condition need to further improve the health of their adrenals before participating in this type of exercise. So why did I bother bringing this up? Well, I am commonly asked about exercise, and, occasionally, I'll have someone with Hashimoto's ask me if it's okay to do high-intensity interval training. I'm not suggesting that everyone with Hashimoto's should avoid this type of exercise until they have achieved a state of remission, but before engaging in high-intensity interval training, it's probably a good idea to consult with a competent healthcare professional about it.

2. Continuous aerobic exercise. Although some will argue that if you do high-intensity interval training, there is no need for regular aerobic exercise, I disagree. Research clearly shows the long-term health benefits of aerobic exercise; thus, I recommend doing both high-intensity interval training and some aerobic exercise. Many people combine high-intensity interval training with continuous aerobic exercise. This is what I routinely do, as when I go to the gym I'll do continuous aerobic exercise on a stationary bike while incorporating short bursts of high-intensity exercise.

My current routine consists of warming up for five minutes on the bike, then, for one minute, I'll exercise at a very high-intensity, and then go at a much slower aerobic pace for two minutes, followed by another one minute of high-intensity exercise, followed by another two minutes of lower intensity cardiovascular exercise, etc. I'll do this for six cycles. If you are a beginner, you can always start out by doing only 10 to 15 seconds of high-intensity bursts and then slowly increase this. However, I would hold off on doing the high-intensity interval training until your adrenal and immune system health have improved.

Should People With Hashimoto's Engage in Continuous Aerobic Exercise?

I recommend many of my patients with Hashimoto's to do continuous aerobic exercise. However, you don't want to overdo it, and you should be able to carry on a conversation while engaging in such exercise. As the health of your adrenals and immune system improve, you can combine continuous aerobic exercise with high-intensity interval training. Of course, if someone is dealing with extreme fatigue, then they might not have the energy to engage in continuous aerobic exercise until their health improves.

What should you do if you are experiencing moderate to severe fatigue? If you have low energy levels throughout the day then I would try to do at least ten to fifteen minutes of mild aerobic exercise a few days per week, and try doing some light weightlifting twice per week. Then, as your energy levels improve, you can increase the intensity and duration of exercise; although, when you reach this point, you still want to make sure not to overexert yourself.

3. Resistance exercise. It's important for just about everyone to do some resistance exercise at least two to three times per week. Keep in mind that resistance exercise doesn't necessarily mean heavy weightlifting. For many people reading this, I would recommend doing some light weightlifting. Others can do more moderate weightlifting. I'm not going to discuss what you specifically should do, as this is beyond the scope of this book, and everyone is in a different situation. I will say that you want to try working out all of the major muscle groups each week.

Should People With Hashimoto's Engage in Resistance Training?

I recommend for most of my patients with Hashimoto's to engage in resistance training. If you haven't done this before, it probably would be a good idea to work with a certified personal trainer for at least a session or two in order to make sure you are doing the exercises correctly and are not overexerting yourself.

Regular Movement Is Important

Although it's great to engage in regular exercise, it's important to keep in mind that going to the gym three to five times per week, or even going for a morning jog isn't enough to overcome the risks associated with sitting most of the time. In other words, if you have a desk job and spend most of your day sitting, this can be detrimental to your health, even if you exercise regularly. Thus, besides exercising frequently, you also want to make sure that you're not sitting for prolonged periods without incorporating some type of movement.

But how can you accomplish this if you have a desk job? Well, if you happen to work from home you can consider investing in a treadmill desk, as this will allow you to keep moving throughout the day. If this isn't practical, then perhaps you can get a standing desk so that you're not sitting down all of the time.

If you don't work from home, then you'll want to make sure to take frequent breaks. This doesn't necessarily mean leaving your desk, as every 30 to 45 minutes, you can stand and stretch for two minutes, or perhaps you can do a few jumping jacks and then go back to work. If you can't remember to do this every 30 to 45 minutes, you can set a timer on your cell phone.

How Does Exercise Affect the Immune System?

Overall, regular exercise seems to have a healthy effect on the immune system, as regular aerobic exercise appears to be associated with a reduction in chronic inflammation.[376] Since regular exercise has a positive effect on the immune system and can help reduce chronic inflammation, then this might suggest that it could benefit those with autoimmune thyroid conditions such as Hashimoto's. Most people with Hashimoto's should engage in continuous aerobic exercise along with some light resistance training.

However, is there a risk of overtraining? Although no studies confirm that excessive exercise causes thyroid autoimmunity, without question, overtraining does have a negative effect on the health of the immune system by increasing proinflammatory cytokines, which play a role in different autoimmune conditions, including Hashimoto's.

Most cases of Hashimoto's are Th1 dominant conditions. However, this isn't always the case, and the only way to know for certain is to test the cytokines. A few years ago, such testing was more common, as many natural healthcare professionals would test the cytokines through the blood to determine if someone was Th1 or Th2 dominant and then recommend specific nutrients or herbs to balance these pathways. Although some healthcare professionals continue to do such testing on their patients, cytokine testing isn't as commonly utilized these days.

So how does exercise specifically affect the cytokines and the Th1/Th2 balance? Well, exercise of moderate intensity seems to cause a slight shift towards a Th1 profile, thus reducing the risk of infections.[377] However, it appears that acute exercise, as well as chronic moderate exercise, shifts the immune response towards a Th2 profile.[377,378] Prolonged intense exercise may shift the balance towards Th2 to an even greater extent.[377,378] Since Hashimoto's is usually a Th1 dominant condition, on the surface, this might appear to benefit those with this condition.

However, as I'll discuss shortly, overtraining can decrease secretory IgA. Secretory IgA is found on the mucosal surfaces of the body and serves as a form of protection, as it binds to antigens such as bacteria, preventing them from entering the body. Thus, low secretory IgA levels can make someone more susceptible to developing an infection, which can be a potential trigger.

More About Excessive Exercise and Infections

Since infections can play a role in the development of autoimmune thyroid conditions, I'd like to further discuss how excessive exercise can make someone more susceptible to developing an infection. Secretory IgA plays an important role in providing protection by binding to pathogens, including viruses and bacteria[379,380] as a first line of defense against them. However, prolonged strenuous exercise can cause a decrease in secretory

IgA,[381] which, in turn, can increase the chances of someone developing an infection.

Thus, there are two mechanisms by which overtraining can increase the risk of developing an infection, which in turn can trigger autoimmunity. The Th1 pathway is important to help prevent someone from getting an infection, but excessive exercise can shift the immune system towards a Th2 dominant state, which can make someone more susceptible to developing an infection. In addition, it can also lead to a decrease in secretory IgA, which plays a big role in providing protection against pathogens, including viruses and bacteria.

Overtraining and Adrenal Insufficiency

The chronic stress that results from overtraining can also cause problems with the adrenal glands, and can even lead to adrenal insufficiency in some cases.[382] However, it appears that excessive exercise alone isn't the only factor, as adrenal insufficiency requires a combination of chronic overtraining along with a triggering stressful event.[382] Of course, many people with Hashimoto's deal with a great amount of stress, and, sometimes, they overtrain as a way of managing their stress. They might initially feel better when overtraining, not realizing that they are actually worsening their health.

Adrenal insufficiency is an extreme condition, and I think it's safe to say that most people who exercise excessively won't develop adrenal insufficiency. However, overtraining still is a stressor; therefore, it can have a negative effect on your immune system and adrenal health over a prolonged period.

How Much Exercise Is Too Much?

The question you might have at this point is "How much exercise is considered to be too much?" Well, further research is still needed in this area, but if you engage in continuous aerobic activity, then you should be able to hold a conversation while exercising. Most people with Hashimoto's should avoid engaging in high-intensity interval training until their adrenals and immune system health improves. In most cases, it's fine to do some light resistance training.

An Overtraining Case Study

Compromised adrenals were a big factor when I was dealing with Graves' Disease. But what causes compromised adrenals? Although two big factors are high levels of prolonged chronic stress and poor stress-management skills, excessive exercise can also be a culprit. And prior to my Graves' Disease diagnosis I was definitely overtraining, as I would exercise almost to the point of exhaustion. This very well could have played a role in my autoimmune thyroid condition. Some of my patients with Hashimoto's have fit under this category, and while I could have included the information on overtraining in Chapter 7 where I spoke about stress and the adrenals, I felt that it deserved its own chapter. So please don't underestimate the impact that overtraining can have on your health.

Chapter Highlights:

- Exercise can benefit cardiovascular health, help with weight loss, reduce stress and anxiety, and increase bone density.
- Short-term high-intensity interval training involves repeatedly exercising at a high intensity for 30 seconds to several minutes, separated by five minutes of recovery.
- Many people with Hashimoto's should be cautious about engaging in high-intensity interval training while restoring their health.
- I recommend that most people with Hashimoto's engage in continuous aerobic exercise.
- Most people with Hashimoto's should also engage in mild to moderate resistance training.
- Besides exercising frequently, you also want to make sure that you're not sitting for prolonged periods of time without incorporating some type of movement.
- Overtraining affects the cytokines of the immune system, which can decrease secretory IgA and make someone more susceptible to developing an infection, which can be a potential trigger.
- For those who aren't currently exercising routinely I would highly suggest hiring a certified personal trainer, even if it's only for a few sessions.

CHAPTER 16

POSTPARTUM THYROIDITIS

W HILE YOU HAVE LEARNED about many environmental factors that can trigger Hashimoto's, many women develop this condition during the postpartum period. Thus, in this section, I decided to include postpartum thyroiditis, as many consider this to be a trigger of Hashimoto's. However, thyroid autoimmunity isn't directly triggered by giving birth. The process actually starts months or years before, and during postpartum, there is an "immunologic flare" that usually leads to overt symptoms. While many women with postpartum thyroiditis become euthyroid (have normal thyroid function) after one year, this isn't the case with everyone, and approximately 25% of childbearing women will develop permanent hypothyroidism within 10 years.[383]

Although some consider the postpartum period to be an autoimmune trigger, most women already have elevated thyroid antibodies well before developing postpartum thyroiditis. Why do many women not experience symptoms until after giving birth? In the Chapter 1, I discussed the silent autoimmune stage when someone has elevated thyroid autoantibodies, but no symptoms. Someone with Hashimoto's might be in this stage for many years before developing overt symptoms.

In addition, pregnancy usually will suppress the autoimmune response in those with Hashimoto's because pregnancy is characterized by a shift towards a Th2 dominant state, which can benefit those with Hashimoto's, which is usually a Th1 dominant condition. This is why many people with Hashimoto's will seem to go into remission during pregnancy.

Postpartum Thyroiditis Symptoms

Although one might expect to experience hypothyroid symptoms when dealing with postpartum thyroiditis, this isn't always the case. In fact, transient hyperthyroidism is very common with postpartum thyroiditis. This hyperthyroid state can lead to symptoms such as increased resting heart rate, heart palpitations, tremors, anxiety, hair loss, increased appetite, loose stools, and/or weight loss. While transient hyperthyroidism is common, most people with this condition will experience a period of hypothyroidism.

How should transient hyperthyroid symptoms be managed? Because the hyperthyroid symptoms are usually temporary, you wouldn't want to take antithyroid medication, and you probably would also want to avoid antithyroid herbs such as bugleweed. Sometimes, beta blockers are prescribed by medical doctors to help manage the cardiac symptoms, including the increased heart rate and palpitations. You can also consider natural alternatives, including hawthorn and motherwort. For those with postpartum thyroiditis who are nursing, master herbalist Kerry Bone considers motherwort to be compatible with breastfeeding.[384]

Should Thyroid Hormone Replacement Be Taken?

As for whether thyroid hormone replacement should be taken in someone with postpartum thyroiditis, if the person is switching back and forth between hyperthyroidism and hypothyroidism, then they wouldn't want to take thyroid hormone replacement. Most of the time, the transient hyperthyroidism period will appear first, followed by a longer period of hypothyroidism. If the thyroid hormone levels are low or depressed for a prolonged period, then it usually is a good idea to take thyroid hormone, while, at the same time, addressing the cause of the problem.

Are High Prolactin Levels A Factor?

Prolactin is a hormone secreted by the pituitary gland, as well as other organs, and evidence shows that it is a factor in promoting autoimmunity.[385] Elevated prolactin levels (hyperprolactinemia) have been described in the active phase of a number of different autoimmune conditions, including Hashimoto's.[386,387]

Prolactin levels normally increase during pregnancy, and they reach a peak at delivery. However, this is considered a period of "physiological" hyperprolactinemia, and the studies I just mentioned seem to suggest that hyperprolactinemia is a factor in autoimmunity. If someone is already in the silent autoimmune phase, then this transient period of hyperprolactinemia might be a factor in postpartum thyroiditis.

How to Prevent Postpartum Thyroiditis

It's very common for women who test positive for thyroid antibodies during pregnancy to develop postpartum thyroiditis. Thus, if someone has elevated thyroid peroxidase or thyroglobulin antibodies during pregnancy, can anything be done to prevent postpartum thyroiditis from occurring? Although I don't commonly give my patients with Hashimoto's nutrients and herbs to make them more Th2 dominant, this is something to consider for a woman who is pregnant and tests positive for thyroid antibodies.

However, rather than using specific nutrients and herbs to balance the Th1 and Th2 pathways, what I would focus on is the following:

1. Detect and remove the autoimmune triggers. This of course is what this book focuses on, and it admittedly can be challenging to remove certain triggers in pregnant women. For example, if stress or gluten are factors, then one can address these triggers. However, if a pregnant woman's autoimmunity is caused by a gut infection, or an environmental toxin such as mercury, then this can be more challenging to treat. This is especially true in the case of an environmental toxin such as mercury, as, for obvious reasons, it's not advised to be aggressive with detoxification during pregnancy. In the case of mercury amalgams, removal isn't advised for pregnant or nursing women.

2. Promote gut healing. Since a leaky gut is a factor in autoimmunity, it is essential to focus on healing the gut. Removing the factor that is causing the leaky gut (the leaky gut trigger) is the first step of the 5-R protocol. I'll discuss the 5-R protocol in Chapter 28.

3. Decrease proinflammatory cytokines and increase regulatory T cells. Decreasing proinflammatory cytokines and increasing regulatory T cells (Tregs) during pregnancy, along with removing the autoimmune trigger and healing the gut, will reduce the likelihood of postpartum thyroiditis from developing. In the first section of this book, I mentioned some different things you can do to increase Tregs and reduce proinflammatory cytokines.

Many women already have elevated thyroid antibodies well before developing postpartum thyroiditis. Yet, some women test negative for thyroid antibodies, but then develop postpartum thyroiditis. In this situation, can we conclude that the birth process is what triggered the autoimmune response? We need to keep in mind that not everyone who has Hashimoto's will have elevated thyroid antibodies. It's possible for people with autoimmune conditions to test negative for antibodies. Thus, even if someone with postpartum thyroiditis had negative thyroid antibodies during pregnancy, we can't assume that the birth process itself was a trigger.

Can Postpartum Thyroiditis Be Treated Naturally?
With postpartum thyroiditis, the goal is to do what is necessary to improve the health of the immune system, which is the same situation with any other case of Hashimoto's. While taking thyroid hormone replacement or herbs to manage the thyroid symptoms is important, postpartum thyroiditis is an immune system condition, not a thyroid condition. Thus, the goal is to find the autoimmune triggers, which this book is all about. It is also necessary to take measures to heal the gut, along with correcting other imbalances, which I discuss in section four.

I will add that there is evidence that taking selenium in the form of selenomethionine during pregnancy can help prevent postpartum thyroiditis.[388,389] This makes sense, as selenium has been shown to decrease thyroid antibodies. The author of one of the journal articles referenced mentioned that "replication of the findings is needed before the recommendation can be made that all pregnant thyroid peroxidase antibody-positive women receive selenium."[389] Nevertheless, I think the benefits of taking 200 mcg of selenium during pregnancy outweigh the risks for those with elevated thyroid antibodies.

Chapter Highlights:

- Although many women develop Hashimoto's during the postpartum period, the autoimmune process usually starts months or years before the birth process.
- During the postpartum period there is an "immunologic flare" that causes the overt symptoms associated with Hashimoto's.
- Pregnancy is characterized by a shift towards a Th2 dominant state, which is why many people with Hashimoto's will show a significant improvement in their health when becoming pregnant.
- Transient hyperthyroidism is very common with postpartum thyroiditis, although the majority of people with this condition will experience a period of hypothyroidism.
- Although women who are in a transient state of hyperthyroidism won't want to take thyroid hormone medication, once they become hypothyroid, they will want to address the low thyroid hormone levels.
- Prolactin levels increase during pregnancy and reach a peak at delivery, and elevated prolactin levels has been described in the active phase of Hashimoto's, as well as other autoimmune conditions.
- Three things pregnant women with elevated thyroid antibodies can do to prevent the development of postpartum thyroiditis include 1) find and remove the autoimmune trigger, 2) heal the gut, and 3) decrease proinflammatory cytokines and increase regulatory T cells.
- One study showed that taking selenium during pregnancy significantly decreased the incidence of postpartum thyroiditis.

• CHAPTER 17 •

BLOOD SUGAR IMBALANCES

MANY PEOPLE HAVE BLOOD sugar imbalances. While most people wouldn't consider blood sugar imbalances to be a potential trigger of Hashimoto's, hyperglycemia and insulin resistance can be factors. In this chapter, I'll discuss four specific mechanisms involved. While hypoglycemia is also common, the main focus here will be on hyperglycemia and insulin resistance, as these are more likely to cause a proinflammatory state and be a factor in the development of thyroid autoimmunity.

Before I discuss the four mechanisms involved, I'll briefly discuss why many people have hyperglycemia and insulin resistance. Not surprisingly, eating a poor diet consisting of plenty of refined foods and sugars is a big factor. However, poor diet isn't the only thing responsible for blood sugar imbalances. Being inactive can also play a role, and even stress can be a contributing factor. Later in this chapter, I'll discuss in greater detail some of the different causes of hyperglycemia and insulin resistance.

Understanding the Difference Between Insulin and Glucose
Many people seem to get confused when it comes to understanding the difference between insulin and glucose; thus, I will briefly discuss this before describing the different causes of blood sugar imbalances.

Glucose is a simple sugar, and it is essential for tissue energy production. The key hormones that regulate glucose homoeostasis include insulin, glucagon, epinephrine, norepinephrine, cortisol, and growth hormone.[390] Thus, imbalances in these other hormones can affect the production and utilization of glucose.

Glycemia refers to the presence of glucose in the blood. As the name implies, hypoglycemia is a condition characterized by low blood sugar levels, whereas insulin resistance is more characteristic of hyperglycemia, which involves high blood sugar levels. The solution might seem simple, as if someone has high blood sugar levels, then they obviously want to reduce their sugar intake, and if someone has low blood sugar levels, they will want to eat more regularly, right? Although dietary factors are obviously important with both hypoglycemia and insulin resistance, these conditions are frequently complex and require more than simple dietary changes.

Insulin is a hormone produced by the beta cells of the pancreas. Insulin has a number of different roles, but one of the primary roles is the regulation of blood glucose levels. When someone eats a meal, this will cause their blood sugar levels to rise, and the beta cells will secrete insulin to help the body utilize or store the glucose.

Insulin reduces blood glucose by inducing glucose uptake into insulin-sensitive tissues such as skeletal muscle, fat, and heart.[391] Insulin also inhibits glucose production in the liver, kidney, and small intestine in the control of blood glucose.[391] Insulin has other functions, as it stimulates the synthesis of fatty acids and glycogen,[392] and it plays a role in mitochondrial function. With insulin resistance the cells are no longer responsive to the effects of insulin.

6 Factors That Cause Insulin Resistance

Although eating a poor diet and a lack of exercise are definitely factors in many people, the development of insulin resistance is usually more complex. Here are some of the factors that are thought to cause or contribute to insulin resistance:

1) Inflammation. Inflammation is one of the biggest factors associated with insulin resistance, and it is primarily why losing weight is so challenging for many people with Hashimoto's. How specifically will inflammation cause insulin resistance? Essentially, the activation of certain immune system cells will cause insulin resistance, while the activation of others will increase insulin sensitivity. Research shows that Th1 dominant conditions are more commonly associated with insulin resistance, whereas Th2 dominant conditions involve an increase in insulin sensitivity. Since most people with Hashimoto's are Th1 dominant, they are more likely to become insulin resistant.

2) Mitochondrial dysfunction. Mitochondria are located in the cytoplasm of our cells where cellular respiration occurs. How can damage to the mitochondria cause insulin resistance? Adipocytes (fat cells) play an important role in regulating energy metabolism and glucose homeostasis, and it appears that free radicals, which are caused by mitochondrial dysfunction, cause impairment of the function of adipocytes in maintaining glucose homeostasis.[393] Thus, the mitochondria help to regulate glucose homeostasis in fat cells, but mitochondrial dysfunction causes free radicals, which, in turn, impairs the fat cells. Thus, if you have insulin resistance, then you want to make sure you have healthy mitochondria.

3) Lipotoxicity. Lipotoxicity refers to an excess of free fatty acids in certain tissues, which can include skeletal and cardiac muscle cells, hepatocytes (liver cells), and pancreatic beta cells.[394,395] This can be a factor in insulin resistance and metabolic syndrome, and it will typically show up as elevated triglycerides on a lipid panel. A good example of a condition associated with lipotoxicity is nonalcoholic fatty liver disease (NAFLD), which is usually associated with insulin resistance. Keep in mind that these fatty acids can accumulate in other cells as well, and not just the liver cells.

4) Intestinal dysbiosis. Accumulating evidence indicates that the gut microbiota play a significant role in the development of obesity, obesity-associated inflammation, and insulin resistance.[396] Many people with Hashimoto's have intestinal dysbiosis. Evidence indicates that intestinal dysbiosis can cause activation of the immune system, thus interfering with insulin receptor function, increasing serum insulin levels.[397]

5) Circadian disruption. Circadian rhythms follow a 24-hour cycle. For example, cortisol is normally at the highest levels when a person first wakes up, and should be at the lowest levels right before going to bed. The opposite is true with melatonin, as this hormone should be at the lowest levels upon waking up, and at the highest levels upon going to bed. Many hormones that modulate insulin secretion and glucose homeostasis are regulated by the circadian system. In addition to cortisol, these include leptin, glucagon, growth hormone, and the catecholamines.[398] Disruptions in the circadian rhythm can lead to an increase in body weight, elevated leptin levels, and increased insulin secretion.[399,400] If you are having problems with sleep, you most likely have problems with the circadian rhythm, which can be a cause of insulin resistance.

6) Genetics. Studies have shown that common genetic variations are associated with insulin resistance and metabolic syndrome, with many of these genetic variants being directly involved in glucose metabolism.[401] However, just as is the case with most other chronic health conditions, lifestyle and environment usually are greater factors. Although some people are more susceptible to developing insulin resistance due to genetic factors, the good news is that it is possible to change the expression of our genes by modifying our lifestyle and environment.

Four Ways Hyperglycemia/Insulin Resistance Can Lead To Thyroid Autoimmunity

Now that you have a better understanding about how insulin resistance develops, let's look at four mechanisms in which hyperglycemia and insulin resistance can be a factor in the development of thyroid autoimmunity:

Mechanism #1: Hyperglycemia (high blood sugar) can cause a decrease in regulatory T cells (Tregs) and increase in Th17 cells. Autoimmune conditions such as Hashimoto's involve proinflammatory cytokines. Hyperglycemia can also increase proinflammatory cytokines as well.[402] One way it seems to increase proinflammatory cytokines is through the nonenzymatic glycosylation of proteins.[403] Glycosylation is a process that involves a carbohydrate attaching to a larger molecule, such as a protein or lipid. What's important to understand is that this can lead to an increase in oxidative stress and proinflammatory cytokines.[404]

This doesn't necessarily mean that proinflammatory cytokines that result from hyperglycemia will directly trigger autoimmunity. However, the research shows that certain proinflammatory cytokines can influence the activity and number of Tregs.[405] Having a decrease in Tregs is a factor in the development of autoimmune conditions. In addition, the presence of the cytokines IL-6 and TGF-Beta supports the development of Th17 cells, which are also associated with autoimmunity.[405]

Mechanism #2: Hyperglycemia can cause a leaky gut. Circulating zonulin in the blood is considered to be a useful marker of intestinal permeability.[406,407,408] In other words, if you have high levels of zonulin in your bloodstream, then you most likely have a leaky gut. Elevated levels of circulating zonulin is commonly found in those people with high fasting insulin and fasting triglycerides, and is negatively correlated with insulin sensitivity.[408] To summarize, having high blood sugar levels and/or insulin resistance is highly associated with a leaky gut, which is part of the triad of autoimmunity discussed in Chapter 1.

However, a more recent study showed that an increase in intestinal permeability results in insulin resistance, along with metabolic endotoxemia and systemic inflammation.[409] So, perhaps the leaky gut makes someone more susceptible to having insulin resistance, and not the other way around. Either way, since a leaky gut is a factor in autoimmunity, this needs to be addressed, and we know from the first mechanism I discussed that hyperglycemia and insulin resistance can increase proinflammatory cytokines. And even if hyperglycemia and/or insulin resistance doesn't directly cause a leaky gut, evidence suggests that high levels of proinflammatory cytokines can cause an increase in intestinal permeability.[410,411]

Mechanism #3: Those with hyperglycemia are more likely to be overweight and obese, which is associated with an increase in proinflammatory cytokines. Even though I listed this as a separate mechanism, there is some overlap with the previous two I listed. Some of the studies I mentioned earlier were conducted in obese men and women. However, not everyone who has hyperglycemia and insulin resistance is overweight, which is why I am discussing this third mechanism. In those people who are overweight and obese, there is an increased secretion of proinflammatory cytokines in adipose tissue.[412,413] Once again, these proinflammatory cytokines can decrease Tregs and increase Th17 cells, which can set the stage for autoimmunity. They can also cause an increase in intestinal permeability.

Mechanism #4: Leptin resistance. Leptin is one of the most important hormones secreted by adipocytes, and it has a number of roles related to the control of metabolism and energy homeostasis.[414] Leptin has also been shown to regulate the immune response, and evidence shows that increased leptin levels are involved in the pathogenesis of autoimmune conditions such as Hashimoto's.[414,415] Leptin itself can induce a proinflammatory Th1 immune response[416] and can increase Th17 cells,[417,418] and it is a mediator of inflammation. In addition to inducing inflammation, leptin can also perpetuate the inflammatory response. A journal article I came across mentioned that, on average, women are 2-3 times higher in serum leptin levels than men, which possibly can contribute to women being more susceptible to autoimmunity.[419]

Many people have leptin resistance, which is a key factor in obesity. One of the main functions of leptin is to regulate appetite, which, in turn, can help to maintain a healthy weight. But leptin resistance can lead to a voracious appetite, which contributes to the weight gain and inflammation; thus, another vicious cycle develops. Fortunately, many of the same strategies that can help overcome insulin resistance will also help someone with leptin resistance. This includes eating well, exercising regularly, and doing things to reduce inflammation.

Testing For Blood Sugar Imbalances

In section three, I'll discuss some of the tests to help determine if someone has hyperglycemia or insulin resistance.

How Can Hyperglycemia/Insulin Resistance Be Corrected?

Here are a few things that can help correct blood sugar imbalances:

Improve insulin sensitivity through diet. Eating a diet consisting of whole, healthy foods can help to increase insulin sensitivity. You already know that you should eat whole foods, and minimize the refined foods and sugars. You also want to minimize your overall carbohydrate intake, and, with hyperglycemia and insulin resistance, it usually is best to consume less than 150 grams of carbohydrates per day, and eating less than 100 grams is sometimes necessary. In addition, you want to eat sufficient protein and healthy fats, and try to eat at least 25 to 30 grams of fiber per day.

Speaking of healthy fats, avocados are one of the best sources, and studies do show that they can help with insulin resistance due to the high amounts of monounsaturated fatty acids.[420,421] Avocados are also a good source of fiber, which can help with insulin sensitivity.[422] However, you won't get enough fiber just from eating avocados, as you'll need to rely on other food sources. One of the problems with following an autoimmune Paleo diet is that many of the foods that are high in fiber are excluded, including legumes and grains. However, fruits and vegetables can provide a lot of fiber, and some of the best sources include apples, avocados, raspberries, winter squash, and cruciferous vegetables such as broccoli, Brussels sprouts, and cabbage.

Improve insulin sensitivity through nutritional supplements and herbs. Although eating well is essential, nutritional supplementation can be beneficial at times. Some of the nutrients that can help to increase insulin sensitivity include chromium,[423,424] magnesium,[425,426] and alpha lipoic acid.[427,428] Vanadium[429,430] and bitter melon[431] can also increase insulin sensitivity. Berberine can benefit those with insulin resistance and type 2 diabetes by lowering blood glucose levels, and it might do this by modulating the microbiota.[432] The herb gymnema sylvestre can help to lower blood glucose levels.[433,434]

Improve insulin sensitivity through exercise. We all know that regular exercise is beneficial. Although many nutrients can increase insulin sensitivity, many studies show that exercise can also help to accomplish this as well.[435,436] A big problem is that many people who exercise regularly also spend a good part of their day sitting. For example, someone might have a job that involves sitting behind a desk for most of the day, and then they expect three or four sessions of exercise each week to offset all of this inactivity. Unfortunately, that won't work, as regular movement is very important.

Improve insulin sensitivity through sleep. Numerous studies show that sleep deprivation is a risk factor for insulin resistance.[437,438] Thus, you want to make sure you get sufficient sleep each night, which I discuss in section four.

Improve insulin resistance by reducing inflammation. Earlier I discussed how inflammation is a big factor in insulin resistance; thus, it's important to take measures to reduce the inflammatory process. Eating a healthy diet can help to reduce inflammation. However, it frequently is necessary to take nutritional supplements to help break the inflammatory cycle. The way to reduce proinflammatory cytokines is by downregulating the transcription factor called Nuclear Factor Kappa B (NF-kB). Certain nutrients that can help with this include vitamin D, fish oils, turmeric, resveratrol, gamma-linolenic acid, ginger, and green tea.

Correct intestinal dysbiosis. Since intestinal dysbiosis can play a role in inflammation and insulin resistance, it is necessary to address this problem. While many people take probiotic supplements to support the microbiota, this is only one piece of the puzzle when trying to correct intestinal dysbiosis. I'll discuss correcting intestinal dysbiosis and healing the gut in Chapter 28.

Chapter Highlights:

- Hyperglycemia and insulin resistance are factors in the development of Hashimoto's.
- Glucose is a simple sugar and is essential for tissue energy production, while insulin is a hormone that is produced by the beta cells of the pancreas.
- Some of the factors that can cause or contribute to insulin resistance include inflammation, mitochondrial dysfunction, lipotoxicity, gut dysbiosis, circadian disruption, and genetics.
- Hyperglycemia (high blood sugar) can cause a decrease in regulatory T cells and increase in Th17 cells.
- Hyperglycemia can cause an increase in intestinal permeability (a leaky gut).
- Those with hyperglycemia are more likely to be overweight and obese, which is associated with an increase in proinflammatory cytokines.
- Leptin has also been shown to regulate the immune response, and evidence shows that increased leptin levels are involved in the pathogenesis of autoimmune conditions such as Hashimoto's.
- Eating a diet consisting of whole, healthy foods can help to increase insulin sensitivity; although, sometimes, taking nutritional supplements and herbs is necessary
- Other factors that can improve insulin sensitivity include exercise, proper sleep, reducing inflammation, improving mitochondrial dysfunction, and correcting intestinal dysbiosis.

CHAPTER 18

CAN ROOT CANALS, MERCURY AMALGAMS, AND TITANIUM IMPLANTS TRIGGER HASHIMOTO'S?

I THINK IT'S SAFE TO say that most people with Hashimoto's wouldn't consider problems with oral health to be related to their condition. However, having poor oral health can increase the risk of developing certain chronic conditions, and very well might also play a role in the development of an autoimmune thyroid condition such as Hashimoto's. I'm not suggesting that most cases of Hashimoto's are caused by problems with oral health, but this is a factor that is overlooked by most people, and it should be considered. Fortunately, many natural healthcare professionals, including biological dentists, realize that mercury amalgams (also known as silver fillings) can cause problems, and some are aware of the potential risk factors of root canals.

It should make sense when you think about the connection between oral health and the rest of the body. This is especially true with mercury amalgams, which I already discussed in Chapter 8. However, many people don't make a similar connection with root canals. Part of this has to do with the approach of most dentists, since, while many dental clinics avoid the use of mercury amalgams (although not all of them), most still perform root canals frequently.

The Relationship Between Hashimoto's and Gum Inflammation

Although the main focus of this chapter will be on mercury amalgams, root canals, and titanium implants, the potential consequences of periodontitis (gum inflammation) shouldn't be overlooked. Some research points to a relationship between periodontitis and Hashimoto's,[439,440] although it shows that Hashimoto's is more likely to cause periodontitis than the other way around. However, what's interesting is that the researchers discussed probable common autoimmune mechanisms in periodontitis and Hashimoto's.

While there is no evidence that periodontitis directly causes Hashimoto's, periodontitis results in an increase in proinflammatory cytokines,[441,442,443] which are also associated with Hashimoto's. In addition, evidence shows the presence of Th17 cells in periodontal disease,[444] which are associated with autoimmunity. There is also an association between Porphyromonas gingivalis and increased intestinal permeability,[445] and a leaky gut can make someone more susceptible to developing Hashimoto's. A stronger link exists between gum disease and other autoimmune conditions such as rheumatoid arthritis, but based on the evidence I provided here, it wouldn't be surprising if periodontitis were a factor in the development of thyroid autoimmunity.

Mercury Amalgams and Hashimoto's

Although I already discussed mercury Chapter 8, I'd like to expand on this here. First, there is no doubt that having mercury amalgams results in the release of mercury vapors during the act of chewing. What's controversial is the effect that the mercury vapors have on our health, and whether these vapors can serve as a trigger for Hashimoto's, as well as other health conditions.

While some studies show that there is no relationship between dental amalgams and Hashimoto's,[446] other studies have shown that the removal of dental amalgam decreases TPO and thyroglobulin antibodies.[447] Both the FDA and Centers for Disease Control (CDC) consider mercury amalgams to be safe in most cases. However, the World Health Organization (WHO) considers mercury to be one of the top ten chemicals of major public health concern, and mentions how exposure to mercury, even in small amounts, may cause serious health problems.[448]

Several different studies demonstrate a negative effect of mercury on the thyroid gland. Keep in mind that not all of these studies involve inorganic mercury, which is the mercury found in dental amalgams. Methylmercury is found in fish, and both inorganic mercury and methylmercury can negatively impact the thyroid gland.

One study looked at the role of environmental factors in autoimmune thyroiditis, and showed that replacement of dental amalgams in mercury-allergic subjects resulted in improvement of health in about 70% of patients, and, in some cases, will result in a normalization of anti-thyroid autoantibodies. Another study looked at the relationship between mercury and thyroid autoantibodies, and showed that there is an association between mercury and thyroglobulin antibodies, but not thyroid peroxidase antibodies.[449] Although these studies focus on the effects of mercury and the immune system, a few studies have shown that mercury can also have a direct effect on the thyroid hormones.[450,451]

Does this mean that everyone who currently has mercury amalgams should get them removed? This remains controversial, as, while mercury undoubtedly shouldn't have been used as fillings in the first place by most dentists, sometimes, getting them removed can do more harm than good. In some cases, removing these amalgams can exacerbate the auto-immune response of someone who has Hashimoto's.

Anyone who is considering getting their mercury amalgams removed should hire a dentist who takes the proper precautions when removing them, such as a biological dentist. You can find one of these dentists by visiting the website of the International Academy of Oral Medicine and Toxicology or International Academy of Biological Dentistry & Medicine. Their respective websites are **www.iaomt.org** and **www.iabdm.org**.

What's the Deal With Root Canals?

Although the American Dental Association (ADA) claims that root canals are safe simply because there is no scientific evidence that proves they are harmful, it's important to keep in mind that no scientific studies prove that root canals are completely safe. As of writing this book, the ADA also considers mercury amalgams to be safe, as if you visit their website they state that "dental amalgam has been studied and reviewed extensively, and has established a record of safety and effectiveness."

In this chapter, along with the chapter on environmental toxins, I provided evidence demonstrating why mercury amalgams aren't completely safe. While some dentists still recommend mercury amalgams to their patients, over the years, thousands of dentists who once considered mercury amalgams to be safe no longer use mercury in their practice. Thus, we can't rely on the ADA's claims about the safety of root canals. Without question, this is a controversial topic, as while some people have had their health improve upon removing their root canals, most dentists will probably continue to routinely recommend root canals to their patients until scientific studies demonstrate this.

Before discussing the potential risks of root canals, it probably would be a good idea to briefly explain what a root canal entails. A root canal is usually recommended when the nerve of the tooth becomes infected or the pulp becomes damaged. I'm not going to get into the details of the procedure, but, essentially, they will drill a hole into the tooth and remove the dental pulp, the decayed nerve tissue, and they will try their best to sterilize the area to kill the bacteria. Once this has been accomplished, the tooth will be sealed, and, oftentimes, a crown will be placed over the tooth.

I left out a number of details, but the main controversy is whether all of the bacteria can successfully be eradicated. In other words, can the canals be permanently sterilized? Many reading this may be familiar with Dr. Weston Price, a dentist who looked at the relationship between dental health and nutrition, and how it impacted our overall health. Dr. Price took one thousand extracted teeth and sterilized the canals with forty different chemicals in order to see if permanent sterilization could be achieved. After 48 hours, he broke the teeth apart and cultured them, and found that all but one of the teeth had bacteria. Other biological dentists have confirmed Dr. Price's findings.

Although no research studies I'm aware of show a correlation between root canals and specific health conditions, numerous people with different health conditions had their health improve dramatically upon removing their root canals. The Weston A. Price website has an article on root canals written by Dr. Hal Huggins (a dentist), who states that "the bacteria in root canals favor destruction of the nervous system and many other systems, resulting in the creation of autoimmune reactions." While root canals aren't the trigger for most cases of Hashimoto's, if someone who is following a natural treatment protocol has one or more root canals and doesn't see an improvement in their health, then they might want to consider having these removed. At the very least, I'd consider consulting with a biological dentist and get their opinion.

Diet vs. Oral Hygiene

Dr. Price was a big advocate of a whole foods diet, as his research discovered that primitive people who didn't incorporate any oral hygiene (e.g., brushing their teeth or flossing) were almost 100% free of tooth decay because they ate a diet devoid of refined foods and sugars. This doesn't mean that you shouldn't practice proper oral hygiene, but those who eat a poor diet are more likely to have oral problems, regardless of how much they brush or floss daily.

More on the Risks of Root Canals

Dr. George Meinig was one of the founders of the American Association of Endodontists. An endodontist is a dentist who specializes in saving teeth. Their additional training focuses on performing root canals and other treatment procedures.

Dr. Meinig wrote a book entitled *Root Canal Cover Up,* which is based on Dr. Weston Price's 25 years of research. In this book, he writes about how Dr. Price removed infected teeth from humans who suffered from certain health conditions (i.e., arthritis), and then implanted the tooth beneath the skin of healthy rabbits. Not only did the health of the human improve upon removal of the infected tooth, but the rabbit with the implanted (and infected) tooth soon developed the same health condition.

Dr. Meinig claims that ALL root canals harbor bacteria. We need to keep in mind that teeth are similar to other organs in that they require a blood supply, along with lymphatic and venous drainage. Thus, when someone has a root canal performed, they are essentially left with a dead tooth in their mouth. This dead tooth has thousands of side canals, which is where the bacteria reside. According to Dr. Meinig and other dentists, having a single root canal can significantly reduce the health of the immune system.

The Focal Infection Theory

The focal infection theory suggests that many chronic diseases are caused by focal infections, which are usually asymptomatic and commonly occur in areas such as the teeth, sinuses, adenoids, tonsils, genitourinary tract, gall bladder, and kidneys.[452] This theory doesn't only apply to root canals, but infections in other areas of the body. A 2002 journal article mentioned that there isn't sufficient evidence that shows a relationship between dental, tonsillar, and urogenital focal infections and allergic or autoimmune diseases.[453] However, a more recent study found a high incidence of focal infections in patients with psoriasis and urticaria.[452]

If the focal infection theory is true, then you might wonder why everyone who has at least one root canal doesn't develop a chronic health condition. It depends on the health of the person's immune system. As you know, having a root canal isn't the only factor that can potentially compromise the immune system. If someone who has a root canal is otherwise in a good state of health, then they very well might not develop any health problems, at least not over the short term. Also, keep in mind that the focal theory of infection is still only a theory, although it's supported by many knowledgeable healthcare professionals, including most biological dentists.

Should You Remove Your Root Canals?

A few years ago, I had a cavity in the back of my mouth that was between my teeth. While I felt some discomfort at times, over a period of years none of the dentists were able to spot it on the on the dental x-rays. By the time one of the dentists discovered the cavity it was too late to get it filled. Because it was towards the back of my mouth, I decided I didn't want a root canal, and I had it extracted.

However, the decision isn't as easy if someone has a similar problem with a tooth in the front of their mouth. If a dentist recommends that someone gets a root canal in one of their front teeth and the person instead chooses to get an extraction, it probably is a good idea to get this replaced. It might also be wise to get it replaced if it's towards the back of the mouth, but it's arguably even more important to get some type of replacement for an extracted tooth in the front of the mouth. The two options usually given are bridges and dental implants. There are pros and cons with each of these.

A dental bridge involves a non-removable prosthesis that is attached to the surrounding teeth. The problem with these is that the healthy teeth surrounding the replacement tooth will usually need to be filed. Regarding dental implants, many people receive these and seem to do fine. However, there are a few drawbacks.

First, they are very expensive, and if someone doesn't have dental insurance then they will be spending thousands of dollars on this procedure. Second, it's an extensive procedure that will take months to complete. Finally, most dental implants are made out of titanium, and, while most people do fine with these implants, a small percentage of people will react to titanium. I'll further discuss titanium dental implants shortly.

Thus, if someone currently has a root canal on a tooth that is towards the back of the mouth it might be best to get it extracted and not get a bridge or implant. However, if someone has one or more root canals in the front or side teeth, then the decision to get the tooth removed can be more difficult. Obviously, the decision is ultimately up to the person, but regardless of where the root canal is, it probably would be a good idea to seek the opinion of a biological dentist to discuss the different options you have.

For those who are considering getting their root canals extracted, I need to mention that, according to Dr. Meinig, simply extracting the tooth isn't sufficient. He also recommends removing the periodontal ligament and the first millimeter of bone that lines the socket of the tooth, as this usually is infected as well. He writes about the extraction procedure in his book, but if you go to a biological dentist, they should know how to appropriately remove the tooth.

Can Titanium Dental Implants Trigger Hashimoto's?

When someone gets a dental implant, it is commonly made out of titanium. Titanium is also used in other procedures, as some hip replacements use titanium alloys. While many people with these implants seem to do fine, over the years, some of my patients with Hashimoto's have asked me whether titanium can be a trigger.

Before I answer this, you might wonder why titanium is commonly used in the first place. One reason is its high resistance to corrosion.[454] Another reason is that most people seem to have a low sensitivity to titanium when compared to other metals. One study showed that all casting alloys seem to have a potential for eliciting adverse reactions in individual hypersensitive patients, although it listed titanium as being a possible exception.[455]

The truth is that some people do react to titanium, which can be a big problem for someone who has a dental implant or titanium as part of a hip or knee replacement. As you read the following information, please keep in mind that I'm not suggesting that people avoid getting titanium implants. However, I recommend being tested for a titanium allergy before getting an implant.

Why Is Titanium Problematic in Some People?

Although most people don't have a problem with titanium implants, a small percentage of people react to titanium. A clinical study involving 1,500 people who received dental implants showed that nine of these patients demonstrated a titanium allergy.[456] The good news is that only 0.6% of these patients experienced problems with the dental implants. However, even a small percentage of negative reactions might be too high.

Another study involved 56 patients who developed clinical symptoms after receiving titanium-based implants, and 21 of these tested positive for a titanium allergy, with another 16 showing ambiguous results.[457] Sometimes, someone will experience symptoms caused by these implants but they won't make the connection, and many times, their doctors also won't be able to figure this out.

For example, in the past, it was revealed that the actor Dick Van Dyke had experienced severe headaches that affected his sleep and caused chronic fatigue. Over a seven-year period, he saw a number of different healthcare professionals, received a CAT scan, MRI, and a spinal tap, along with other tests, but everything came back negative. It wasn't until his dental implants were removed that he finally received relief from his symptoms.

Once again, most people do fine with titanium implants. But these patient experiences I mentioned show that, in some cases, titanium can lead to severe symptoms. In some cases, the symptoms can be debilitating. Many times, people live with these symptoms for years before they figure out that the problem is due to titanium.

Is There a Relationship Between Titanium and Hashimoto's?

Currently, no evidence I'm aware of suggests that having titanium implants can be a trigger for Hashimoto's or any other autoimmune condition. However, we already know that other metals, such as mercury and nickel, have been associated with thyroid autoimmunity.[458,459] Therefore, if someone with Hashimoto's was diagnosed with their condition after getting a titanium implant, then this factor should be considered.

Keep in mind that it can be difficult to make such a connection, as someone can be in the "silent" autoimmune stage I discussed in Chapter 1 for years, which means they might have elevated thyroid autoantibodies for many years, yet have no positive lab markers or symptoms. Thus, even if someone with Hashimoto's began presenting with symptoms shortly after getting a titanium implant, this doesn't necessarily mean the implant was responsible for the development of their condition. Therefore, if you have a titanium implant and then eventually developed Hashimoto's, it might be worth doing some testing to see if you have an allergy to titanium.

What Other Options Are There?

Before someone gets a dental implant, or a hip or knee replacement that involves titanium, it probably would be a good idea to get a metal allergy assessment along with some allergy testing. Skin testing is an option, as the sensitivity of patch tests has been shown to be about 75% for a type IV metal allergy, although, so far, no study related to dental implant allergies has used this method.[460] A lymphocyte transformation test is another option, although false-positive results are possible.[460]

A Memory lymphocyte immunostimulation assay (MELISA) test[461] can determine if someone has an allergy to a metal such as titanium. In my opinion, it should be routine to get such testing before getting a metal implant. After all, even if titanium doesn't act as an autoimmune trigger, if someone is allergic to it, I think it's safe to say that it would be best to use a different material for the implant.

If someone tests positive for a titanium allergy then zirconium implants should be considered. Zirconia is a ceramic, has been used to replace hip joints, and can be an option to consider with dental implants. Even though an allergy to zirconia is unlikely, it is still possible to be allergic to zirconia. Once again, if you need a dental implant then this is something to discuss with your dentist.

Chapter Highlights:

- There is some evidence of a relationship between periodontitis and Hashimoto's in the literature.
- Some studies have shown that the removal of dental amalgam decreases TPO and thyroglobulin antibodies in patients with autoimmune thyroiditis.
- Dr. Weston Price states that "the bacteria in root canals favor destruction of the nervous system and many other systems, resulting in the creation of autoimmune reactions.
- Although most people don't have a problem with titanium implants, a small percentage of people are sensitive.
- There is no concrete evidence that having titanium implants can trigger an autoimmune response and lead to a condition such as Hashimoto's.
- If you have a titanium implant and then eventually developed an autoimmune thyroid condition, then it might be worth doing some testing to see if you have an allergy to titanium.
- A Memory lymphocyte immunostimulation assay (MELISA) test can determine if someone has an allergy to a metal such as titanium.

• CHAPTER 19 •

IS THERE A LINK BETWEEN VACCINES AND HASHIMOTO'S?

NITIALLY, I WASN'T PLANNING on dedicating a chapter to vaccines, as, while there are few controversial topics in this book, vaccines are perhaps the most controversial of them all. The goal of this chapter isn't to convince you that vaccinations are harmful in all situations, but, instead, to provide you with some information so that you can make an informed decision. The truth is that vaccines have benefits, but just as is the case with everything else, you need to consider both the risks and benefits. While most of the vaccinations are given during childhood, I'm also going to discuss vaccines in adults, including the flu shot.

I'm not going to discuss all of the different types of vaccines, as this is too much to cover in a single chapter. If this is a topic that interests you, a number of good books have been published on this, along with some documentaries. For more information you can visit **www. naturalendocrinesolutions.com/resources**.

What Are Vaccines, and Why Are They Given?

A vaccination involves the injection of a killed or weakened organism that causes the body to produce antibodies against that organism. In other words, vaccines are given to prime the immune system with the organism that causes the disease, so that if you are exposed to it, the immune system will react quickly. For example, the MMR vaccine is designed to protect people against measles, mumps, and rubella, and it does this by injecting weakened forms of the live viruses that cause these conditions.

According to the CDC website, "after injection the viruses cause a harmless infection in the vaccinated person, and the person's immune system fights the infection caused by these weakened viruses, and immunity develops."[462] It's also worth noting that according to the same website, about 3 out of 100 people who get two doses of the MMR vaccine will still get measles if exposed to the virus, although they are more likely to have a milder illness.

How Do Vaccines Work?

Vaccines use either live attenuated (weakened) pathogens (i.e., viruses), or inactivated pathogens. The MMR vaccine is an example of a vaccine using an attenuated pathogen. Attenuated vaccines elicit strong and cellular antibody responses and usually result in immunity against the pathogen that lasts for decades.[463] However, many vaccines that use inactivated pathogens include substances called adjuvants.

An adjuvant is an ingredient added to a vaccine to help create a stronger immune response by the person who receives the vaccine. This is especially true when a vaccine consists of an inactivated bacteria or virus, which is the case with most vaccines. Thus, the adjuvant helps to enhance the immune response against the inactivated virus that is in the vaccine, which, in turn, will cause the person to develop antibodies against the virus. Not all inactivated vaccines use adjuvants. For example, although the flu vaccine uses inactivated viruses, as of writing this book, only one type (Influenza FLUAD) uses an adjuvant.

The Three Main Adjuvants Currently Used In Vaccines

Aluminum. Aluminum gels and aluminum salts are commonly used as adjuvants in vaccines. Some argue that aluminum is safe because it is present in very low amounts, and it has been used in vaccines since the 1930s. I'll further discuss this shortly.

Monophosphoryl lipid A. This substance was isolated from the surface of bacteria, as it is a detoxified form of the endotoxin lipopolysaccharide.[464] It has been used since 2009 in the Human Papillomavirus (HPV) vaccine.

MF59 adjuvant. This is an oil-in-water emulsion of squalene oil, and is in one of the flu vaccines (FLUAD) that is approved for people 65 years and older.

Of these three adjuvants, aluminum is the most controversial one. While the current research doesn't show a direct correlation between aluminum and Hashimoto's, aluminum is considered to be a toxic metal. Numerous studies show that it is neurotoxic, as its free ion is highly biologically reactive and can cause damage to our neurons.[465,466] This is why aluminum toxicity has been linked to neurodegenerative diseases such as Alzheimer's disease.[467] One study I came across showed that aluminum inhibits more than 200 biologically important functions and causes various adverse effects in plants, animals, and humans.[467]

Regarding aluminum's effect on the immune system, one study showed that administration of as little as two to three immune adjuvants can overcome genetic resistance to autoimmunity.[468] Other studies also show that aluminum adjuvants have the potential to trigger autoimmunity.[469,470] This doesn't mean that most people who receive vaccines will develop autoimmunity, or that vaccines will exacerbate the autoimmune response in most people who currently have Hashimoto's, but even if only a very small percentage of people will be affected, this still needs to be considered.

Dr. Chris Exley, a professor of bioinorganic chemistry, has been researching aluminum for over 30 years. In the documentary *Injecting Aluminum*, he mentioned that aluminum has never been demonstrated to be safe as an adjunct in vaccines. Of course this doesn't prevent the use of aluminum in certain vaccines. The same can be said about other chemicals, as many harmful chemicals are assumed to be safe in small amounts.

Which Vaccines Include Adjuvants?

- Hepatitis A
- Hepatitis B
- Diphtheria-tetanus-pertussis (DTaP)
- Haemophilus influenzae type b (Hib)
- Human papillomavirus (HPV)
- Pneumococcal vaccine
- FLUAD

All of these include aluminum as an adjuvant, with the exception of the HPV vaccine and FLUAD. FLUAD is an influenza vaccine given to adults 65 years and older.

Vaccines That Are Recommended for Adults
Although the majority of vaccines are administered to children, a few vaccinations are recommended for adults. Since most people with Hashimoto's are adults, I figured it would be beneficial to list some of the vaccines recommended to adults.

Influenza vaccine. This is recommended annually for adults of all ages, and I'll discuss this vaccine in greater detail shortly.

Meningococcal conjugate vaccine. This helps to protect against bacterial meningitis. First year college students living in residence halls should be vaccinated for this virus.

Tdap vaccine. This offers protection against tetanus, diphtheria, and pertussis. Although a single dose of this vaccine is usually recommended for preteens and teens, it is recommended for adults 19 or older who haven't received it. Pregnant women are especially encouraged to receive this vaccine, with some sources suggesting that pregnant women should receive a dose of Tdap during each pregnancy.

HPV vaccination. This helps to protect against the human papillomavirus, which is the major cause of cervical cancer, as well as genital warts. Like the Tdap vaccine the HPV vaccine is recommended for preteens and teenagers, although young adults who haven't received this vaccine as a teenager are encouraged to receive it.

Which Ingredients Are Present in Vaccines?
In addition to the adjuvants listed earlier, here are some other ingredients commonly found in vaccines. Just as a reminder, not all of the ingredients are included in all of the different vaccines:

Octoxynol-10 (TRITON X-100). This is an ethoxylated alkyl phenol found in some personal care products. Speaking of which, according to the Skin Deep website from the Environmental Working group, this ingredient has a moderate overall hazard.

Thimerosal. This is an ethyl mercury-based preservative used in vials that contain more than one dose of a vaccine to prevent germs, bacteria and/or fungi from contaminating the vaccine. According to the CDC, while flu vaccines in multi-dose vials contain thimerosal to safeguard against contamination of the vial, most single-dose vials and pre-filled syringes of the flu shot do not contain a preservative because they are intended to be used only used once. Material Safety Data Sheets (MSDS) are produced by companies that manufacture hazardous substances, and they provide information that includes the physical properties, toxicity, and reactivity of many different chemicals. The MSDS says that thimerosal may be toxic to the kidneys, liver, spleen, bone marrow, and central nervous system.

Formaldehyde. The MSDS lists formaldehyde as being very hazardous in case of eye contact or ingestion. It also lists it as a probable human carcinogen. This ingredient is also listed on the Skin Deep website, and its overall hazard is high, and the Environmental Working Group also lists it as being a high risk in cancer formation, along with organ system toxicity. Some will argue that formaldehyde can be broken down when ingested, which is true, but it apparently can remain in its whole form when injected.

β-propiolactone. According to the MSDS, this is very hazardous in case of ingestion or inhalation, and is hazardous in case of skin contact or eye contact.

Neomycin. This is an antibiotic, and is added to some inactivated influenza virus vaccines to prevent the growth of bacteria during production and storage of the vaccine.

Polysorbate 80. This is a surfactant and emulsifier used in cleaners and personal care products. The Environmental Working Group lists the overall hazard as low. The MSDS lists it as being slightly hazardous in case of skin contact, of eye contact, of ingestion, or inhalation. On the surface, it doesn't seem to be as bad of an ingredient when compared to the others, although apparently it is used by the pharmaceutical industry to help drugs get past the blood brain barrier, and there is a concern that it can also bind to some of the ingredients that are present in the vaccine.

Ovalbumin. This is the main protein found in egg whites. If someone has an egg allergy, then getting a vaccine with this ingredient can be problematic; although, if the ovalbumin concentration is low, then those with egg allergies might be able to get it without a problem.[471]

Are Small Amounts of These Ingredients Safe?

According to the CDC and other sources, the amount of these chemical additives found in vaccines is very small. While this may be true, this doesn't mean that they are safe. For example, the amount of mercury used in mercury amalgams is very small as well, but there is a relationship between thyroid autoimmunity and mercury amalgams in some people.

Another thing to keep in mind is that, according to the US Food and Drug Administration, safety assessments for vaccines have often not included appropriate toxicity studies because vaccines have not been viewed as inherently toxic. In other words, comprehensive toxicity studies haven't been conducted because it is assumed that the amount of chemicals included in vaccines is so small that they can't possibly cause any problems.

In addition, there is a difference between ingesting or inhaling certain chemicals and having them injected. For example, some will mention that we are exposed to chemicals such as aluminum, mercury, and formaldehyde through sources other than vaccines. While this is true, this doesn't mean that it's safe to add these chemicals to vaccines. Some healthcare practitioners and researchers also express concern about these chemicals being more harmful when injected.

This last point shouldn't be taken lightly, as, when discussing certain ingredients in vaccines, some will argue that the amounts of these chemicals are so small that they won't cause any harm. But besides the fact that small amounts of some of these chemicals can potentially cause harm if ingested or inhaled, they might cause more harm when injected. In addition, one also needs to consider the synergistic effects of these chemicals. In toxicology, synergism refers to the effect caused when exposure to multiple chemicals at a time results in health effects that are greater than the effects of the individual chemicals. In Chapter 20, when discussing the harmful effects of glyphosate, I'll discuss how the combination of glyphosate with other chemicals in Roundup can make the formulation even more toxic. And this is true with other chemicals as well.

Should You Get the Flu Shot?

The influenza (flu) shot is unique when compared with other vaccines in that this vaccine needs to be updated periodically to match the vaccine strains with the current influenza strains. Thus, every year or two, different influenza vaccines need to be formulated with different virus antigens. However, the main concern isn't with the virus antigens that are in the vaccine, but the other ingredients.

Two main arguments exist in favor of getting the flu shot. One argument is that influenza can sometimes be very serious, leading to hospitalization in some cases, and, in rare cases, death. According to the CDC website, flu-related hospitalizations since 2010 ranged from 140,000 to 710,000, while flu-related deaths are estimated to have ranged from 12,000 to 56,000. However, this apparently includes cases of pneumonia because some deaths related to influenza are due to secondary complications, although not all cases of pneumonia are related to influenza.

Another reason to consider getting the flu shot is that, in some cases, getting this vaccine will reduce your risk of getting the flu virus, as well as spreading it to others. However, many different strains of the flu exist, and if you are exposed to a strain of influenza that is not in the flu vaccine, then there is a good chance that you will get the flu.

5 Reasons to Consider Avoiding the Flu Shot

1. There are different strains of the flu. Getting the flu shot won't completely protect you from getting the flu if you are exposed to a strain of influenza that isn't in the vaccine. Unfortunately, there is a greater chance of being exposed to a strain that isn't in the vaccine, which is why it's common for people who get the flu shot to get the flu.

2. There are harmful ingredients in the flu vaccine. Of course, this is the case with all vaccines, and I listed a number of them earlier. While it is true that these ingredients are present in small amounts, this doesn't mean they are safe. Also, we can't dismiss the potential synergistic effects of the chemicals included in the vaccine.

3. Side effects are common when getting the flu vaccine. Most of the time, the side effects are minor, such as local swelling, redness, and pain at the site of the injection. Other symptoms include headaches, nausea, fatigue, muscle pain, and neuropathy.

4. Vaccines can potentially trigger or exacerbate the autoimmune response. I'll discuss the research shortly, and, while this does seem to be rare, it still should make anyone with an existing autoimmune thyroid condition think twice about getting the annual flu vaccine.

5. You can protect yourself naturally from the flu. While it's true that doing things to improve your immune system health won't guarantee that you won't get the flu, the same is true when getting the flu vaccine. Plus, it won't hurt to eat a good diet, improve your stress-management skills, take measures to improve the health of your gut (where most of your immune system cells are located), make sure you have healthy levels of vitamin D, take vitamin C and other nutrients and herbs that can improve your immune system health, etc.

Is There Evidence That Vaccines Can Trigger Hashimoto's?

It can be difficult to make a direct link between vaccines and autoimmunity, and correlation doesn't always mean causation. While it's probably safe to say that in most cases getting a vaccine won't trigger an autoimmune response, a few studies suggest that vaccines can occasionally stimulate autoantibody production, and, in some cases, the ingredients in the vaccines can cause a condition known as autoimmune/inflammatory syndrome.[472,473,474]

A journal review article looked at the relationship between autoimmune/inflammatory syndrome caused by vaccine adjuvants and autoimmune thyroid conditions.[475] Other than a few case reports, there honestly isn't a lot of evidence showing a direct link between vaccine adjuvants and autoimmunity, although the authors concluded that physicians need to be aware that thyroiditis and other thyroid conditions can be induced by vaccine adjuvants, and, therefore, should reconsider nonessential vaccination.[475] Keep in mind that autoimmune conditions, such as Hashimoto's, can take many years before someone presents with noticeable symptoms after receiving a vaccine, which is why it is difficult to prove a direct relationship.

What Alternatives Are There to Vaccines?

Improve your immune system health. Just remember that your immune system was designed to naturally fight off infections, without the use of drugs and vaccines. While I realize that there is a time and place for medical intervention, it's crazy to think we need dozens of vaccines throughout our life to protect ourselves from viruses and other pathogens, just as it would be crazy to think that we need to take an antibiotic every time we have a bacterial infection.

This entire book is designed to help improve your immune system health. While the primary goal is to show you how to find and remove your autoimmune triggers, other information is included to help you to optimize the health of your immune system. While it is true that you will need to take responsibility for your health in order to accomplish this, doing so is necessary in order to increase your chances of living a long and healthy life.

Consider homeopathy. Some reading this might also be familiar with nosodes, which is a homeopathic alternative to vaccines. I can't say that I have a great deal of knowledge in this area, and, while you can find some information about this online, if this interests you, then it probably would be best to work with a homeopathic practitioner. A journal article entitled "'Nosodes Are No Substitute for Vaccines," mentions that there is scant evidence in the medical literature for either the efficacy or safety of nosodes.[476] Unfortunately, there will probably never be any research that shows how effective homeopathy is compared to vaccines. With regards the safety of nosodes, I would rather receive homeopathy than to be injected with chemicals such as aluminum, mercury, and formaldehyde.

Whether or not you decide to get any vaccines is up to you, but, hopefully, you will do some research first, and, if you have children, you might want to consider reading the book *The Vaccine Friendly Plan* by Dr. Paul Thomas and Dr. Jennifer Margulis.

Chapter Highlights:

- A vaccination involves the injection of a killed or weakened organism that causes the body to produce antibodies against that organism.
- An adjuvant is an ingredient that is added to a vaccine in order to help create a stronger immune response by the person who receives the vaccine.
- The three main adjuvants currently used in vaccines include aluminum, Monophosphoryl lipid A, and the MF59 adjuvant.
- Although the amount of these chemical additives found in vaccines are very small, this doesn't mean that they are safe.
- In addition, there is some concern about the safety of these chemicals when they are injected.
- Every year or two, different influenza vaccines need to be formulated to match the vaccine strains with the current influenza strains.
- 5 reasons to consider avoiding the flu shot include 1) there are different strains of the flu, 2) there are harmful ingredients in the flu vaccine, 3) side effects are common, 4) vaccines can potentially trigger or exacerbate the autoimmune response, 5) you can take measures to protect yourself naturally.
- Although no evidence in the research shows that vaccines can trigger Hashimoto's, some studies demonstrate the formation of autoantibodies when vaccines are administered.
- Two alternatives to vaccines include improving your immune system health and homeopathic remedies.

· CHAPTER 20 ·

GLYPHOSATE AND GMOS

'M ALWAYS ENCOURAGING MY patients to eat foods that are organic. Some of the reasons for this are to avoid the hormones and antibiotics given to the livestock, and the pesticides and herbicides sprayed on fruits and vegetables. Another reason is to avoid GMOs (genetically modified organisms). Certain foods are genetically modified, and evidence shows that this can lead to many different health issues, including Hashimoto's.

Before further discussing GMOs, I'd like to say that, as of writing this book, no direct studies show that consumption of GMOs can lead to the development of Hashimoto's. However, this doesn't mean that there isn't a relationship between GMOs and autoimmunity, and, after reading this chapter, I'm hoping you'll understand the potential mechanisms involved.

These are currently the primary genetically modified foods as of autumn 2017:

- Corn
- Soybeans
- Canola oil
- Cottonseed oil
- Papaya
- Alfalfa
- Sugar beet

- Squash
- Potatoes
- Flax
- Apple
- Salmon

Please keep in mind that this list will grow in the upcoming years. Also, some of the foods listed are more commonly genetically modified than others. For example, as of writing this book, most of the corn and soy in the United States are genetically modified. This isn't necessarily the case with the other foods listed, but assuming you don't eat a 100% organic diet, then you want to try avoiding non-organic forms of these foods and oils I just listed.

In addition, you need to be careful when reading ingredients, as it's obvious that corn meal, corn syrup, and corn starch are all derived from corn. However, other ingredients may not be as obvious, such as caramel and baking powder (from corn starch). Most people don't know that ascorbic acid is made from corn syrup; thus, if you're taking a vitamin C supplement in the form of ascorbic acid then this can include genetically modified ingredients; thus, you'll want to confirm that any ascorbic acid supplement you're taking is from a non-GMO source.

Why Does Genetic Modification of Foods Take Place?

Foods that are genetically modified have changes made to the DNA. What they are doing is essentially taking genes from one species and inserting them into another species. This leads to crops that are able to be resistant to herbicides, as well as crops that are actually able to produce their own pesticides to kill organisms.

Why are foods genetically modified? A big reason is because GMO crops make it easier for farmers to kill weeds. Genetic modification allows the crops to be resistant to herbicides such as Roundup. Crops that can produce their own pesticides sounds like a great idea, until you realize that it not only kills organisms that may be harmful to the plant but also can cause harm to the animals and humans that ingest these crops. Obviously, it all comes down to making a greater profit. Even though FDA scientists have issued warnings about the risks associated with GMOs, these has been ignored.

How Are We Exposed to GMOs?

Diet is the primary way that we are exposed to genetically modified foods. The best way to avoid exposure to GMOs is to eat food that is certified organic. People who eat a lot of processed foods and/or non-organic foods are susceptible to developing health issues associated with GMOs. Approximately 90% of the corn and soy in the United States is genetically modified. Many processed foods include corn and soy as ingredients. For example, many breakfast cereals have corn as an ingredient. Many adults and children eat these sugary cereals every morning. To make matters worse, some will add non-organic soy milk to this.

This is just one example, but many other processed foods include corn and/or soy. Many years ago (when I didn't know any better), I often ate vegetarian chicken nuggets, which primarily consisted of soy and other unhealthy ingredients. I know many people reading this realize how unhealthy such foods are, but some still aren't aware of this, which is why I'm giving these examples. Many people eat soy nuggets and soy burgers and drink soy milk, thinking this is benefiting their health, when the exact opposite is true.

Here's another example. For those who eat meat, it's important to realize that most of the livestock are fed genetically modified foods. Many of these animals eat the plants treated with Roundup, which leads to the development of nutrient deficiencies, and then we eat these unhealthy animals. Thus, even if we avoid processed foods but continue to eat non-organic beef, pork, chicken, etc., then we still will be impacted by GMOs.

Why Do GMOs Cause so Many Health Issues?

First, the body doesn't process these genetically modified foods the same way as non-GMO foods. Once again, when you genetically modify corn, soy, or other foods, this will change the DNA, and the immune system sees the proteins in these foods as being foreign. So there will be an immune system response, resulting in inflammation.

Genetically modified foods can be harmful in other ways as well. For example, Bacillus thuringiensis is a gram positive bacteria, used as a microbial insecticide. The genes of these bacteria have been incorporated into several major crops, making them resistant to insects. So, essentially, the crop's DNA has been altered to produce what's called the Bacillus thuringiensis (Bt) toxin, which, in turn, breaks open the stomachs of insects, thereby killing them. Although we were initially told that only insects would be negatively affected by the Bt toxin, some are concerned about it potentially harming some of the cells of the human digestive system, perhaps contributing to an increase in intestinal permeability (a leaky gut), which is part of the triad of autoimmunity I discussed in Chapter 1.

What You Need to Know About Glyphosate

Another reason to avoid GMOs is glyphosate, which is the active ingredient in the herbicide Roundup. It is used primarily on genetically modified crops, and can be a big factor in the increased prevalence of chronic health conditions, including autoimmune conditions such as Hashimoto's. If you are eating any type of processed or refined foods, then there is an excellent chance that you are being exposed to the negative health consequences of glyphosate. This is especially true if these foods are not organic.

Many reading this have heard of Monsanto, a corporation that is the leading producer for Roundup and genetically engineered seeds. An example of this is "Roundup ready soybeans," which are soybeans that were made to be resistant to the effects of Roundup. In other words, Roundup kills everything with the exception of the genetically engineered crop. While this might sound like a good idea to some people, the problem is that these crops contain high levels of glyphosate, which can be a factor in the increase of chronic health conditions.

Why is glyphosate used on these crops if they can potentially cause chronic health problems? The main reason has to do with making a large profit. It's unfortunate that some businesses will do whatever it takes to make a lot of money, even if it means risking the health of millions of people.

What Does the Research Show With Regards to Glyphosate?

Neurotoxicity and oxidative stress. Evidence shows that glyphosate can lead to neurotoxicity and oxidative stress. One study conducted on rats showed that Roundup might lead to excessive extracellular glutamate levels and glutamate excitotoxicity and oxidative stress.[477] In other words, Roundup can cause excessive levels of the neurotransmitter glutamate, which, in turn, can cause damage to the neurons. Another study showed that glyphosate could cause toxicity to the cells, oxidative effects, and apoptosis on human cells.[478] Yet another study showed that inhalation of glyphosate may cause DNA damage.[479]

Cardiovascular health. Glyphosate might also have a negative effect on cardiovascular health, leading to direct cardiac electrophysiological changes, conduction blocks, and arrhythmias.[480]

Breast cancer. Evidence shows that low and environmentally relevant concentrations of glyphosate possesses estrogenic activity and can induce the growth of human breast cancer cells.[481] This doesn't mean that glyphosate will cause breast cancer in most individuals exposed to it, but it might increase the risk in susceptible individuals. Thus, while everyone should try to minimize their exposure to GMOs, those with a family history of breast cancer might want to make a greater effort to avoid these foods.

Impaired liver detoxification and bile metabolism. Glyphosate can inhibit cytochrome P450 enzymes,[482] which play an important role in detoxification. The cytochrome P450 enzymes play an important role in the production of bile acids;[483] thus, glyphosate also can disrupt bile acid homeostasis,[483] which can be one reason why many people have gallbladder issues. Also evidence shows that disrupting the production of bile acid can also promote the toxic accumulation of the mineral manganese in the brainstem, which can cause or be a contributing factor to conditions such as Parkinson's disease.[484]

Gut dysbiosis. Glyphosate disrupts something called the shikimate pathway through the inhibition of 5-enolpyruvylshikimate-3-phosphate synthase,[485] which is an enzyme produced by plants and microorganisms. One reason why glyphosate isn't supposed to be harmful to humans is because we don't have a shikimate pathway.

The problem is that the bacteria present in our body have this pathway, including our gut bacteria. This is how glyphosate can cause intestinal dysbiosis. In addition, it appears that while glyphosate harms the good bacteria in our gut, many pathogenic bacteria are resistant to glyphosate.

A few animal studies demonstrate this effect, as one study looked to determine the impact of glyphosate on potential pathogens and beneficial members of poultry microbiota.[486] The study showed that pathogenic bacteria such as salmonella and clostridium are highly resistant to glyphosate, while most of the beneficial bacteria were found to be moderate to highly susceptible. Another study showed that glyphosate had an inhibitory effect on some of the good bacteria in the gut, but increased the population of pathogenic species.[487] Thus, these studies show how glyphosate can lead to intestinal dysbiosis by killing the good bacteria, while not harming any bad pathogens that may be present.

Some people may argue that some of these studies were conducted on animals, and you can't assume that humans will experience the same health effects. While this is true, we also can't assume that glyphosate won't have the same health effects, and it's also worth mentioning that other animals also don't have a shikimate pathway. Although I agree that we can't always rely on animal studies, we also can't ignore them and conclude that none of this research applies to humans.

Mineral deficiencies. Glyphosate is a chelating agent, as studies show that at physiologically relevant pH levels, copper and zinc can be relatively strongly complexed with glyphosate, whereas iron, calcium, magnesium, and manganese are complexed to lesser degrees.[488] Speaking of manganese, it is an overlooked nutrient, but it has many important functions in the body. For example, manganese superoxide dismutase protects the mitochondria from oxidative damage.

In addition, lactobacillus depends on manganese for antioxidant protection,[489] and reduced lactobacillus can lead to the overgrowth of certain pathogens. While manganese (and a few other nutrients) weren't complexed strongly with glyphosate, glyphosate has been shown to result in severe depletion of manganese in cows and plants,[488] and some claim that it has big impact on manganese in humans as well.

Glyphosate kills the good bacteria in the gut by disrupting the shikimate pathway. This also can result in amino acid deficiencies because bacteria use the shikimate pathway to produce the aromatic amino acids, including tryptophan and tyrosine. Tryptophan is a precursor to the neurotransmitter serotonin, and tyrosine is necessary not only for the production of dopamine and the catecholamines but also for thyroid hormone formation.

Glyphosate Affects More Than Our Food and Water Supply

Although the primary concern when it comes to glyphosate is the impact it has on the food we eat, there are other concerns as well. For example, some studies show that glyphosate can have a negative impact on honeybees.[490] The results suggested that glyphosate at concentrations found in standard spraying can reduce sensitivity to nectar reward and impair associative learning in honeybees. I know that some reading this might not think this is too big of a deal, but while many people realize the problems that herbicides and pesticides cause with regards to our food and water supply, most people have a tendency to overlook the harmful impact of herbicides and pesticides on other areas of our environment.

Glyphosate Is Even More Toxic When Combined With Other Chemicals

One of the flaws of most research studies that test for the toxicity of different chemicals is that they frequently will test these chemicals in isolation. The problem with this approach is that most herbicides and pesticides, as well as other chemicals (i.e., household cleaners) include multiple chemicals, which, when combined, make the product even more toxic.

Most of these pesticide and herbicide formulations also contain adjuvants, which are labeled as being inert by most manufacturers, to enhance the herbicidal action of the formulation. Roundup contains not only glyphosate but also ethoxylated adjuvants, which makes the formulation even more toxic.[491,492] Thus, while glyphosate alone can cause health issues, the combination of glyphosate with these adjuvants makes it even more toxic.

Another issue with most of the research studies regarding certain chemicals has to do with the frequency of exposure and duration of the studies. For example, one can make the argument that consuming genetically modified foods occasionally might not be as bad as eating genetically modified foods every day, which many people do. In addition, if someone were to eat genetically modified foods daily for one year, this probably would be worse than eating genetically modified foods daily for three months.

Don't get me wrong, as eating these foods daily for three months might cause health issues. The point I'm trying to make is that it's very easy to manipulate the findings of research studies, as, if they do a study and determine that a pesticide formulation causes obvious health issues after one year, they can easily design another study that only lasts six months and, therefore, demonstrates no harmful effects.

That's a big issue with many of the research studies on toxic chemicals. Most of them are short-term studies, and most of these chemicals are tested individually. However, in most cases, people are exposed to these chemicals for many years, and most of these formulations include more than one chemical.

How Does Glyphosate Directly Affect Those With Hashimoto's?

Glyphosate can affect those people with Hashimoto's in a few different ways. First, lactobacillus converts inorganic selenium into more bioavailable forms such as selenocysteine and selenomethionine.[493] However, lactobacillus is negatively impacted by glyphosate,[494] which, in turn, can lead to a depletion of selenomethionine and selenocysteine. Selenium plays an important role in the formation of thyroid hormone[495] and can help to lower thyroid antibodies.[496,497,498]

In addition, having a leaky gut and intestinal dysbiosis are other factors in Hashimoto's. Glyphosate can cause intestinal dysbiosis, and evidence shows that glyphosate can also disrupt the barrier properties of intestinal cells.[499] In other words, exposure to glyphosate might cause a leaky gut in some people, increasing their risk of developing Hashimoto's, as well as other autoimmune conditions.

Testing for Glyphosate

Although I have dedicated a separate section on testing, since I don't routinely have all of my patients test for glyphosate, I figured I'd briefly discuss this here. I don't think it's necessary for everyone with Hashimoto's to test for glyphosate because it's safe to say that most people have glyphosate in their tissues. However, if someone lives in an agricultural area, there is a good chance they have higher levels of glyphosate than others; thus, perhaps in this case, it would make sense to test for this. One can also argue that it might not be a bad idea for those who aren't eating mostly organic food to get a baseline reading, as high levels of glyphosate might encourage them to eat a cleaner diet.

As for how glyphosate is tested, a few different companies offer urinary testing. The one I'm most familiar with is Great Plains Laboratory, although others offer this as well. In addition to testing glyphosate in the urine, Great Plains Laboratory also offers water testing for glyphosate; thus, whether or not you have a water filter, you can see if high levels of glyphosate are in your drinking water. For other resources on how to test glyphosate please visit **www.naturalendocrinesolutions.com/resources**.

The Difference Between Organic and Non-GMO Foods

In order to try to avoid GMOs, I recommend to eat mostly organic foods. However, some foods aren't organic but are labeled as "non-GMO." This label should confirm that the product doesn't include genetically modified ingredients. However, this doesn't mean that it is free of glyphosate. For example, some non-GMO crops are sprayed with glyphosate right before they are harvested,[500] which allows farmers to harvest their crops more efficiently. Unfortunately, glyphosate can't simply be washed off.

In addition, other synthetic herbicides and pesticides can be used on non-GMO crops. Thus, while it's definitely better to eat foods that have a non-GMO label than foods that you suspect might have genetically modified ingredients, eating organic is the only way to avoid glyphosate, along with other synthetic herbicides and pesticides.

Is the Problem With Gluten or Glyphosate?

In this section, I dedicated an entire chapter (Chapter 5) on the health risks associated with gluten, and I recommend that those with Hashimoto's avoid gluten while trying to get into a state of remission. Many healthcare professionals recommend that people with Hashimoto's permanently avoid gluten, which seems to make sense, since gluten has been shown to cause a leaky gut in everyone. However, some non-GMO crops are sprayed with glyphosate right before they are harvested, including wheat and other grains. Thus, some speculate that many people don't necessary have a problem with gluten but, instead, have a problem with wheat and other grains due to the glyphosate.

It's common to hear stories about people who have problems eating wheat in the United States, but who have no problem eating wheat in other countries where glyphosate isn't sprayed on the crops. Hybridization of wheat is also something to consider, but perhaps glyphosate is the primary culprit. The truth is that I don't know if the widespread spraying of crops with glyphosate is the main reason why gluten is a problem in so many people.

In Chapter 5, I asked whether someone with Hashimoto's who doesn't have celiac disease can safely reintroduce healthier forms of wheat or other forms of gluten (i.e., rye and barley) upon improving their digestive and lymphatic systems. Based on the evidence provided so far, if someone does choose to reintroduce gluten after they get into remission, it probably is best to make sure to stick with organic grains. In October 2017, I attended a nutritional conference that focused on environmental toxins, and one of the presenters mentioned that many of his patients who have problems with conventional wheat don't seem to have a problem with einkorn (ancient) wheat. He also mentioned that many of his patients tolerate organic barley.

However, you also need to remember that the lack of symptoms doesn't necessarily mean these foods aren't having a negative effect on intestinal permeability in some people, which makes it difficult to know if someone can safely reintroduce these foods. Thus, there is always a risk with reintroducing gluten, regardless if it is organic and/or you have healed your gut, improved the health of your lymphatic system, etc. Some people are willing to take this risk and might do fine, while others might not do well and perhaps even suffer a relapse.

Is Changing Your Diet Enough?

Of course, it is important to modify your diet and try to eat foods that aren't genetically modified, but is doing this enough to reverse the potential damage caused by GMOs? It depends on the person, as sometimes just changing one's diet alone is sufficient. Numerous stories exist of adults and children who had different health issues that were resolved just by eliminating GMOs from their diet. In some cases, their health condition wasn't completely resolved, but the person's symptoms significantly improved.

However, if consuming genetically modified foods caused problems with the gut flora or the lining of the intestines, then, many times, just stopping the consumption of GMOs won't be sufficient. Thus, while changing one's diet is important, if significant damage has been done, then some additional support might be required.

What You Can Do to Minimize Your Exposure To GMOs and Glyphosate?

Although you probably have a pretty good idea on how to reduce your exposure to GMOs and glyphosate, to make it easier I'll include a brief summary:

- **Eat only certified organic foods.** If you do this, then you will greatly reduce your exposure to GMOs and glyphosate.

- **If you don't eat organic, avoid the genetically modified foods I discussed earlier.** I realize that not everyone can eat 100% organic, and I'd be lying if I told you that I eat a 100% organic diet. However, when not eating organic try your best to avoid the genetically modified foods I mentioned earlier.

- **Be aware that non-organic meat will most likely consist of GMOs.** The reason for this is because many of these animals will be fed genetically modified corn and soy. This is why it's best to try to eat organic meat whenever you can.

- **Consider testing your drinking water for glyphosate.** Even if you eat a 100% organic diet, there is a chance that your drinking water has glyphosate. If you have a water filter, it still might be a good idea to test the filter to ensure that it is doing a good job of filtering out the glyphosate.

- **If you don't eat mostly organic, or if you live in an agricultural area, then consider doing a urinary test for glyphosate.** The main advantage of this is getting a baseline reading, and if the test reveals very high levels of glyphosate, then this might help encourage you to eat more organic foods and/or detoxify glyphosate from your body.

- **Detoxify glyphosate from your body.** Dr. Stephanie Seneff is a senior research scientist who is a well-known expert on glyphosate. She mentions a paper that shows how the application of charcoal, sauerkraut juice and humic acids in feed of cows can result in a significant reduction of glyphosate.[501] Some suggest that infrared sauna can help with the excretion of glyphosate, although I wasn't able to come across any studies which demonstrated this.

Chapter Highlights:

- Some of the genetically modified foods include corn, soybeans, canola oil, cottonseed oil, papaya, alfalfa, sugar beet, squash, and white potatoes.
- Foods that are genetically modified have changes made to the DNA, which leads to crops that are resistant to herbicides as well as crops that are actually able to produce their own pesticides to kill organisms.
- Diet is the primary way that we are exposed to genetically modified foods.
- When you genetically modify corn, soy, or other foods, this will change the DNA, and the immune system sees the proteins in these foods as being foreign.
- Glyphosate is the active ingredient in the herbicide Roundup and can be a big factor in the increased prevalence of chronic health conditions, including autoimmune conditions such as Hashimoto's.
- Glyphosate disrupts something called the shikimate pathway, and, while humans don't have this pathway, the bacteria present in our body have this pathway. This is how glyphosate can cause intestinal dysbiosis.
- Glyphosate is a chelating agent and, as a result, can lead to nutrient deficiencies.
- Some non-GMO crops (i.e., wheat) are sprayed with glyphosate right before they are harvested, and some speculate that many people don't necessary have a problem with gluten, but, instead, have a problem with wheat and other grains due to the glyphosate.
- In order to minimize your exposure to GMOs and glyphosate you want to 1) eat only certified organic foods, 2) be aware that non-organic meat will most likely consist of GMOs, 3) consider testing your water for glyphosate, and 4) detoxify glyphosate from your body.

CHAPTER 21

SMALL INTESTINAL
BACTERIAL OVERGROWTH

S MALL INTESTINAL BACTERIAL OVERGROWTH, also known as SIBO, can lead to symptoms such as bloating, gas, and abdominal pain, along with diarrhea and/or constipation. Over the last few years, I have seen more and more cases of SIBO in my patients with Hashimoto's. However, can SIBO be an autoimmune trigger?

Different pathogens have been associated with thyroid autoimmunity. These include H. pylori, Yersinia enterocolitica, Lyme disease, Epstein-Barr, and Blastocystis hominis. Of course, I have discussed all of these in Chapter 9. However, it's important to understand that SIBO isn't a pathogenic infection. This condition involves having good bacteria in the wrong place, as most of the bacteria should be located in the large intestine, and only a small amount of bacteria should be located in the small intestine. However, for numerous reasons, an overgrowth of bacteria can occur in the small intestine.

SIBO itself doesn't seem to be a direct trigger of Hashimoto's. However, some cases of SIBO are a result of an autoimmune process, and having one autoimmune condition can make someone more susceptible to having another autoimmune condition. So perhaps having SIBO can lead to another autoimmune condition such as Hashimoto's, but the connection hasn't been made yet. However, even if this isn't the case, SIBO can cause a leaky gut, which, in turn, can set the stage for the development of an autoimmune thyroid condition.

4 Potential Causes of SIBO

Four different factors can cause someone to develop SIBO:

1. Dysfunction of the migrating motor complex (MMC). This is the main reason why people develop SIBO. The MMC is a small wave that cleanses the small intestine of debris. If the MMC isn't working properly, then bacteria and other debris are no longer swept through the lumen of the small intestine, which can lead to SIBO.[502,503] Food poisoning is the most common cause of a dysfunctional MMC, but other causes include hypothyroidism, diabetes, or an infection such as C. difficile, giardia, or Lyme disease. Certain drugs such as opiates and antibiotics can also affect the MMC.

2. Altered anatomy. This can interfere with the clearance of bacteria. For example, adhesions due to surgery or endometriosis are potential causes of SIBO. Other anatomical anomalies include a narrowing of the small intestine, fistulas, and diverticuli.

3. Hypochlorhydria (low stomach acid). Millions of people take acid blockers, which is a huge problem. Besides being necessary to break down nutrients, stomach acid also can help to eradicate harmful pathogens, and prevent the overgrowth of bacteria. However, you don't need to take acid blockers to have low stomach acid, as having a hypothyroid condition alone can decrease production of stomach acid. Stress can also decrease the production of stomach acid.

4. Absent or inefficient Ileocecal valve. The ileocecal valve is the barrier that separates the small intestine from the large intestine. It prevents backflow from the large intestine into the small intestine. If this is absent or dysfunctional, it can cause the bacteria from the large intestine to migrate into the small intestine, thus leading to SIBO.

The Relationship Between IBS and SIBO

Infectious gastroenteritis, more commonly known as food poisoning, can result in the production of toxins by bacteria that can damage the nerves that play an important role in gut motility. The specific name of the toxin is cytolethal distending toxin (CDT). The immune system forms antibodies to this toxin (called anti-CDTb antibodies), but anti-vinculin antibodies are also produced.[504] Vinculin is a protein that helps connect the interstitial cells of Cajal (ICC) so that they can communicate properly to help the MMC. The CDT toxins harm the ICC, and, in a case of mistaken identity, the immune system attacks vinculin, which has a negative effect on gut motility.

To summarize, food poisoning is the most common cause of irritable bowel syndrome with diarrhea (IBS-D). The food poisoning causes an autoimmune process involving anti-vinculin antibodies, which has a negative effect on gut motility, and the problem with gut motility leads to SIBO. In the past, a blood test called IBSchek by Commonwealth Laboratories determined if someone had IBS-D associated with anti-CDTb and anti-vinculin antibodies. Unfortunately, Commonwealth Laboratories went out of business in 2017, but a few other labs offer similar testing, including Quest Diagnostics and Cyrex Labs.

How Is SIBO Diagnosed?

Although one's symptoms can provide a lot of valuable information, if SIBO is suspected, then one should do a breath test that measures hydrogen and methane. I discuss this in greater detail in Chapter 25. I will say here that the breath test is looking for bacterial fermentation, and it determines this fermentation by measuring the levels of hydrogen and methane. In other words, if someone has SIBO, there will be more fermentation, which will lead to higher levels of hydrogen, methane, or both gases.

Other Health Conditions Are Associated With SIBO

Here are some other health conditions associated with SIBO:

- Acne Rosacea
- Chronic fatigue syndrome
- Fibromyalgia
- Gastroesophageal Reflux Disease (GERD)
- Inflammatory bowel disease (Crohn's disease, ulcerative colitis)
- Interstitial Cystitis
- Pancreatitis
- Restless legs syndrome
- Rheumatoid arthritis
- Scleroderma

Dietary Options for SIBO

Although I prefer that most of my patients with Hashimoto's start on an autoimmune Paleo (AIP) diet, no diet fits everyone perfectly. The same concept applies with SIBO. While all cases of SIBO involve the overgrowth of bacteria in the small intestine, the bacteria will differ from person to person. Thus, one person with SIBO might be able to tolerate foods that someone else with SIBO can't tolerate, and vice versa.

In addition, some people might be able to eat small quantities of a certain food, but if they eat larger quantities, they experience bloating and gas. However, there are certain diets people with SIBO should consider following, although there will be some modifications depending on the person.

I'm going to discuss the different diets that are recommended for patients with SIBO. The primary goal of each of these diets is to feed the person while starving the bacteria.

Low FODMAP diet. FODMAP stands for fermentable oligosaccharides, disaccharides, monosaccharides, and polyols. Examples of high FODMAP foods include fermented foods (i.e., sauerkraut), starch (grains, beans, starchy vegetables), soluble fiber (grains, beans, fruits, vegetables), sugar (fruit, agave), and resistant starch (legumes, whole grains).

This doesn't mean that everyone with SIBO needs to avoid all of these foods. For example, some people with SIBO are able to tolerate sauerkraut, while others can't eat any fermented foods without experiencing gas, bloating, and other symptoms. Some people are able to eat small amounts of these foods, while others are unable to tolerate certain foods altogether. Thus, you need to listen to your body.

Specific Carbohydrate Diet. The Specific Carbohydrate Diet (SCD) is similar to a Paleo diet in that it allows meat, fish, eggs, nuts, seeds, vegetables, and fruit. It differs in that it does allow some lactose-free dairy and certain beans. The dairy products that are allowed include yogurt, aged cow and goat cheeses, butter, ghee, and cottage cheese. The allowed beans include white beans, navy beans, lentils, split peas, lima beans, kidney beans and black beans. In order to make the beans easier to digest, you soak them overnight.

GAPS diet. GAPS stands for Gut and Psychology Syndrome, and the diet was developed by Dr. Natasha Campbell-McBride. The diet is very similar to the Specific Carbohydrate Diet, and involves minimal supplementation. The only legumes allowed on the GAPS diet include lentils, split peas, and white navy beans, and they need to be soaked first.

Dairy is initially eliminated, but the person is then allowed to slowly reintroduce ghee, followed by butter, yogurt, sour cream, kefir, hard cheese, and cream. One of the main differences between the GAPS diet and the Specific Carbohydrate Diet is that the GAPS diet involves going through a 6-stage introduction diet before moving onto the "full" GAPS protocol, which is usually followed for one or two years.

SIBO Specific Diet. This diet, created by Dr. Allison Siebecker, is a combination of the Specific Carbohydrate Diet and the low FODMAP diet. While it's a great diet for those who have SIBO, it's important to understand that this is a very restrictive diet, so you can always try one or more of the other diets first. If you don't do well with the other diets, then you might want to consider trying this diet. For more information, I would visit **www.siboinfo.com/diet**.

SIBO Bi-Phasic Diet. This is a protocol put together by Dr. Nirala Jacobi, and is based on the SIBO Specific Food Guide created by Dr. Allison Siebecker. This uses a phased approach to the diet and treatment for SIBO patients, and, according to Dr. Jacobi, it helps to limit side effects associated with die-off. In addition, this diet focuses on gut healing prior to having the patient take antimicrobials, which is the opposite of the "5-R Protocol," which I'll discuss in Chapter 28.

The first phase focuses on reducing foods that feed the bacteria (fermentable starches and fiber), and repairing the gut while doing things to improve digestive health. Phase 2 then focuses on using antimicrobials to remove the remaining bacteria and fungi from the small intestines, while restoring the motility of the small intestines, usually by giving the person a prokinetic. I'll discuss prokinetics in Chapter 33.

Elemental diet. Although this is referred to as a "diet," it is also considered to be an antimicrobial treatment. Thus, I'll discuss the elemental diet in Chapter 33." In that chapter, I'll discuss treating not only SIBO, but also Lyme disease and toxic mold.

Should Someone With Hashimoto's Also Follow an AIP Diet?

Many people with Hashimoto's follow an AIP diet, and they might want to know if they should continue following an AIP diet when trying to address SIBO. So for example, should they follow an AIP diet and at the same time follow a specific diet for SIBO? Doing this is extremely difficult, and what you usually want to do is prioritize the eradication of SIBO.

In other words, it's usually okay to stray from the AIP diet while trying to address SIBO, which falls into the "Remove" category of the 5-R protocol. Then once the bacterial overgrowth has been "removed" you can focus more on gut healing by following the AIP diet, along with eating gut-healing foods and taking certain nutrients. I'll discuss the 5-R protocol in greater detail in Chapter 28.

Conventional and Natural Treatment Options for SIBO

In section four, I'll discuss both conventional and natural treatment options for eradicating SIBO. In this chapter, I briefly mentioned the elemental diet, which can be a very effective treatment option for SIBO, although most people prefer to follow one of the other two options, which are prescription antibiotics and natural antimicrobials. In Chapter 33, I'll discuss the pros and cons of both conventional and natural treatment options.

What Is SIFO?

Whereas SIBO is *small intestinal bacterial overgrowth*, SIFO stands for *small intestinal fungal overgrowth*, and is characterized by the presence of an excessive number of fungal organisms in the small intestine associated with gastrointestinal symptoms.[505] The most common symptoms associated with SIFO include belching, bloating, indigestion, nausea, diarrhea, and gas.[505] Two recent studies showed that approximately one quarter of patients with unexplained GI symptoms had SIFO.[505] Keep in mind that someone with SIFO can also have extra-intestinal symptoms such as fatigue, joint pain, brain fog, headaches, and other symptoms that can improve with treatment.

How can one differentiate SIBO from SIFO? Although there is no diagnostic test currently available that evaluates for SIFO, if someone has symptoms similar to SIBO but has a negative breath test, then this can be suggestive of SIFO. Or if someone with a confirmed or suspected case of SIBO doesn't respond to treatment, then SIFO should be suspected. This is especially true if the person took Rifaximin and didn't respond.

Of course, when this is the case, there is always the chance that a second round of treatment with the antibiotics is necessary, or perhaps a different treatment approach (i.e., natural antimicrobials) is warranted. But there is also a chance that the person has SIFO, and not SIBO.

Can Treating SIBO Help Reverse Hashimoto's?

SIBO doesn't seem to be a direct trigger of Hashimoto's. However, SIBO can cause an increase in intestinal permeability. Because of this, if someone has SIBO and a leaky gut, then in order to heal the gut, it is necessary to get rid of SIBO, and, if the trigger is also removed, then this can put the person into remission. Thus, while eradicating SIBO might be necessary for healing a leaky gut, in order to get someone with an autoimmune thyroid condition into remission, it is still necessary to find and remove the trigger.

SIBO Case Study

Sarah was experiencing a lot of gas and bloating, especially after eating certain foods. She worked with a couple of different natural health-care professionals prior to consulting with me, and while following an AIP diet for her Hashimoto's condition helped with some of her symptoms, it didn't do much for her digestive symptoms, and on top of the gas and bloating, she started getting some bouts of pain. Before working with me she was diagnosed with H. pylori. She took antibiotics to eradicate the H. pylori, but this didn't help with her digestive symptoms. Based on her symptoms, during our initial consultation I suggested for Sarah to get a lactulose breath test, and sure enough she tested positive for small intestinal bacterial overgrowth. She chose to take the antibiotic Rifaximin, and it seemed to work well initially, although eventually its effectiveness diminished, and so she switched to an herbal protocol. After a few additional months her symptoms greatly improved, and eventually resolved, and I then put her on a prokinetic. This in itself was great news, but even better news was that this seemed to put her on the road to recovery, and eventually she was able to achieve a state of remission with her Hashimoto's condition. While I'm not 100% certain that the H. pylori that was previously eradicated was an autoimmune trigger, it does seem likely, but either way it's clear that the SIBO was a leaky gut trigger that needed to be addressed before she was able to achieve a state of remission.

Chapter Highlights:

- Although SIBO itself doesn't seem to be an autoimmune trigger, some cases of SIBO are a result of an autoimmune process, and SIBO can cause a leaky gut, which is a factor in thyroid autoimmunity.
- Four potential causes of SIBO include 1) dysfunction of the migrating motor complex, 2) altered anatomy, 3) low stomach acid, and 4) an absent or inefficient ileocecal valve.
- Many people with irritable bowel syndrome will develop SIBO.
- SIBO is detected through either a lactulose or glucose breath test.
- Some other health conditions associated with SIBO include acne rosacea, chronic fatigue syndrome, fibromyalgia, inflammatory bowel disease, interstitial cystitis, restless legs syndrome, and rheumatoid arthritis.
- The different diets that can benefit people with SIBO include the low FODMAP diet, the specific carbohydrate diet, the GAPS diet, the SIBO Specific Diet, the SIBO Bi-Phasic diet, and the elemental diet.
- Prescription antibiotics, herbal antimicrobials, and the elemental diet can help with the eradication of SIBO.
- SIFO stands for small intestinal fungal overgrowth, and it is characterized by the presence of excessive number of fungal organisms in the small intestine associated with gastrointestinal symptoms.

• SECTION THREE

DETECTING YOUR SPECIFIC TRIGGERS

I N THIS SECTION, I will show you what you need to do in order to find your specific triggers. Chapter 22 will show you how to detect triggers through a thorough health history. Chapter 23 will help you find your specific food triggers. I dedicated Chapter 24 to the most important blood tests, including the optimal reference ranges. In Chapter 25, I will talk about all of the different "alternative" tests available, including saliva testing, stool panels, leaky gut testing, organic acids, etc.

However, the goal isn't just to list all of the different tests that are available, as when I put these chapters together I wanted to help you understand which tests you should consider getting to find your specific triggers. And while I do recommend testing to my patients, you can use other methods to assist in detecting your specific triggers. For example, in Chapter 22, I show you how digging into your history can sometimes help to identify your triggers. And Chapter 23 also doesn't rely on testing.

Where Can You Get The Recommended Tests?

With regards to the blood tests I discuss, you probably will need to visit a local lab to get the blood drawn. In most cases, you will need a lab order from your doctor, although most of states allow patients to order their own blood tests. There are both walk-in labs and online ordering options available. For more information, visit **www.naturalendocrinesolutions. com/testing**.

If you need an ultrasound, you will need to visit an imaging center for this, along with an order from a doctor.

As for "alternative" testing options such as saliva testing, comprehensive stool panels, and other tests, most conventional medical doctors and endocrinologists don't order these tests. However, it still doesn't hurt to ask your primary care physician (if you have one), as there is a small percentage of medical doctors who will order some of these alternative tests. Chiropractors, naturopaths, and holistic medical doctors are more likely to order these for you. If you are unable to find a doctor who will order these tests for you, please visit **www.naturalendocrinesolutions.com/testing**.

CHAPTER 22

DETECTING YOUR TRIGGERS THROUGH A COMPREHENSIVE HEALTH HISTORY

WHEN IT COMES TO trying to find out the cause of your Hashimoto's condition, testing can play a very important role. This is why I recommend testing to just about all of my patients. However, one shouldn't underestimate the importance of a comprehensive health history. While, many times, doing a thorough health history alone won't identify your autoimmune triggers, it can still provide some important clues.

In this chapter, I'll discuss some of the more important components of a health history. While I hope that most people reading this are working with a natural healthcare professional who will conduct a thorough health history, if this isn't the case, I would go through each of these components on your own. Regardless of whether or not you are working with an expert, I think it's a good idea to read this information, as doing so might help to identify certain triggers. Another benefit of a thorough health history is that it can help determine which tests are required to find certain imbalances that are either directly or indirectly responsible for your condition.

It's also important to understand that completing a thorough health history might require you to fill out multiple forms. It depends on the healthcare professional you're working with, as some doctors will have all of the information on a single form, while others will require multiple forms to be completed. Some offices will allow you to fill out all of the patient information electronically, while this won't be the case for others.

Components of a Comprehensive Health History

Let's go ahead and look at the more common components included in a health history:

Lifestyle factors. This is one of the main reasons that more and more people are developing autoimmune conditions such as Hashimoto's, and I have discussed most of these factors in this section. Here are some of the more common lifestyle factors that can either directly trigger Hashimoto's, or make someone more susceptible to developing this condition:

- Common allergens (gluten, dairy, etc.)
- High amounts of stress
- Low stress handling skills
- Drinking alcohol regularly
- Eating a lot of sugar
- Overtraining
- Insufficient sleep

Medications and supplements. Certain medications such as antibiotics, NSAIDs, and acid-blockers can make someone more susceptible to developing Hashimoto's by having a negative effect on the health of the gut. While most nutritional supplements and herbs won't trigger or exacerbate Hashimoto's, there are possible exceptions. For example, some natural healthcare professionals recommend that people with Hashimoto's avoid Echinacea out of fear that this herb will further stimulate the immune system, thus exacerbating the autoimmune response.

However, some healthcare professionals regularly give their patients with Hashimoto's Echinacea without a problem. I can't say that I commonly recommend Echinacea to my patients with Hashimoto's, but, over the years, I have had some patients take this herb, and I can't say that I've seen it exacerbate someone's condition, but, of course, everyone is different. In 2014, I released a blog post entitled "Echinacea: Harmful for Hashimoto's, Beneficial for Graves' disease?," and if you visit my website and check out the comments from this post you'll see mixed results, as a few people found Echinacea to be beneficial, while others thought that it might have worsened their condition.

Past procedures and surgeries. While most medical procedures and surgeries won't trigger Hashimoto's, certain procedures may make someone more susceptible to developing this condition. For example, while there is a concern over estrogen dominance, estrogen also has a protective effect on immune system health. While I didn't find any evidence of a correlation between getting a hysterectomy and developing Hashimoto's, there is evidence that a hysterectomy can be a factor in other autoimmune conditions, such as systemic lupus erythematosus.[1]

Other surgical procedures might also increase the risk of autoimmunity, such as bariatric surgery.[2] Keep in mind that I'm not suggesting that women should never get a hysterectomy, as there is a time and place for these and other surgical procedures. I think it's safe to say that most of the time these and other medical procedures won't trigger Hashimoto's, but it's still a factor we need to consider when gathering information.

Infections (current and past). Certain infections can play a role in the development of Hashimoto's. Thus, it's good to know if someone with Hashimoto's had a previous infection. Of course, just because someone had a previous infection prior to developing Hashimoto's doesn't mean that the infection was the trigger. However, it still can be beneficial to know if someone had an infection.

Family history. Although genetics isn't the most important factor in the development of an autoimmune condition, it is a factor. While you can't change your genes, I still think it is beneficial to find out if there is a family history of a thyroid or autoimmune thyroid condition in someone who has Hashimoto's. Although the natural treatment approach might not differ much for someone who does have a strong family history of thyroid autoimmunity, if a person with Hashimoto's has multiple family members with this condition, then they might want to be a little more strict with the diet and other lifestyle factors not only while restoring their health but also while trying to maintain a state of wellness. It also is worth finding out if there is a family history of an autoimmune condition other than Hashimoto's.

Signs and Symptoms. While you can't rely on signs and symptoms for detecting the autoimmune trigger, this doesn't mean that your signs and symptoms should be ignored. For example, many people with Hashimoto's are overweight, but some people with this condition have the opposite problem and have difficulty gaining weight. If this is the case, then one possible cause is a malabsorption problem, which, in turn, can be due to a pathogenic infection, or a condition such as small intestinal bacterial overgrowth. If someone has extreme fatigue, along with migrating muscle and joint pain, then Lyme disease might be the culprit; thus, this is another example where paying attention to symptoms can be important.

Of course, certain symptoms can have multiple causes. For example, if someone with Hashimoto's has extreme fatigue, this can be due to low thyroid hormone levels, adrenal problems, one or more nutrient deficiencies, a pathogenic infection, or even blood sugar imbalances. While testing might be necessary to determine the cause of the fatigue, asking the right questions can also help.

Here are some of the signs and symptoms people with Hashimoto's commonly have:

- Trouble concentrating/memory difficulties/brain fog
- Fatigue
- Cold hands and feet
- Weight gain
- Bloating/belching/gas
- Constipation
- Hair loss
- Lowered libido
- Hot flashes and/or night sweats

These are other signs and symptoms some people with Hashimoto's can experience:

- Sweet cravings
- Caffeine cravings
- Headaches/migraines
- Muscle pain/joint aches
- Bloating/belching/gas
- Stomach burning
- Dry eyes and/or dry skin
- Increased frequency of food reactions
- Intolerance to smells

- Multiple smell and chemical sensitivities
- Indigestion and fullness lasting 2-4 hours after eating
- Sense of fullness during and after meals
- Coated tongue
- Dizziness when standing up quickly

Exposure to Environmental Toxins. We live in a toxic world, and most people are exposed to hundreds, if not thousands of different chemicals regularly. Because of this, if an environmental toxin is the trigger, then many times it can be challenging to find out what the triggering chemical is. While you can spend money to test for certain environmental toxins, including heavy metals, as well as other chemicals, you can't test for all of the chemicals you're exposed to. Thus, rather than spend a lot of money testing for environmental toxins, sometimes, the best approach is to 1) minimize your exposure to environmental toxins, and 2) take measures to eliminate chemicals from your body.

However, sometimes, you can find out valuable information about environmental toxins during a thorough health history. For example, mercury is a potential trigger of Hashimoto's. Thus, a natural healthcare professional who conducts a health history should find out if their patients with Hashimoto's have mercury amalgams. The presence of these amalgams doesn't mean that mercury is the trigger, although there is a possibility that this is the case.

Recently, I had a patient who had very high cadmium levels. Upon further investigation, the patient told me that his work environment involves exposure to certain chemicals, and cadmium was one of them. While I haven't seen a correlation in the literature between cadmium and Hashimoto's, this doesn't mean that high cadmium levels can't be a factor. For example, even if a certain environmental toxin isn't a direct trigger of Hashimoto's, this doesn't mean that it can't indirectly cause autoimmunity by compromising the immune system (i.e., causing a decrease in regulatory T cells).

The truth is that we don't know everything about environmental toxins and autoimmunity. Thus, when conducting a health history, it's foolish to just focus on the environmental toxins that have been proven to trigger autoimmune thyroid conditions. Keep in mind that being exposed to many environmental toxins can result in a loss of chemical tolerance, which, in turn, can make someone more susceptible to developing an autoimmune thyroid condition.

When conducting a health history, I recommend asking the patient the following questions about environmental toxins (or you can ask yourself if you are conducting your own health history):

- Do you eat conventionally grown fruits and vegetables regularly?
- Do you eat conventionally raised animal products regularly?
- Do you eat fish or seafood frequently?
- Do you eat foods with artificial colors, flavors, and/or preservatives regularly?
- Do you frequently use conventional cleaning chemicals, hand sanitizers, air fresheners, and other scented products?
- Do you smoke or are you often exposed to second-hand smoke?
- Do you have mercury amalgams, root canals, crowns, dental implants, etc.?
- Do you have a history of heavy alcohol use?
- Do you have a history of heavy use of recreational or prescription drugs?
- Have you been exposed to new construction materials or furniture?
- Are you frequently exposed to adhesives, paints, solvents, and other air-borne chemicals?
- Do you live near a cell phone tower or high-voltage power lines?
- Have you been frequently exposed to herbicides, pesticides, and/or fungicides?
- Do you jog or ride your bike along busy streets?

Sex hormones/Reproductive health history. Sex hormone imbalances can be a factor in Hashimoto's, and here is some of the information I ask for on my health history forms:

- Do you currently take, or have you taken oral contraceptives or bioidentical hormones?
- Do you currently take, or have you had an intrauterine device (IUD)? If you answered "yes," was it a copper or hormonal IUD?
- How many live births have you had?
- Were they natural births or Cesarean sections?
- Is there a history of ovarian cysts?
- Is there a history of uterine fibroids?
- Is there a history of endometriosis?
- Is there a history of fibrocystic breasts?

Estrogen dominance can be a trigger of Hashimoto's, and estrogen dominance is also a common factor with ovarian cysts, uterine fibroids, endometriosis, and fibrocystic breasts. Thus, if someone checks off one of these, I will suspect problems with estrogen metabolism. This is also one way to determine if testing of the sex hormones is necessary. For example, if a cycling woman has irregular menstrual cycles, moderate to severe cramping, and a history of ovarian cysts, uterine fibroids, and/or endometriosis, then one can argue that testing the sex hormones might be necessary in this situation.

Consider Completing a Food Diary

I find that putting together a food diary can be valuable. After all, certain foods can act as triggers, or can make someone more susceptible to Hashimoto's by increasing the permeability of the gut. I would recommend putting together at least a one-week food diary because a person's eating habits can vary depending on the day of the week. For example, many people eat well Monday through Friday but indulge on the weekend.

When putting together your food diary, it's also a good idea to list not only the foods you eat, along with any beverages you drink but also the timing of any symptoms you experience. For example, if you experience gas and stomach pain, put this on the food diary, as you might be able to make a correlation between certain foods you eat and the symptoms you're having, although this admittedly can be challenging if you have a delayed food sensitivity, which I discuss in Chapter 23.

Chapter Highlights:

- While many times doing a thorough health history alone won't identify the autoimmune trigger, it can still provide some important clues.
- A good health history can help to determine which tests are necessary to obtain, as well as what diet you should follow, supplements you should take, etc.
- Common components of a comprehensive health history include lifestyle factors, medications and supplements, past procedures and surgeries, infections, family history, signs and symptoms, exposure to environmental toxins, and reproductive health history.
- In addition to completing a health history, putting together a food diary can be valuable.
- If you choose not to work with a healthcare professional, I would recommend that you conduct your own health history.

CHAPTER 23

DETECTING FOOD TRIGGERS

A S YOU LEARNED IN section two, certain foods can be a potential trigger of Hashimoto's. Accordingly, I have most of my patients follow an elimination diet initially. Alternatively, some healthcare professionals have all of their patients do food sensitivity testing to see what specific foods they are reacting to. Both of these procedures have benefits and limitations, and in this chapter, I'll discuss the pros and cons of each so that you can better make an informed decision.

Before comparing the elimination diet with food sensitivity testing, I'll discuss how food can cause autoimmunity in the first place. Certain foods, such as gluten, can lead to autoimmunity by causing an increase in proinflammatory cytokines and a decrease in regulatory T cells.[3,4,5] Molecular mimicry can also play a role, and certain food allergens can result in a decrease in oral tolerance. This, in turn, triggers an immune system response against various components of food proteins, and cross-reaction with B-cell molecules may trigger autoimmunity.[3] In other words, eating certain foods will result in the immune system attacking the food proteins, and, in the case of mistaken identity, the immune system can also attack body tissues with a similar amino acid sequence.

In addition to causing an increase in proinflammatory cytokines or resulting in a molecular mimicry mechanism, certain food allergens can also cause an increase in intestinal permeability, which is synonymous with a leaky gut. According to the triad of autoimmunity, a leaky gut is one of three factors required for the development of an autoimmune condition. It can also lead to food sensitivities through a loss of oral tolerance.

What Are The Most Common Allergens?

While it is possible to have a sensitivity to any food, the following are the most common allergens:

- Gluten
- Dairy
- Corn
- Eggs
- Soy
- Shellfish
- Peanuts

In addition, the following foods are commonly problematic in some people:

- Beef
- Pork
- Coffee
- Tea
- Citrus fruits
- Chocolate

The Elimination Diet vs. the Autoimmune Paleo Diet

Just as a reminder, the autoimmune Paleo (AIP) diet is similar to a standard Paleo diet, but also requires people to avoid eggs, the nightshades, nuts, and seeds. The primary reason why these and other foods such as grains and legumes are excluded is because they have compounds that can potentially increase intestinal permeability and/or interfere with healing of the gut. However, the AIP diet also serves as an elimination diet, as you would essentially be eliminating the most common allergens, although some healthcare professionals do allow their patients to eat shellfish because, while shellfish is considered to be a common allergen, shellfish is AIP-friendly.

The Benefits of an Elimination Diet

There are a few reasons why I like to have my patients do an elimination diet initially. First, I find that many patients can identify their food triggers if they follow this type of diet carefully. Essentially, you want to follow a strict AIP diet for a minimum of 30 days, and then after 30 days, you can choose to reintroduce certain foods one at a time, every three days, and pay close attention to symptoms.

Another benefit of the elimination/reintroduction diet is that it is more cost effective than doing food sensitivity testing. Testing for food allergens can be expensive, which would be fine if the information provided was completely accurate. However, as you'll read shortly, food sensitivity testing is far from perfect.

The Flaws of an Elimination Diet

Although I start most of my patients with Hashimoto's on an elimination diet, this admittedly does have certain limitations. First, while many people are able to identify foods they are sensitive to, this isn't always the case. For example, someone who follows an elimination diet and reintroduces a certain food might experience obvious symptoms, such as bloating and gas, headaches, an increase in fatigue, brain fog, or other symptoms. However, some people don't experience any symptoms upon reintroducing foods, and the lack of symptoms doesn't always rule out a food sensitivity.

I will add that most people will notice symptoms upon reintroducing foods they are sensitive to if they pay close attention. Many times, people are only focusing on digestive symptoms, but other symptoms can develop as well. How do you know if a specific symptom is related to the food you introduced? For example, if someone reintroduces eggs, and they experience headaches, how do they know if the headaches were caused by the eggs?

Perhaps it was a coincidence and the person might have experienced the headaches regardless. This admittedly can be challenging, but in a situation where you are unsure if the symptom experienced was a result of the food that was reintroduced, what you would want to do is take a break from that food for a few additional weeks, and then you can try reintroducing the food again. If you experience the same symptom, then you can almost be certain that the food is responsible for that specific symptom.

Another limitation of an elimination/reintroduction diet is that it is possible for someone to be sensitive to one or more of the "allowed" foods. For example, someone can be sensitive to AIP-friendly foods such as broccoli, asparagus, avocados, chicken, blueberries, and other foods that are not part of an elimination diet. This, admittedly, can be a major limitation of the elimination diet, and it is a good argument for doing food sensitivity testing.

How to Reintroduce Foods

After someone has gone on an elimination diet for 30 days, the next step is to consider the reintroduction of foods. Before I discuss this, I will add that some people with Hashimoto's will thrive on a strict AIP diet, and if this is the case with you, then please feel free to stick with it for a longer period. For example, if you are experiencing an improvement in your symptoms upon following the diet, and if following a restrictive diet isn't stressful, then it makes sense to continue with the diet for a few additional months. However, it's common for people to struggle when following this diet, and many people are ready to reintroduce foods after 30 days.

How should you go about reintroducing foods? Well, you always want to reintroduce one new food at a time. The obvious reason is because if you were to reintroduce more than one food simultaneously and then experienced a negative reaction, you wouldn't know which food was responsible.

You also want to eat the food you reintroduce a couple of times on the same day, starting with a smaller serving the first time, and then you should eat a full serving the second time. You then should wait at least an additional two days before reintroducing the next food because it is possible to have a delayed reaction to a food. If all goes well when reintroducing a certain food, then you can continue eating that food regularly and can reintroduce the next food.

For example, let's say you followed the elimination diet for 30 days. On day #31, you decide to reintroduce egg yolks, and have half of a scrambled egg yolk for breakfast and an entire egg yolk with lunch. If by the end of day #33 (the third day after reintroducing the food) you experience no negative symptoms, then on day #34 you can reintroduce a new food. However, if you did experience a negative reaction to the eggs, then you would wait until the symptoms subsided before reintroducing the next food.

Which Foods Should You Reintroduce First?

While some healthcare professionals will recommend reintroducing foods in a specific order, others don't think this is necessary. I fall somewhere in between, as, while I would never have someone initially reintroduce foods that have dairy and gluten, I don't have a specific order of foods that I have my patients reintroduce. One of the main reasons for this is because not everyone likes the same foods. For example, I commonly recommend that my patients first reintroduce egg yolks, but some people don't like eggs, and if someone is a vegan, this also wouldn't be an ideal first food to reintroduce.

What I usually do is ask my patients the following question when they are ready to reintroduce foods: "If you had to choose 3 to 5 foods to reintroduce, which ones would you choose?" Some of the common responses include foods such as eggs, nuts and seeds, dark chocolate, and nightshade vegetables. Others want to know if they can reintroduce legumes and gluten free grains.

For those looking for a specific order of foods to reintroduce, Sarah Ballantyne has put together a very helpful PDF entitled "The Paleo Approach Quick-Start Guide to Reintroducing Foods." You can easily find this upon doing a Google search, although I'll also include a link on my resources page (**www.naturalendocrinesolutions.com/resources**). Once you get this list, you will see that Sarah Ballantyne separates the foods into four different stages. Ideally, you would want to start with the foods in stage #1, and this is the order she has them listed:

- Egg yolks
- Legumes with edible pods
- Fruit- and berry-based spices
- Seed-based spices
- Seed and nut oils
- Ghee from grass-fed dairy

I can't say I have all of my patients with Hashimoto's follow this list strictly. For example, I usually recommend for my patients to reintroduce nuts and seeds before legumes. Also, while Sarah Ballantyne doesn't recommend for nightshades to be reintroduced until Stage #3, some of my patients reintroduce nightshades sooner than later. Now to be fair, on her reintroduction handout she does mention that there is no right or wrong way to choose what foods to reintroduce first. Her suggested order is based on the likelihood that someone will react to a certain food, along with the inherent nutritional value of the food.

Symptoms You Might Experience When Reintroducing Foods

If all goes well, then you won't experience a negative reaction when reintroducing a specific food. However, if you do have a negative reaction then you want to look out for symptoms such as bloating, gas, abdominal discomfort, headaches, fatigue, muscle or joint pain, insomnia, skin problems, sinus congestion, etc. One question you might have is, "If I experience a specific symptom, how do I know for certain it's related to the food I reintroduced?"

For example, if you reintroduce a new food and shortly thereafter, you experienced severe gas and bloating, then there is a good chance that these symptoms were related to the food. However, if you experienced a headache or an increase in fatigue, then these symptoms might be related to the food, but there is also a chance that they weren't related.

If you're not certain if a symptom is related to the food being reintroduced, then I would recommend stop eating the food for a few weeks and then reintroducing it again in the future. If you do this and experience the same symptoms again, then chances are the specific food is responsible for the symptoms.

Using Food Sensitivity Testing To Detect Food Triggers

Now that I have discussed the elimination diet in detail, along with how to reintroduce foods, I'd like to go ahead and discuss food sensitivity testing. I'll first explain the pros and cons of such testing, and then I'll discuss the different methods used to detect food allergens.

The Benefits of Food Sensitivity Testing

One of the main benefits of food sensitivity testing is that it has the potential to identify specific foods you are reacting to. While I can't say that I'm a big fan of such testing due to some of the limitations I'll discuss shortly, I have had some patients successfully identify foods that were causing problems. In some of these cases, the foods were allowed on an elimination/AIP diet.

Another potential benefit of food sensitivity testing is that it might prevent the person from having to eliminate certain foods, although this is controversial. For example, if someone is eating gluten or dairy regularly and tests negative for both of these, does this mean it's safe to eat these foods, even though they are excluded from an AIP diet, as well as many other diets? We need to keep in mind that false negatives are possible with this type of testing. I personally recommend that my patients avoid gluten and dairy while restoring their health, regardless of what a food sensitivity panel shows. With regards to some of the other "excluded" foods, we need to keep in mind that some foods are excluded not because they are common allergens but because they have compounds that can affect the healing of the gut.

For example, nightshades are excluded from an AIP diet due to the compounds that can potentially cause inflammation and/or an increase in intestinal permeability. Solanine is one example, as it's a glycoalkaloid found in the nightshade foods, especially eggplant and white potatoes, although it's also found in tomatoes and peppers. However, if someone tests negative for eggplant, white potatoes, tomatoes, and peppers on a food sensitivity panel, this doesn't mean that these foods won't cause problems.

Getting back to the potential benefits of food sensitivity testing, one additional benefit that comes to mind is that if someone tests positive, and if it is a "true" positive, then this serves as a baseline. In other words, if someone tests positive for one or more foods, and if they decide to reintroduce the food in the future when their gut is healed and immune tolerance has been restored, they can do another food sensitivity panel after reintroducing the food to see if they are still reacting to that specific food.

The Disadvantages of Food Sensitivity Testing

While it might sound great to do food sensitivity testing to determine the specific foods you are reacting to, unfortunately, this type of testing has many disadvantages. Here are a few of the main ones:

- False results are common.
- You need to either be eating the foods, or have recently eaten the foods you're testing for to get an accurate result.
- Doing this type of testing can be expensive.
- Most food sensitivity panels are incomplete, meaning that most panels don't test for all of the foods a person eats.
- There can be differences between raw and cooked foods, yet most food sensitivity panels don't test for both of these.

Comparing the Different Types of Testing for Food Allergens

Now that you know some of the pros and cons of food sensitivity testing, let's look at some of the different types of testing available for food allergens.

IgE testing. A food allergy usually results in immediate symptoms. Skin prick testing is still used initially by many doctors to determine the presence of an IgE allergy. The way this test works is by introducing a needle into the upper layers of the skin and using a drop of the allergen, and then the release of histamine from mast cells will lead to the development of a wheal greater than 3 mm in diameter if the person is sensitive to the allergen.[6,7] However, there is the possibility of false positive results with this test.[8,9] Serum IgE can also be used in some cases to detect food allergies.[10] Although this also has some limitations, this does seem to be more accurate than the skin prick test.

IgG testing. Serum IgG testing is commonly used to determine whether someone has a food sensitivity. Unlike IgE food allergies, which involve an immediate response, IgG testing for food sensitivities involve a delayed response. In other words, the person with one or more IgG sensitivities might not experience symptoms for a few hours or, in some cases, a few days after eating a certain food.

Many different companies offer this type of testing. However, just as is the case with IgE testing for food allergies, IgG testing for food sensitivities has the potential of giving a false negative or a false positive result. It's also important to keep in mind that an increase in intestinal permeability can increase the incidence of food sensitivities. Thus, if someone has many food sensitivities on a panel then this is good indication of an increase in intestinal permeability, along with a loss of oral tolerance. Therefore, if someone has many food sensitivities, then it makes sense to take measures to heal the gut and restore oral tolerance, which I discuss in the fourth section.

How to Choose a Company for Food Sensitivity Testing

When choosing a company for food sensitivity testing, keep in mind that they are testing food proteins, and the purity and quality of these purified proteins are very important because if there are any contaminants, then it's possible for a positive reading to be false due to the contaminant and not the food protein.

In addition, some people might react to a certain food when eaten raw, but they might do fine when eating that same food cooked. This is one of the advantages of certain food sensitivity panels such as the Multiple Food Immune Reactivity Screen from Cyrex Labs, as this panel tests a number of different foods both raw and cooked, including asparagus, broccoli, carrots, and mushrooms. I have run this test on some of my patients and have seen some people test positive for a raw food, and test negative for the same food when cooked, and vice versa.

You also want to choose a lab that runs every sample through twice, as it's important for the results to be reproducible. There have been some cases with certain labs when two separate blood samples from the same person were submitted and the two reports gave different findings.

Although I like Cyrex Labs a lot and recommend their panels at times due to some of the reasons discussed here, other food sensitivity tests from different companies can also be valuable. If your doctor is using a specific company and has been doing so for a long time, chances are they are doing so because they are getting good results with their patients. I admit that I have used other labs for food sensitivity testing as well such as Alletess Medical Laboratory.

Leukocyte activation testing. The ALCAT test from Cell Science Systems utilizes this technology, and, as mentioned on their website, "The ALCAT test measures food/immune reactions through stimulation of leukocytes. The leukocytes, which comprise five classes of white blood cells, including monocytes, lymphocytes, eosinophils, basophils and neutrophils can be challenged with individual food or chemical extracts".[11] The patient's unique set of responses help to identify substances that may trigger potentially harmful immune system reactions.

This is different than IgG testing, but is it more accurate? Some healthcare professionals question whether leukocyte activation testing is reproducible. Many healthcare professionals use other labs for IgG testing and receive great results with their patients, although some healthcare professionals have successfully used leukocyte activation testing in their practice for many years.

Mediator Release Testing (MRT). Just as is the case with leukocyte activation testing, there isn't much research on mediator release testing. However, some healthcare professionals frequently use this type of testing and receive great results with their patients.

Can You Do Both Food Sensitivity Testing AND Follow an Elimination Diet?

Since neither an elimination diet nor food sensitivity testing is a perfect method for detecting food sensitivities, in some cases, it might make sense to combine both. You can choose to do a food sensitivity panel initially, and combine this with an elimination diet. For example, before starting the elimination diet, the person would get the blood draw for the food sensitivity panel. Then, while waiting for the results, they can follow an elimination diet for 30 days, and then upon receiving the results of the food sensitivity test they would stop eating any foods they test positive for. For example, if they tested positive on the food sensitivity panel for broccoli, carrots, and a few other "allowed" foods, they will not only stop eating these foods, but they won't reintroduce these foods until their gut has been healed.

An advantage of this approach is that not only are you following an elimination diet but you also are eliminating other foods that you might be reacting to that you wouldn't otherwise eliminate if you were following an elimination diet alone. The downside is that this can be challenging for someone whose food sensitivity panel shows that they are reacting to dozens of foods that are allowed on an elimination/AIP diet, as it can get to the point where the diet becomes too restrictive.

Another challenge is that false negatives are possible with food sensitivity testing. Thus, the person might continue eating foods they are reacting to. This is why it's important to choose a lab that does a good job of purifying the food antigen, and preferably runs through each sample twice in order to make sure the results are reproducible. While doing this won't guarantee that the results are accurate, it will greatly minimize the incidence of false results.

In addition, false negative results on an IgG food sensitivity test can be due to depressed immunoglobulin G, which is why some healthcare professionals will recommend that their patients have the serum immuno-globulins tested before conducting a food sensitivity test. Most well-known labs (i.e., Labcorp and Quest Diagnostics) offer this type of testing.

Finally, remember that if you are concerned about reacting to a specific food, you must have recently eaten that food in order to get accurate results. For example, if you want to find out if you have a sensitivity to eggs, but you haven't eaten eggs for at least a few months, then the test results would most likely come back negative for eggs, even if you have an egg sensitivity.

What Approach Do I Take in My Practice?

I have most of my patients with Hashimoto's follow an elimination diet initially in the form of the AIP diet. I have them do this for the first month, and if they are doing well, I'll encourage them to follow this diet for a longer period. Eventually, I'll have them reintroduce some of the excluded foods, as the goal isn't to keep them on this diet permanently. However, at times, I will order an IgG food sensitivity panel. If someone insists on ordering this type of testing, then I'm fine ordering it.

Another situation when I might order such testing is if the patient started out with an elimination diet and followed my other recommendations, but a few months later they still aren't progressing. Another scenario where I might order a food sensitivity panel is if the patient is progressing but then they hit a roadblock and don't show further improvement. Thus, I'm not completely opposed to doing food sensitivity testing, but it's not a test that I recommend to all of my patients.

Can Applied Kinesiology Detect Food Triggers?

Some doctors choose to use applied kinesiology to detect food sensitivities. This is a type of manual muscle test founded by Dr. George Goodheart, and many chiropractors and other natural healthcare professionals use this on their patients. I'm not going to discuss this in detail here, mainly because it's something that I don't do in my practice. However, other doctors successfully use it in their practice to detect food sensitivities and other imbalances; thus, I wanted to briefly mention it here.

I did come across a pilot study that compared the findings of applied kinesiology with serum immunoglobulin levels for food allergies and sensitivities.[12] It was a small study involving only seventeen subjects who showed muscle weakness upon oral provocative testing of one or two foods, using a total of 21 positive food reactions. So just to clarify, some applied kinesiology practitioners have their patients hold a food or supplement in their hand when muscle testing them, but this study involved oral administration of the foods. The serum tests, which involved both IgE and IgG, confirmed 19 of the 21 food allergies suspected based on the applied kinesiology techniques.

Of course, this is only a single study involving a small number of participants; nevertheless, it still provides some credibility towards using applied kinesiology in helping to detect food allergies and sensitivities. One of the drawbacks of this technique is that it depends on the skill of the practitioner. Thus, if you rely on applied kinesiology to help you detect certain food triggers for your Hashimoto's condition then it's probably best to work with someone who has a good amount of experience.

How Should YOU Detect Food Triggers?

After reading this, you still might not be sure what approach you should take. Of course, ultimately the decision is up to you, and if you are working with a natural healthcare professional, then you might leave the decision making up to them. Some healthcare professionals recommend food sensitivity testing to all of their patients. Others never recommend food sensitivity testing to their patients. Practitioners like myself recommend an elimination diet initially, but are open to food sensitivity testing. Some healthcare practitioners utilize other techniques such as applied kinesiology, while others use a biomeridian device to detect food sensitivities.

What I recommend is to find a doctor who is compatible with what you're looking for. For example, if you decide that you don't want to do food sensitivity testing, then it's probably not a good idea to work with a healthcare professional who does food sensitivity testing on every patient. If you want to get a food sensitivity panel done, it doesn't make sense to work with someone who is unwilling to order one for you.

Chapter Highlights:

- Certain foods can set the stage for Hashimoto's by causing an increase in proinflammatory cytokines and a decrease in regulatory T cells.
- Molecular mimicry is another mechanism that explains how food allergens can result in Hashimoto's.
- Some of the most common food allergens include gluten, dairy, corn, soy, eggs, shellfish, and peanuts.
- I have most of my patients with Hashimoto's follow an elimination diet initially in the form of the autoimmune Paleo diet.
- After someone has gone on an elimination diet for 30 days, the next step is to consider the reintroduction of foods.
- If someone is thriving on the elimination/autoimmune Paleo diet after 30 days, it is fine to continue with it for a few additional months.
- Some of the symptoms you might experience upon reintroducing foods you are sensitive to include bloating, gas, abdominal discomfort, headaches, fatigue, muscle or joint pain, insomnia, skin problems, and sinus congestion.
- Concerning the different tests for food allergens, IgE testing is specific for food allergies, while IgG testing is for delayed food sensitivities.
- Leukocyte activation and mediator release testing are two other options.
- A food allergy usually results in immediate symptoms, while a food sensitivity usually results in a delayed reaction.

CHAPTER 24

CAN BLOOD TESTS HELP TO DETECT YOUR TRIGGERS?

NEARLY EVERYONE WITH HASHIMOTO'S will get some type of thyroid-related blood tests, and many will have other blood tests done. But can blood tests help to detect your autoimmune triggers? In most cases, blood tests won't be enough to detect the underlying cause of Hashimoto's. However, there are a few exceptions, and certain blood tests can provide some valuable information that plays a role in helping you to get into remission and achieve optimal health.

Thus, in this chapter, I'm going to discuss some of the different blood tests I recommend to my patients with Hashimoto's.

An Important Note About the Reference Ranges

I'll be using the reference ranges from Labcorp and Quest Diagnostics, which are two common labs in the United States, and, in some cases, I will list the reference range from a "random lab." You need to keep a few things in mind regarding the reference ranges. First, different labs use different reference ranges, and some labs also use different units of measurement. For example, for the 25-OH vitamin D test, in the United States they typically use ng/ml, whereas in many other countries they use nmol/L. Second, there is also an "optimal" range for each lab marker, and I'm going to include the optimal reference range for most of them.

Also, I'm not suggesting that everyone needs to obtain all of these blood tests I'll be listing in this chapter. The more information you can get the better, but I realize that not everyone can order all of these tests due to various reasons. For example, some people don't have health insurance and are unable to afford all of these tests. Others might be able to afford these tests, but they are unable to get an order from a doctor. While there are online websites in the United States (and in some other countries) where you can order blood tests on your own and bring a requisition to a local lab, some other countries don't have this option.

Let's look at the different blood tests.

Thyroid Panel With Autoantibodies. Everyone with Hashimoto's should receive a thyroid panel that consists of the following:

Thyroid stimulating hormone (TSH). This is a pituitary hormone and is usually elevated in those with Hashimoto's. In fact, the diagnosis of Hashimoto's is usually based on an elevated TSH, along with elevated thyroid autoantibodies. TSH is a pituitary hormone, and while it's important to measure this marker in everyone, one shouldn't rely on the TSH alone.

> **Labcorp:** 0.450-4.50 uIU/ml
> **Quest:** 0.40-4.50 uIU/ml
> **Other Lab**: 0.34-4.82 uIU/ml
> **Optimal reference range**: 1.0 to 2.0 uIU/ml

Free thyroxine (T4). Thyroxine, also known as T4, is a type of thyroid hormone. The free T4 represents the free form of thyroxine in the blood, whereas the total T4 represents both the free and bound form of thyroxine. T4 is converted into T3. In hypothyroid conditions, the free T4 and total T4 are low or depressed.

> **Labcorp**: 0.82-1.77 ng/dL
> **Quest**: 0.8-1.8 ng/dL
> **Other Lab**: 0.59-1.61 ng/dL
> **Optimal reference range**: 1.1 to 1.5 ng/dL

Free triiodothyronine (T3). Free T3 is the active form of thyroid hormone, meaning it is the form of thyroid hormone that binds to the thyroid receptors. Unfortunately, many endocrinologists don't test the free T3, but will only test the TSH and free T4. However, many people have problems converting T4 into T3, and while sometimes this will show up as a slightly high TSH and a normal T4, at other times both the TSH and free T4 will be within the optimal reference range, while the free T3 is low or depressed.

Labcorp: 2.0-4.4 pg/ml
Quest: 2.3-4.2 pg/ml
Other Lab: 2.3-4.2 pg/ml
Optimal reference range: 3.0 to 3.7 pg/ml

Note: Although I'm not listing total T4 and total T3 in this chapter, it's not a bad idea to measure these as well. These look at mostly the bound form of thyroid hormone. However, if you have to choose between testing the total and free hormones, I find it more valuable to measure the free hormones.

Thyroid peroxidase (TPO) antibodies. TPO antibodies are associated with Hashimoto's, and if these antibodies are elevated, it means the immune system is damaging thyroid peroxidase, which is an enzyme that's necessary for the production of thyroid hormone.

Labcorp: 0-34 IU/ml
Quest: <9 IU/ml
Other Lab: <35 IU/ml
Optimal reference range: <9 IU/ml

Thyroglobulin antibodies. These antibodies are also associated with Hashimoto's. If these are elevated, it means the immune system is attacking and damaging thyroglobulin, which is a protein produced by the thyroid gland.

Labcorp: 0.0-0.9 IU/ml
Quest: <1 or = 1 IU/ml
Other Lab: <20 IU/ml
Optimal reference range: <1 IU/ml

Note: While some will argue that these antibodies should be zero, the research shows that these and other autoantibodies are abundant in all human serum, and might even have some important physiological function.[13] Thus, having a very small amount of thyroid antibodies might be normal, even in healthy individuals.

Reverse T3. Reverse T3 is manufactured from thyroxine (T4), and its role is to block the action of T3. When someone is dealing with frequent chronic stress, the adrenals will initially produce an excess amount of cortisol. The cortisol, in turn, will inhibit the conversion of T4 to T3, and can result in elevated reverse T3 levels. Other factors that can lead to elevated reverse T3 levels include liver and gut problems, as well as a moderate to severe selenium deficiency.

> **Labcorp**: 9.2-24.1 ng/dL
> **Quest**: 8-25 ng/dL
> **Other lab**: 10-24 ng/dL
> **Optimal reference range**: 10-18 ng/dL

Note: In addition to looking at the value of reverse T3, it might be helpful to look at the ratio between the free T3 and reverse T3. *Stop the Thyroid Madness* has some wonderful information on this, including a calculator you can access by visiting **https://stopthethyroidmadness.com/rt3-ratio/**. They recommend that the free T3/reverse T3 ratio be greater than 20. If you've had the total T3 tested instead of the free T3, you can still use their calculator to find out the ratio.

Complete Blood Count (CBC) With Differential. The main purpose of the test is to see if there are any disorders related to the red and white blood cells. This can provide a lot of information, including if someone has anemia, polycythemia, a possible infection, clotting disorders, nutrient deficiencies, etc. However, you usually can't rely on this test alone for diagnosing specific health conditions. For example, if someone had elevated or depressed white blood cells, this might indicate an infection, but further testing is frequently required to determine this. Depending on the positive finding, sometimes the best option is to do another CBC with differential in two to four weeks to see if the out of range markers are getting better or worse.

I'm not going to discuss all of the markers and list all of the reference ranges, but the panel tests for the following markers: Hematocrit; hemoglobin; mean corpuscular volume (MCV); mean corpuscular hemoglobin

(MCH); mean corpuscular hemoglobin concentration (MCHC); red cell distribution width (RDW); percentage and absolute differential counts; platelet count; red cell count (RBC); white blood cell count (WBC).

Some of the more common findings I see with my patients on this panel include a low white blood cell count (WBC) and neutrophils, high mean corpuscular volume (MCV), high red cell distribution width (RDW), and low red blood cell count (RBC), hemoglobin, and hematocrit. If someone has low WBCs and neutrophils, this commonly means they have a chronic infection, although there can be other causes. MCV is the average size of a red blood cell, and a high MCV usually relates to a vitamin B12 or folate deficiency. A high RDW usually relates to an iron deficiency, while low RBC, hemoglobin, and/or hematocrit are commonly found with anemia.

Comprehensive Metabolic Profile. I'm not going to discuss all of the markers and list all of the reference ranges, but this panel tests for the following markers: alanine aminotransferase (ALT/SGPT); albumin:globulin (A:G) ratio; albumin, serum; alkaline phosphatase, serum; aspartate aminotransferase (AST/SGOT); bilirubin, total; BUN; BUN:creatinine ratio; calcium, serum; carbon dioxide, total; chloride, serum; creatinine, serum; eGFR calculation; globulin, total; glucose, serum; potassium, serum; protein, total, serum; sodium, serum.

Some of the more common findings I see with my patients on this panel include high fasting glucose and a low serum potassium and sodium. A high fasting glucose can mean that someone has insulin resistance or diabetes, although other markers need to be tested to confirm this. Low serum potassium and sodium levels can relate to the health of the adrenals.

Sometimes bilirubin will be high, which, in some cases, can be due to a condition called Gilbert's syndrome, which is an inherited conjugation defect that results in a mild increase in the bilirubin levels. Elevated serum calcium can be due to a vitamin D toxicity or hyperparathyroidism. While I commonly see elevated liver enzymes (ALT and AST) in my patients with hyperthyroidism and Graves' disease, I don't see them frequently high in my patients with Hashimoto's. If they are high, then this is a sign of liver damage.

Lipid Panel. I'm not going to discuss all of the markers and list all of the reference ranges, but this panel tests for the following markers: total cholesterol; high-density lipoprotein (HDL) cholesterol; low-density lipoprotein

(LDL) cholesterol; triglycerides; very low-density lipoprotein (VLDL) cholesterol

Some of the more common findings I see with my patients on this panel include high total cholesterol, high LDL levels, and high triglycerides. Total cholesterol and LDL is commonly elevated in those with hypothyroidism. In other words, those with a high TSH and low thyroid hormone levels will typically have a high total cholesterol and LDL. As for high triglycerides, this frequently is related to eating too many carbohydrates, although hypothyroidism can also play a role. Some other factors that can lead to elevated triglycerides include alcohol consumption, kidney disease, pregnancy, certain medications, and nonalcoholic fatty-liver disease.[14]

Serum Iron, Ferritin, TIBC, % Saturation. I recommend for most of my patients with Hashimoto's to not only test serum iron, but other iron-related markers as well. As is the case with other markers, keep in mind that you can't just pay attention to the lab reference range for these markers, as you also want to look at the optimal reference range.

Serum iron. This relates to the amount of iron in the blood, and these levels are decreased when someone has an iron deficiency and are increased in iron overload.

> **Labcorp**: 27-159 mcg/dL
> **Quest**: 45-160 mcg/dL
> **Optimal reference range**: 80 to 130 mcg/dL

Ferritin. Ferritin relates to the iron stores, and is decreased when someone has an iron deficiency and increased in iron overload. However, ferritin can also increase in response to inflammation. Thus, if someone has elevated ferritin levels but the serum iron and iron saturation are either normal or depressed, then the high ferritin levels usually are related to inflammation.

> **Labcorp**: 15-150 ng/ml
> **Quest**: 10-232 ng/ml
> **Optimal reference range**: 45-120 ng/ml

Note: When going through my masters in nutrition course, I was taught that the ferritin levels should be at least 40 to 45 ng/ml, although some sources claim they should be between 70 and 90 ng/ml, especially if some-one is experiencing hair loss. However, one important thing to keep in mind is that inflammation can raise the ferritin levels, which is why you can't rely on this test alone for determining iron status.

Iron Saturation. This is also referred to as transferrin saturation or % sat-uration. Iron saturation tells us how much serum iron is actually bound to a protein called transferrin. For example, if someone has a value of 20% then this means that 20% of the iron-binding sites of transferrin are being occupied by iron. A low value is common in an iron deficiency. Oral contraceptives and pregnancy can also increase this value.

> **Labcorp**: 15-55%
> **Quest**: 11-50%
> **Optimal reference range**: 30 to 40%

Total iron binding capacity (TIBC). When iron moves through the blood, it is attached to transferrin. TIBC measures how well transferrin can carry iron in the blood. A high TIBC means that the iron stores are low.

> **Labcorp**: 250-450 ug/dL
> **Quest**: 250-450 ug/dL
> **Optimal reference range**: 300 to 350 ug/dL

25 Hydroxy Vitamin D. Vitamin D is commonly deficient in those with Hashimoto's. In fact, vitamin D is deficient in most people overall. While vitamin D is important for bone health, it also plays an important role in immune system health. This is why I recommend that all of my patients get vitamin D tested through the blood.

> **Labcorp**: 30–100 ng/ml
> **Quest**: 30–100 ng/ml
> **Optimal reference range**: 50–80 ng/ml

Note: Since 1,25(OH) vitamin D is the active form, some practitioners recommend testing this marker. And while it's fine to test both vitamin D markers, according to Dr. Alan Gaby, author of the well-researched text-book "Nutritional Medicine," serum 1,25(OH) vitamin D is not a reliable indicator of vitamin D status because a vitamin D deficiency causes a compensatory increase in the concentration of parathyroid hormone, which, in turn, increases the renal production of 1,25(OH) vitamin D.[15] Thus, these levels can be normal or even elevated in those with a vitamin D deficiency. The American Academy of Family Physicians also mentions how serum levels of 1,25-dihyroxyvitamin D have little or no relationship to vitamin D stores but rather are regulated primarily by parathyroid hormone levels, and that with a vitamin D deficiency, 1,25-dihydroxyvitamin D levels go up, not down.[16] The vitamin D Council also agrees that 25-OH vitamin D should be tested, and not 1,25(OH) vitamin D.[17]

Vitamin B12. Many people are deficient in vitamin B12. Although doing a serum vitamin B12 test isn't the best method of determining if someone has a vitamin B12 deficiency, I commonly recommend a serum vitamin B12 because 1) if it is low then this does seem to confirm a deficiency, and 2) many medical doctors are willing to order a serum B12 test. The major drawback of this test is that a normal or high serum B12 doesn't rule out a vitamin B12 deficiency. This is why some healthcare professionals don't test for serum B12 and only will test for methylmalonic acid.

> **Labcorp**: 211-946 pg/ml
> **Quest**: 200-1100 pg/ml
> **Other Lab**: 211-911 pg/ml
> **Optimal reference range**: >700 pg/ml

Note: Optimal levels of serum B12 won't always rule out a vitamin B12 deficiency

Methylmalonic Acid (MMA). This is another marker that can determine if someone has a vitamin B12 deficiency. Vitamin B12 is an important cofactor for the conversion of MMA to succinate; thus, if someone has a vitamin B12 deficiency this will lead to high MMA levels. Although I'm listing the serum reference range, MMA seems to be more accurate when tested through the urine.

> **Labcorp**: 79-376 nmol/L
> **Quest**: 87-318 nmol/L
> **Optimal reference range**: <250 nmol/L

RBC Folate. When someone has low folate levels, this usually is related to low dietary intake of folate, malabsorption, and chronic alcoholism. Having an MTHFR defect can also have a negative effect on folate metabolism.

> **Labcorp**: >498 ng/ml
> **Quest**: >280 ng/ml
> **Optimal reference range**: >498 ng/ml

C-reactive protein (CRP). This is one of the main inflammatory markers commonly tested for. It increases as interleukin 6 (IL6) is secreted by immune system cells. CRP is not a specific test. Thus, if it is positive, it means you have inflammation, but it won't tell you where the inflammation is located. When getting this test, it's best to order "high sensitivity" C-Reactive protein, also known as hs-CRP.

> **Labcorp**: 0.0–4.9 mg/L
> **Quest**: <8.0 mg/L
> **Optimal reference range**: <1.0 mg/L

Hemoglobin A1C. Hemoglobin A1C gives an average of the blood glucose levels over a period of 2 to 4 months. It is high in prediabetes and diabetes, although, if someone has diabetes, then self-monitoring of blood glucose is also recommended.

> **Labcorp**: 4.8-5.6%
> **Pre-diabetes**: 5.7-6.4%
> **Diabetes**: >6.4%
> **Optimal reference range**: less than 5.3%

Insulin. Although testing the fasting glucose and hemoglobin A1C can both be valuable to determine if someone has blood sugar imbalances, doing a fasting insulin can provide some value as well. Some will suggest that a fasting insulin is far more valuable than either a fasting glucose or hemoglobin A1C.

> **Labcorp**: 2.6-24.9 uIU/ml
> **Quest**: 2.0-19.6 uIU/ml
> **Optimal reference range**: <5.0 uIU/ml fasting

Leptin. In the blood sugar imbalances chapter in section two, I discussed how high circulating leptin levels could not only induce a proinflammatory response and increase Th17 cells but also perpetuate inflammation. If someone is having problems losing weight then not only will they want to consider doing a fasting insulin blood test, but a leptin test as well. In Chapter 11, I also mentioned how this marker can be elevated in those with chronic inflammatory response syndrome.

Note: Reference ranges depend on the age, gender, and body mass index (BMI)

Homocysteine. Homocysteine is a sulfur amino acid, and its metabolism requires folate, vitamin B6, and vitamin B12.[18] There seems to be an association between high homocysteine levels and hypothyroidism.[19]

> **Labcorp**: 0-15 umol/L
> **Quest**: <10.4 umol/L
> **Optimal reference range**: 4.0 to 8 umol/L

Note: Although you don't want homocysteine to be too high, you also don't want this marker to be too low, as if someone has very low homocysteine levels then this can lead to a glutathione deficiency.

Ceruloplasmin. This is a liver-derived circulating protein that is important for iron release from certain tissues.[20] In other words, ceruloplasmin plays a role in iron metabolism. One of the causes of hereditary iron overload is a genetic polymorphism in the ceruloplasmin gene.[21] While elevated levels of ceruloplasmin may indicate a copper toxicity, it's also important to keep in mind that ceruloplasmin is an acute phase reactant, and like ferritin, it can be elevated in the presence of moderate to severe inflammation. However, ceruloplasmin can be too low in some people, which can be related to a vitamin A or a magnesium deficiency or, in some cases, taking too much vitamin D.

> **Labcorp**: Men: 11-31 mg/dL; women: 19-39 mg/dL
> **Quest**: Men: 18-36 mg/dL; women: 18-52 mg/dL
> **Optimal reference range**: 25 to 35 mg/dL

Gamma Glutamyl Transferase (GGT). Elevated GGT is an indication of liver disease. Elevated values can indicate obstructive jaundice, cholangitis, and cholecystitis. GGT also plays a role in glutathione homeostasis, and high levels are correlated with glutathione depletion in the liver.[22]

> **Labcorp**: 0-60 IU/L
> **Quest**: 3-70 U/L
> **Optimal reference range**: <20 IU/L

RBC Magnesium. Although there is no perfect test for measuring tissue levels of magnesium, RBC magnesium can be a good indication, providing that you don't pay attention to the standard lab reference ranges. However, serum magnesium is almost useless, as like serum calcium, the body will do everything it can to maintain healthy serum levels of magnesium, even if it means pulling it from the bone.

> **Labcorp**: 4.2–6.8
> **Quest**: 4.0-6.4 mg/dL
> **Optimal reference range**: 6.0 to 6.5 mg/dL

Which Blood Tests Are the Most Important to Order?

While all of these blood tests can be valuable, I realize that not everyone will be able to order all of them. Regarding your thyroid health, I would prioritize the following markers:

- TSH
- Free T3
- Free T4
- Thyroid peroxidase antibodies
- Thyroglobulin antibodies

As for the other blood tests, at minimum I would order the following:

- Complete blood count with differential
- Comprehensive metabolic panel
- Lipid panel
- Iron panel (serum iron, ferritin, iron saturation, TIBC)
- 25-OH vitamin D
- High sensitivity CRP

Other Tests to Consider Ordering

There are too many different blood tests to discuss in this chapter, but I wanted to cover some of the more important ones. However, I'll list some others that might be worth testing for in some cases. I'm not going to include the reference ranges:

- RBC zinc
- Estradiol
- Progesterone
- Total testosterone
- Free testosterone
- Sex hormone binding globulin (SHBG)
- Methylenetetrahydrofolate Reductase (MTHFR)
- Celiac Antibodies Profile tTG IgA, tTG IgG, DGP IgA, DGP IgG, EMA IgA, and Total IgA
- Epstein-Barr Virus (EBV) Profile, Chronic, Active Infection IgG, IgM
- Cytomegalovirus Profile, IgG, IgM
- Lipoprotein Analysis (LDL-P, HDL-P, LDL Size)
- Lipoprotein A
- Lipoprotein-associated Phospholipase A-2 (Lp-PLA2)
- Fatty acid profile with omega-3 index

How Can You Order Specific Blood Tests?

Many people will get a lab order from their medical doctor or endocrinologist for blood tests. Most medical doctors will only order what they feel is necessary, and, unfortunately, this usually excludes most of these tests. For people in the United States who don't have health insurance, or are unable to get a lab order from their doctor, there are online websites where you can order these tests on your own. The way this works is that you purchase the labs online, and then the company will provide you with a requisition form that you can print and bring to a local lab. The downside is that there are usually specific labs you need to visit, and this service isn't available in all states. Since there are always new companies that offer this type of testing, rather than post my current favorites, I'll lead you to the webpage **www.naturalendocrinesolutions.com/testing**.

Chapter Highlights:

- Blood tests not only can help to diagnose Hashimoto's in many cases, but they can also give an idea if someone has an infection, anemia, liver or kidney problems, as well as certain nutrient deficiencies.
- Blood tests can also help to establish a baseline so that you can monitor your progress.
- Different labs use different reference ranges, and some labs also use different units of measurement.
- There is an "optimal" range for each lab marker.
- The different thyroid markers include TSH, free T4, total T4, free T3, total T3, TPO antibodies, thyroglobulin antibodies, and reverse T3.
- Most people should obtain a CBC with differential, a comprehensive metabolic profile, a lipid panel, a full iron panel, and a 25 hydroxy vitamin D.
- Although I commonly recommend a serum vitamin B12 test to my patients, methylmalonic acid is another marker that can determine if someone has a vitamin B12 deficiency.
- Some other blood tests to consider include RBC folate, hemoglobin A1C, fasting insulin, leptin, homocysteine, ceruloplasmin, Gamma Glutamyl Transferase, and RBC magnesium.

CHAPTER 25

DETECTING TRIGGERS THROUGH TESTING

AS YOU NOW KNOW, the first step in detecting the autoimmune triggers of Hashimoto's is through a comprehensive health history. While a thorough health history can provide a lot of valuable information, in my experience, testing is usually required to help detect the triggers. In Chapter 24, I discussed blood tests, but usually some other tests are required to help detect the autoimmune triggers associated with Hashimoto's thyroiditis.

In this chapter, I'll discuss many of the different tests available. I'm not suggesting that you order all of these tests, as, many times, only a few basic tests are needed. Other times, more comprehensive testing is necessary. Some healthcare professionals are conservative when recommending tests to their patients, while others will recommend more comprehensive testing initially to all of their patients. The advantage of doing more comprehensive testing is that there is a greater chance of finding the triggers. The disadvantage is that the patient might end up spending more money than necessary, since not everyone requires comprehensive testing.

For example, many natural healthcare professionals will recommend a comprehensive stool panel to all of their patients. While I utilize stool testing at times, I find that many stool panels will come back negative for triggers such as pathogenic bacteria, yeast, and parasites. Also, while other markers on a comprehensive stool panel can provide some value, I find that many patients with Hashimoto's don't need a comprehensive stool panel in order to find their triggers and, thus, get into remission. However, at times, I will recommend a comprehensive stool panel to my patients. In addition, if I feel that a patient doesn't need a comprehensive stool panel (or a different test), but they still want to order the test, then I'm fine with this.

The Downside of Using Symptoms to Determine the Appropriate Testing

In Chapter 22, I discussed how symptoms can sometimes be helpful in determining whether someone needs to order a specific test. Sticking with the comprehensive stool panel, if someone presents with several digestive symptoms, then it might be a good idea to do some stool testing.

However, there are flaws with relying on symptoms in order to determine which tests are necessary. For example, if someone has digestive symptoms when eating certain foods, some healthcare professionals will suggest doing a food sensitivity panel, since the symptoms are related to eating certain foods. However, having the person follow an elimination diet might provide the solution without ordering such a panel.

Nevertheless, sometimes you can't rely on symptoms when determining if someone needs a certain test, which is why some natural healthcare professionals recommend more comprehensive testing. In this chapter, I included a case study of someone who tested positive for parasites on a stool panel, even though she didn't have digestive symptoms. Upon eradication of the parasites, the person went into remission.

I included this case study not to encourage everyone with Hashimoto's to get a comprehensive stool panel, but only to remind you that symptoms aren't always a reliable indicator when deciding what test is necessary. While I don't recommend a comprehensive stool panel to all of my patients, I recommend such testing more frequently these days than in the past, and if someone isn't progressing, I'm definitely more aggressive about recommending more comprehensive testing. Nevertheless, I still take a conservative approach initially, although I give the option to do more comprehensive testing for those who prefer this.

A Breakdown of the Different Tests That Can Help Detect Your Hashimoto's Triggers

Let's take a look at some of the different tests that can help identify your Hashimoto's triggers. In order to make it easier, I will list a specific category of testing (e.g., adrenal testing), and then discuss some of the different types of tests associated with this category (e.g., blood testing, saliva testing). I'll also list some specific companies I have used for each type of test.

ADRENAL TESTING

Adrenal saliva panel. Many natural healthcare professionals utilize saliva testing to determine the health of the patient's adrenals. For many years, I have conducted saliva testing on my patients. One of the main advantages of saliva testing is that it allows the patient to collect a few different samples throughout the day. The reason why this is important is because cortisol follows a circadian rhythm, as it should be at the highest level upon waking up, and at the lowest level when you are ready to go to bed. Testing for cortisol through the blood doesn't provide the same information since it only looks at a single sample.

Another downside of serum testing for cortisol is that, in many cases, the blood draw itself can cause a false elevation of the cortisol levels because cortisol elevates in response to stress, and many people become stressed when getting blood drawn. This is another advantage of saliva testing, as it is non-invasive, and you can do it from the comfort of your home.

However, is saliva testing as accurate as blood testing when it comes to evaluating the adrenals? Numerous studies show that using saliva testing to measure the cortisol levels is either just as good or even better than blood testing.[23,24,25] When I went through my certification training through the Institute for Functional Medicine, just about all of the instructors, many of whom were medical doctors, utilized saliva testing in their practice.

While most medical doctors in general don't utilize saliva testing in their practice, many medical doctors who practice functional medicine understand the benefits of saliva testing. When I order a saliva test for a patient I not only want to look cortisol levels throughout the day, but I also like to test for the DHEA, 17-OH progesterone, and secretory IgA in order to get a full picture of their adrenal health.

Companies I have used for saliva testing: Diagnos-Techs Adrenal Stress Index, Genova Diagnostics Adrenocortex Stress Profile, ZRT Laboratory Adrenal Stress Profile, BioHealth HPA Stress Profile.

Blood testing. Although blood testing does have some value, it usually isn't a good option to determine if someone has compromised adrenals in the absence of a severe condition such as Addison's disease or Cushing's syndrome. It's not practical to look at the circadian rhythm with serum cortisol; thus, you would be relying on a single sample to determine the health of the adrenals. This is the main reason why I prefer salivary testing over serum testing, and many other healthcare professionals utilize salivary testing as well.

This doesn't mean that blood testing is completely useless for evaluating the adrenals. While false elevations of cortisol are common with serum testing, cortisol concentrations less than 5μg/dL can be a sign of primary adrenal insufficiency, although additional testing is necessary to confirm this. Adrenocorticotropic hormone (ACTH) is a hormone secreted by the pituitary gland, and it can be useful in diagnosing a condition such as Addison's disease. Values that are greater than 100 pg/ml are usually suggestive of primary adrenal insufficiency, while values that are greater than 500 pg/ml are diagnostic.[26]

Some labs will test for cortisol binding globulin, which has a high affinity for binding to cortisol. This is something I don't commonly test for. You can also test for dehydroepiandrosterone (DHEA) and dehydroepiandrosterone-sulfate (DHEA-S) in the blood. Anti-adrenal antibodies, including 21-hydroxylase antibodies, can also be tested for in the blood, and can be useful in order to determine if someone has an autoimmune condition involving the adrenals, such as Addison's disease.

Urine testing. In the past I wasn't a fan of urinary testing for the adrenals. However, I will admit that I've been impressed with the DUTCH test, which stands for "Dried Urine Test for Comprehensive Hormones." This test looks at the circadian rhythm of cortisol by measuring the free cortisol and cortisone levels throughout the day. In addition, it looks at the cortisol metabolites, along with DHEA-S.

The cortisol metabolites evaluated include a-Tetrahydrocortisol, b-Tetrahydrocortisol, and b-Tetrahydrocortisone. Looking at the cortisol metabolites does have a few advantages. For example, if someone has elevated levels of free cortisol on this test and low metabolites, then this suggests that there is a problem with cortisol metabolism.

In other words, while you are producing sufficient cortisol in this situation, if the metabolites are low, then you have an impaired ability to clear cortisol from your body. This is common in hypothyroid conditions, although poor liver function can also be a cause. If both the free cortisol and the cortisol metabolites are low, then this usually indicates that not a lot of cortisol is being produced.

Many conventional labs offer a 24-hour urine free cortisol test, and you might be wondering what the difference is between this and the DUTCH test. One difference is that the DUTCH test is a dried urine test, and the collection process is easier. In addition, the 24-hour urine free cortisol test isn't looking at the circadian rhythm of cortisol. This confuses some people, as they think this is looking at the circadian rhythm since it requires collection urine samples over a 24-hour period. However, you are collecting all of the urine samples in a single plastic container, and, because of this, it's impossible to evaluate the circadian rhythm.

Companies I have used for urinary adrenal testing: Precision Analytical DUTCH Test

Other tests for assessing adrenal health. A few other tests can help to determine the health of the adrenals. The ACTH stimulation test is one of these, as this differs from the ACTH serum test in that the person gets their baseline cortisol levels measured, then they receive an injection of ACTH, and then the cortisol levels are measured again. Thus, this test is essentially measuring the response of your adrenals to stress, and if there is a significant spike of cortisol, then this is indicative of "normal" adrenals. However, if there isn't a large spike, then the person might have adrenal insufficiency.

Aldosterone is another hormone secreted by the adrenals that can be measured. Aldosterone is a mineralocorticoid, and it increases the absorption of sodium and water, while causing the excretion of potassium. This, in turn, increases blood pressure. Thus, when someone has high blood pressure and/or water retention, this usually is associated with high aldosterone levels.

Ragland's test. This involves testing your blood pressure while lying down and again after you stand up. Under normal circumstances, the number on top (systolic) should increase by 6 to 10 mm. However, if someone has weakened adrenal glands, this number will drop from 5 to 10 mm upon standing. If it drops more than 10 mm, then this is usually an indication of more severe adrenal problems.

GASTROINTESTINAL HEALTH TESTING

Comprehensive stool panel. A comprehensive stool panel is one of the best, and perhaps THE best test, for determining the health of the digestive system. This is why many natural healthcare professionals will recommend this test to their patients, as you can't have a healthy immune system without having a healthy gut. I don't recommend a comprehensive stool panel to all of my patients, although I recommend it at times.

A comprehensive stool panel tests for pathogenic bacteria, yeast, and parasites, and many companies will also test for markers of digestion and absorption (i.e., pancreatic elastase and fecal fat), gut inflammation (i.e., calprotectin), short chain fatty acids (i.e., n-butyrate), and beta-glucuronidase. For greater accuracy, I usually recommend that those who order a stool panel collect a stool sample on three consecutive days. One exception to this is the GI Microbial Assay Plus (GI-MAP), which is a comprehensive stool panel by Diagnostic Solutions Laboratory that uses DNA/PCR technology. Even though this only involves a one-sample test, I find this to be very sensitive due to the technology used.

You might wonder what the difference is between a comprehensive stool panel you would obtain at a specialty lab and a stool panel from a conventional lab such as Labcorp or Quest Diagnostics. The stool panels ordered through local labs usually don't evaluate for the presence of as many microbes as comprehensive stool panels. Thus, a negative finding doesn't always rule out a gut infection. In addition, many doctors will recommend a stool culture, which relies a lot more on the skill of the lab technician when compared to DNA/PCR technology. This also will result in more false negatives when compared to DNA-based testing. However, some of the specialty labs will also do culture testing.

While DNA/PCR technology is great, it's not perfect. There have been healthcare professionals who have submitted different stool samples from the same patient to two different labs at the same time, only to have one panel come back positive, and the other negative. At times, the DNA/PCR has come back negative, whereas other diagnostic methods such as a stool culture or a trichome stain has resulted in positive findings. Thus, if given the choice, I'd go with DNA/PCR technology, but you need to keep in mind that false negatives are possible regardless of the method used.

Companies I have used for stool testing: Genova Diagnostics GI Effects and CDSA, Doctor's Data Comprehensive stool panel, Diagnostic Solutions GI-MAP, BioHealth GI Screen.

Organic acids test. This isn't primarily a "gastrointestinal" test, although it does look at markers of yeast and bacterial overgrowth, which relates to the health of the gut. I'll further discuss organic acids testing shortly.

Companies I have used for organic acids testing: Great Plains Lab Organic Acids Test, Genova Diagnostics Organix

Intestinal permeability test. The classic method of determining whether someone has an increase in intestinal permeability (leaky gut) is through the lactulose-mannitol test, which is a urine test that involves swallowing a solution of lactulose and mannitol. Lactulose is a larger sugar molecule, and if someone has a healthy gut, this molecule shouldn't be absorbed. Therefore, if someone does this test and has large amounts of lactulose in the urine, then this usually confirms that the person has a leaky gut.

How accurate is the lactulose-mannitol test? A study in 2008 concluded that the lactulose-mannitol ratio had the highest diagnostic value to assess intestinal permeability.[27] Another study looked to determine the value of the lactulose-mannitol test in detecting intestinal permeability in those people with celiac disease.[28] The study showed that the sensitivity of the test was 87% in the screening situation and 81% in the clinical situation. Thus, it definitely isn't a perfect test, and while the evidence is strong that everyone with Hashimoto's has a leaky gut, I've seen this test negative in some patients who had elevated thyroid autoantibodies.

Some newer testing methods have been developed in recent years. The company Cyrex Labs has a test called the Intestinal Antigenic Permeability Screen (the Array #2), which is a blood test that measures the immune system response to an increase in intestinal permeability. It specifically tests for the presence of antibodies against actomyosin, occludin/zonulin, and lipopolysaccharides. Before briefly discussing these markers, I want to mention that intestinal permeability can occur through two pathways. With the paracellular pathway, the antigen (e.g., food particle, infection) is transported between the cells of the small intestine, while, with the transcellular pathway, the antigen goes through the body of the cell.

Actomyosin helps to regulate intestinal barrier function, and when there is damage to the cells of the small intestine via the transcellular pathway, this will result in antibodies to actomyosin. This is very common in those who have celiac disease. Occludin and zonulin are considered to be tight junction proteins, as occludin helps to hold together the tight junctions, and zonulin helps to regulate the permeability of the small intestine. If someone has antibodies to occludin or zonulin, then this indicates that the tight junctions between the cells of the small intestine have been compromised.

Lipopolysaccharides (LPS) are large molecules found in gram-negative bacteria, and if they are absorbed, they elicit a strong immune response. These lipopolysaccharides, in turn, can cause an increase in intestinal permeability.[29,30] However, they apparently don't always cause a leaky gut, as I've seen patients who have had antibodies to LPS but not to actomyosin or occludin/zonulin.

Companies I have used for measuring intestinal permeability: Cyrex Labs Intestinal Antigenic Permeability Screen (Array #2), Genova Diagnostics Lactulose-Mannitol Test

Other tests for assessing gastrointestinal health. Although I'm focusing on some of the more alternative tests, sometimes, conventional testing can be beneficial. For example, while I don't think that invasive tests such as a colonoscopy or endoscopy should be the first option, at times, they are necessary. Sometimes, an ultrasound, computed tomography (CT) scan, and/or magnetic resonance imaging (MRI) can be helpful.

Another test that can be useful at times is a barium swallow, which evaluates the esophagus, stomach, and upper part of the small intestine. With this test, barium is swallowed and x-rays are taken.

A fecal occult blood test is a part of some comprehensive stool panels, although it can be tested separately. This checks for hidden blood in the stool. This test can be useful if someone has unexplained anemia, although a positive test can also indicate polyps in the colon or rectum.

TESTING FOR INFECTIONS

Conventional blood testing. Doing blood testing at a local lab can sometimes provide some good information on infections. You can test for certain pathogenic bacteria in the blood, including Yersinia enterocolitica, H. pylori, and the pathogen associated with Lyme disease (borrelia burgdorferi). I discussed testing for Lyme disease in Chapter 10, but I will say here that false negatives are common when testing for Lyme disease in conventional labs.

Candida albicans antibodies can also be tested for through the blood, but, as I'll discuss shortly, I find the organic acids test to be more accurate. Blood testing can provide some valuable information on viruses. This is especially true for Epstein-Barr. Let's take a look at an Epstein-Barr Virus antibody profile:

1. **Viral capsid antigen (VCA)-IgM.** The presence of these IgM antibodies indicates a recent infection with EBV.
2. **VCA-IgG.** The presence of these IgG antibodies indicates a past infection.
3. **Epstein-Barr nuclear antigen (EBNA).** These antibodies will develop 6 to 8 weeks after being infected initially with EBV, and will remain detectable for life.

So just to summarize, the presence of VCA IgM antibodies indicates a recent infection, while the presence of VCA IgG antibodies indicates a past infection. Thus, if someone tests positive for the VCA IgM antibodies, then this usually indicates an active infection, but positive VCA IgG antibodies along with negative VCA IgM antibodies indicates that the person had a past EBV infection. Thus, the EBV is in a dormant state. It's important to point out that over 90% of adults will test positive for IgG antibodies to VCA and EBNA.[31]

Cyrex Labs Pathogen Associated Immune Reactivity Screen (Array #12). This is an immune system test conducted through the blood that measures the IgG antibodies of some of the most common pathogens associated with autoimmunity. Some of the pathogens it tests for include Helicobacter pylori, Yersinia enterocolitica, Entamoeba histolytica, Blastocystis hominis, Mycoplasmas, Cytomegalovirus, Stachybotrys chartarum, Aspergillus, and Streptococcus mutans. Keep in mind that many of these pathogens can be tested through a local lab, although if you are paying out of pocket then it might be more cost effective to do the Array #12.

Although I like the Array #12, this panel has a few drawbacks. One drawback is that it only measures IgG antibodies, which means that a positive finding doesn't confirm an active infection. Second, if someone has depressed serum immunoglobulin G levels, then this can lead to a false negative result; thus, before doing this test, it probably is a good idea to get the serum immunoglobulin G levels tested, which can be conducted at most local labs.

This also applies to other tests that involve measuring immunoglobulins. For example, if you had an active Epstein-Barr infection, but had depressed immunoglobulin M (IgM) levels, then you would most likely get a false negative result of the VCA-IgM marker. The only way you would know that this was a false negative would be by testing serum immunoglobulin M. You can test for the serum immunoglobulins at most well-known labs (e.g., Labcorp and Quest Diagnostics).

Comprehensive stool panel. A comprehensive stool panel can be used to detect certain pathogenic bacteria, yeast overgrowth, and parasites. However, it's important to keep in mind that false negatives are possible, especially with yeast and parasites. Most local labs also offer stool testing, including Labcorp and Quest Diagnostics. While these can provide some value, just keep in mind that these aren't as comprehensive as specialty labs that perform stool testing.

Organic acids test. I find the organic acids test to be the most accurate test for detecting yeast overgrowth, and it also has some value in detecting mold by looking at certain metabolites, including 5-hydroxymethyl-2-furoic, furan-2,5-dicarboxylic, and furancarbonylglycine. These are related to aspergillus and penicillum mold, and are usually the result of consumption of moldy food.

The organic acids test from Great Plains Laboratory also tests for clostridia bacterial markers. While many comprehensive stool panels will test for the presence of clostridia, most aren't able to differentiate between the commensal and pathogenic strains. Genova Diagnostics also offers an organic acids test.

SIBO breath test. Prior to the breath test, the person will follow a "prep" diet for 24 to 48 hours, and then fast 12 hours. Then, in the morning after the fast, they will start with a baseline breath test, followed by the consumption of a substrate (i.e., lactulose or glucose). After the baseline breath test, they will measure a breath sample approximately every 20 minutes. What the lab is looking for is bacterial fermentation by measuring the levels of hydrogen and methane. In other words, if someone has

SIBO, there will be more fermentation, which will lead to higher levels of hydrogen, methane, or both gases. Let's take a look at the two main breath tests used:

Lactulose breath test. Lactulose can't be absorbed by humans, but it can be broken down by bacteria. As bacteria consume lactulose, they produce hydrogen and/or methane gases, which are measured with the breath test. This is most commonly used because it can diagnose SIBO in the distal end of the small intestine.

Glucose breath test. The benefit of using glucose as a substrate is that all bacteria will ferment glucose, which isn't the case with lactulose. However, this test isn't as commonly used because glucose is absorbed in the beginning of the small intestine. Thus, if SIBO is occurring in the distal small intestine, then it is less likely to be detected. However, some bacteria don't ferment lactulose; Therefore, if SIBO is suspected yet the lactulose test comes back negative, then you should consider doing a glucose breath test. Another option is to do both the lactulose and glucose tests initially, although many labs don't offer both types of testing.

Some people reading this might wonder what the difference is between a breath test for SIBO, and a breath test for Helicobacter pylori. Whereas the breath test for SIBO uses either lactulose or glucose as a substrate, the urea breath test is used for diagnosing an active H. pylori infection. Thus, you can't use a urea breath test to determine if someone has SIBO, and you can't use a lactulose or glucose breath test to diagnose H. pylori.

Companies I have used for SIBO breath testing: BioHealth SIBO 3-hour glucose/lactulose test, Aerodiagnostics SIBO test, Genova Diagnostics SIBO test.

Can a Stool Panel Detect SIBO?

Hydrogen and methane are produced by bacteria and measured on the breath tests. The bacterium that accounts for most of the methane production in the body is methanobrevibacter smithii. Some comprehensive stool panels test for this methane-producing bacteria, including the GI Effects from Genova Diagnostics, and elevated levels of this bacteria might suggest that someone has SIBO. However, this is inconclusive, and the breath test remains the gold standard for determining if someone has SIBO.

SEX HORMONE TESTING

Blood testing. This is how most healthcare professionals test the sex hormones (i.e., estrogen, progesterone, testosterone), and I use blood testing at times as well. This is especially true for men and postmenopausal women, as in these a one sample test is sufficient. Although a cycling hormone test is a great option for cycling women, one can do a one-sample blood test in the early second half of the cycle, usually between days 18 through 21, although this may vary depending on the average length of the woman's menstrual cycle.

It's also important to understand that blood testing for the sex hormones usually involves measuring the "total" hormone, unless you specify the free form. For example, regarding blood testing for testosterone, many healthcare professionals will recommend testing for both the total and free testosterone. Total testosterone involves testing for mostly the bound form of the hormone, while free testosterone involves only looking at the free hormone. Although some labs do offer tests for free estradiol and free progesterone, the "total" estradiol and progesterone are usually ordered.

Saliva testing. This looks at the free form of the hormone. Although I recommend one-sample testing through saliva for many of my patients who are men, along with postmenopausal women, a cycling hormone test is preferred for cycling women. This involves collecting a single sample every few days of the cycle, which is more accurate than looking at a single sample in one's entire cycle.

Although I don't have all of my cycling patients do this test, it is a valuable test for those cycling women who are experiencing PMS symptoms, fertility issues, or other symptoms that might suggest a hormone imbalance. In addition to testing for progesterone, estradiol, and testosterone, it usually is a good idea to test for the pituitary hormones, which include follicle stimulating hormone (FSH) and luteinizing hormone (LH).

Companies I have used for salivary testing of the sex hormones: Diagnos-Techs cycling and postmenopausal female hormone panels, ZRT Laboratory saliva test, BioHealth Premenopause Hormone Profile.

Urine testing. The main benefit of urine testing for the sex hormones is the ability to measure the hormone metabolites. Estradiol and estrone both lead to the formation of estrogen metabolites, which include 2-hydroxyestrone (2-OH-E1), 4-hydroxyestrone (4-OH-E1), and 16α-hydroxyestrone (16α-OH-E1). These metabolites have different biological activity, as the 2-OH metabolite has weak estrogenic activity, and thus is labeled as being the "good" estrogen.

In contrast, the 4-OH and 16α-OH metabolites have a greater amount of estrogenic activity. Evidence shows that those with higher amounts of 4-OH and 16α-OH metabolites have an increased risk of developing certain types of cancers.[32] What are the benefits of testing the metabolites? Well, if someone has a greater ratio of the "bad" metabolites to the "good" metabolites, then they can take measures to increase the 2-OH metabolites by eating cruciferous vegetables regularly or taking a DIM supplement.

In addition to these metabolites, some companies test for other hormone metabolites. This includes a-pregnanediol, b-pregnanediol, 5a-androstanediol, 5b-androstanediol, and 2-Methoxy-estrone. Looking at these can also have some benefits. For example, it can help you determine if 2-OH-E1 is converting to 2-Methyoxy-E1.

Companies I have used for urinary testing of the sex hormones: Precision Analytical DUTCH Test, ZRT Urine Metabolites Profile

TESTING FOR ENVIRONMENTAL TOXINS

Provoked urine testing. Many healthcare professionals utilize both pre- and post-provocation testing. In other words, the patient collects a baseline urine sample, then takes some type of oral chelating agent such as dimercaptosuccinic acid (DMSA), dimercaptopropanesulfonate (DMPS), or ethylenediaminetetraacetic acid (EDTA), followed by a second urine collection. The purpose of the chelating agent is to mobilize heavy metals from the tissues, which will greatly increase the chances of one or more heavy metals being elevated on the second urine test.

Provoked urine testing is somewhat controversial. First, while most people seem to do fine when taking an oral chelating agent, adverse effects are possible. While, in some cases, this might be due to a detoxification reaction, in other cases it's due to an immune system reaction to the chelating agent.

In addition, there is some concern that mobilized heavy metals from the tissues might be redeposited in other areas of the body.[33] For example, if someone has a compromised blood brain barrier, then it's possible that these metals will be redeposited in the tissues of the brain, which can lead to neuroinflammation. However, this can be minimized by making sure that you have healthy glutathione levels. Thus, for anyone who takes an oral chelating agent or receives chelation therapy, it probably is wise to take measure to increase glutathione levels, which I discuss in section four.

Although I personally don't do provoked urine testing in my practice, I realize that many healthcare professionals successfully utilize this type of testing. This is just another example of how different practitioners will utilize different testing methods. Many of the same practitioners who recommend provoked urine testing will also use oral chelation therapy to assist with the excretion of heavy metals, which I'll discuss in Chapter 29. Everything comes down to risks vs. benefits, and while the risks of provoked urine testing might be minimal, a valid case can be made that other testing methods might be a better first option.

Companies that offer urinary testing of heavy metals: Genova Diagnostics Comprehensive Urine Element Profile, Doctor's Data Urine Toxic Metals test.

Hair mineral analysis. I like hair testing, although there admittedly are some limitations. Methylmercury is an example of organic mercury, and is the type found in fish. Hair analysis testing does a good job of picking up organic mercury, but does not do as good of a job of evaluating inorganic mercury, which is the mercury found in dental amalgams. However, urine testing is more accurate for inorganic mercury but is not as accurate for organic mercury. Thus, if you eat a large quantity of fish, then you probably want to do a hair analysis test, and if you have many mercury amalgams, then you might want to consider urine testing.

Speaking of eating a lot of fish, I once had a patient who had extremely high levels of mercury on his hair test. When I see high mercury levels on a hair test, one of the first things I ask the patient is if they eat fish frequently, and if so, what type of fish. In this person's case, he had been eating tuna sandwiches daily for many years. Many species of tuna are high in mercury; thus, this explains why his mercury levels were so high on this test.

Companies I have used for hair mineral analysis testing: Analytical Research Labs Hair Tissue Mineral Analysis, Trace Elements Hair Tissue Mineral Analysis.

Blood testing for heavy metals. Blood testing is typically used for acute heavy metal exposure. For example, if you are working in a factory and are constantly being exposed to certain heavy metals, then this is likely to show up in the blood.

Quicksilver Scientific Mercury Tri-Test. This measures both methylmercury and inorganic mercury. This doesn't involve provoked challenge testing, and uses blood, hair, and urine samples as part of the analysis. This can be a great option for determining the body burden of mercury.

Stool testing for heavy metals. Some labs offer stool testing for heavy metals, and while most practitioners (including myself) don't utilize this type of testing, fecal excretion is the major route of elimination for many toxic metals. One study I came across showed that hepatic biliary concentrations of lead and arsenic were higher than urinary concentrations, although some other heavy metals such as cadmium and inorganic mercury were higher in the urine.[34] Not too many labs offer this type of testing, although Doctor's Data is one of them.

GPL-TOX. This is a relatively new test by the company Great Plains Laboratory, as this is a urine test that screens for the presence of 172 different toxic chemicals using 18 different metabolites, including organophosphate pesticides, phthalates, benzene, xylene, vinyl chloride, pyrethroid insecticides, acrylamide, perchlorate, diphenyl phosphate, ethylene oxide, acrylonitrile, and more. This panel also tests for a marker called tiglylglycine, which is a marker for mitochondrial damage. You can also add glyphosate to this panel or can test for this separately.

You might wonder what the point of getting such a test is. After all, why not simply save the money on testing and take measures to support detoxification, which I'll discuss in Chapter 29. This, of course, is an option, and, without question, there are too many environmental toxins to test for; thus, on the surface, it might make sense to bypass the testing and to simply support detoxification. I admit that this is the approach that I take with most of my patients.

However, while increasing glutathione levels and utilizing infrared sauna therapy can be beneficial in most people even without doing any testing, the number one goal is to minimize your exposure to environmental toxins. That's where the value of this test lies. For example, if someone tests positive for perchlorate, the most likely source is water; thus, in this case, the person would want to make sure to use a water filtration device that will remove this, and/or drink from a different source (e.g., spring water out of a glass bottle).

An increase in phenylglyoxylic acid is usually indicative of exposure to styrene, which can be found in automobile exhaust, cigarette smoke, packaging materials, insulation for electrical uses, insulation for homes, styrofoam drinking cups, fiberglass, and other sources. Monoethyl Phthalate (MEP) is the most abundant phthalate metabolite found in urine, and usually comes from plastic products. 3-Phenoxybenzoic Acid (3PBA) is a metabolite of pyrethroid insecticides. These are just a few examples of how we are exposed to these chemicals.

Cyrex Labs Chemical Immune Reactivity Screen (Array #11). Unlike most tests that measure the levels of certain chemicals, the Array #11 is a blood test that measures the immune system response to some of the more common environmental toxins. This can be a very valuable test, as you can have low levels of heavy metals on one of the other tests I discussed, yet have an immune system response to one or more of these. What happens is that certain chemicals can bind to our tissues, and the immune system will not just attack the chemical, but our own tissues as well. This is one mechanism of how an environmental toxin can be a trigger for autoimmunity.

For example, someone can have an entire mouth filled with mercury amalgams, yet not have an immune system response to the mercury. This doesn't mean that there aren't negative health consequences associated with the mercury, but in this situation it means that the mercury isn't an autoimmune trigger. However, someone with only one or two mercury amalgams can have an immune system that is reacting to the mercury.

This is dependent on whether or not the person has what's referred to as chemical tolerance. If the person has a loss of chemical tolerance, also referred to as toxicant-induced loss of tolerance (TILT), then their immune system is likely to react to the mercury and other chemicals. Thus, while one can make a valid argument that having ten mercury amalgams is worse than having two mercury amalgams, if the person with ten mercury amalgams has chemical tolerance, while the person with two mercury amalgams has a loss of chemical tolerance, then the person with only two silver fillings is much more likely to develop an immune system reaction.

But the Array #11 doesn't just test for mercury. It tests for the antibodies to other heavy metals, as well as the antibodies to other common environmental toxins, including bisphenol A (BPA), aflatoxins, formaldehyde, isocyanate, benzene, parabens, and tetrachloroethylene. Because this test measures the antibodies, there is always a possibility of a false negative result; thus, before doing this test, it probably is a good idea to get the serum immunoglobulin G, M, and A levels tested.

TESTING FOR NUTRIENT DEFICIENCIES

Local blood testing. I use local blood testing to measure some of the nutrients. First, I recommend a 25-OH vitamin D test for most of my patients. I also usually recommend a complete iron panel, vitamin B12, and RBC folate. I discussed this in Chapter 24. RBC magnesium and RBC zinc can also provide some value. However, there are limitations when it comes to testing nutrients through the blood, although this is the case with other methods as well.

Micronutrient panels. Some companies focus on micronutrient testing, which involves evaluating all of the vitamins, minerals, and antioxidants. One of the more well-known labs tests the micronutrients through the white blood cells, specifically the lymphocytes. These lymphocytes are supposed to represent a history of an individual's nutrient status and the intracellular deficiencies.
    Companies that offer micronutrient testing: Spectracell Laboratories.

Hair mineral analysis. As I mentioned earlier, I like the hair mineral analysis test, although just as is the case with micronutrient panels, I'd never rely on this test for evaluating all of the minerals. However, this test isn't just evaluating nutrient deficiencies, but it also looks for excess mineral levels (i.e., copper toxicity) and certain patterns. Thus, interpreting this test on the surface might seem easy, but it can be very challenging.
    While hair testing evaluates the heavy metals, it also isn't perfect in this regard. Just as is the case with urine testing, hair testing won't reveal all of the heavy metals because most people have many toxic metals stored in their tissues. This is the reasoning behind provoked urine testing, although this also isn't perfect, and as mentioned earlier, it comes with certain risks. The truth is that there is no perfect test that will give us all

of the answers regarding detecting mineral imbalances and heavy metal toxicities. Nevertheless, hair mineral analysis can provide some valuable information at a very reasonable cost.

Organic acids test. Over the last few years, I've ordered many organic acids tests for my patients, as it's a wonderful test. It does a lot more than test for nutrients, and it only evaluates some of the nutrients. For example, the company I use the most measures methylmalonic acid, which is an excellent marker for vitamin B12. It also evaluates markers related to vitamin B2, vitamin B6, vitamin B5, biotin, vitamin C, CoQ10, and N-acetylcysteine.

TESTING FOR AN IODINE DEFICIENCY

Because testing for iodine can be somewhat complex, I will discuss this separately. A few different methods of iodine deficiency testing exist. Unfortunately, no consensus about which is the most accurate method has been established. Blood testing doesn't seem to be too accurate, as it doesn't test for the levels of iodine in the tissues. Urine testing seems to be the most accurate, although there are limitations with this type of testing as well. In addition, different types of urine tests can make testing for iodine confusing.

You can do a one-sample iodine spot test, a 24-hour urinary iodine test, and a 24-hour urinary iodine loading test. Although I like the iodine loading test, as this is the test I used when I was diagnosed with Graves' disease, the dilemma is that this test involves taking a 50 mg tablet of potassium iodide before collecting the urine samples. While many people do fine when taking this high dose of potassium iodide, there is always a risk of someone having a negative reaction.

A safer option would be to do an iodine spot test, or a 24-hour urinary iodine test. If you choose to do an iodine spot test, I would also recommend testing the bromide levels, as when these levels are elevated, this almost always indicates an iodine deficiency, even in the presence of normal iodine levels. As for what lab to use for iodine testing, a number of different labs conduct urinary iodine testing, although I usually use Hakala Labs (**www.hakalalabs.com**).

Elevated serum thyroglobulin levels can also be an indication of an iodine deficiency.[35,36] Keep in mind that I'm discussing testing for "thyroglobulin," and not the "thyroglobulin antibodies." Some healthcare professionals aren't familiar with the thyroglobulin marker on a blood test, and they commonly order the thyroglobulin antibodies instead; thus, you want to specify when requesting to get this measured. It's also important to realize that elevated thyroglobulin levels can also be an indication for thyroid cancer.[37,38] Keep in mind that I have worked with many patients who had elevated thyroglobulin values and didn't have cancer; nevertheless, it's something to be aware of.

TESTING FOR FOOD ALLERGIES/SENSITIVITIES

Food allergy testing. Food allergies are typically referred to as being IgE-mediated. In other words, they involve something called IgE immuno-globulins. Immunoglobulins are also known as antibodies, as they are produced by your immune system and attach to foreign substances, and then your immune system attacks and destroys these substances. IgE is found in the lung, skin, and mucous membranes, and this immuno-globulin is typically involved in immediate allergic reactions.

For example, if someone is allergic to peanuts and accidentally eats a peanut or is stung by a bee and has a severe allergic reaction within a few seconds or minutes, this is typically an IgE-mediated reaction. IgE-mediated reactions occur within two hours of exposure, although, in most cases, the person reacts much sooner than this. Some of the more common foods that cause allergic reactions include milk, eggs, peanuts, fish, wheat, soy, tree nuts in children, and peanuts, tree nuts, fish, and shellfish in adults.[39,40]

These types of allergies can cause symptoms involving the skin, gastro-intestinal tract, respiratory tract, and other areas.[39] Some of the potential causes of food allergies include a vitamin D deficiency, eating unhealthy dietary fat, obesity, increased hygiene, and the timing of exposure to foods, although genetics and other lifestyle factors can also play a role.[41] And evidence shows that a leaky gut can increase the incidence of IgE allergies due to a loss of oral tolerance.[42]

Food sensitivity testing. Whereas food allergies are IgE-mediated, food sensitivities involve immunoglobulin G (IgG). These immunoglobulins play an important role in fighting bacterial and viral infections. They are involved in delayed-type reactions, and they aren't always accompanied by overt symptoms. While someone who has an IgE-mediated food allergy will present with symptoms within the first two hours of exposure to the allergen, and frequently within a few seconds or minutes, it can take a few days for someone with an IgG food sensitivity to develop symptoms.

I don't recommend IgG testing initially to my patients for a few reasons. One reason is that false results are common. For example, someone might have a false negative for a certain food on one of these panels, and continue to eat that food. Consequently, they will continue to experience inflammation.

A few factors can minimize false results, such as running through the sample twice, and the purity of the antigen. These are also expensive tests for being inaccurate. Nevertheless, I think they have some value, and, at times, I will order food sensitivity testing for my patients, but it's not something I recommend to everyone.

Remember that not everyone with a food sensitivity will develop overt symptoms. Others will develop symptoms, but they won't always be gastrointestinal in nature. In other words, while some people with food sensitivities might experience digestive symptoms such as gas, bloating, and/or stomach pain, others might experience fatigue, brain fog, joint pain, and other extraintestinal symptoms.

Food intolerance testing. Unlike food allergies and food sensitivities, food intolerances don't involve immunoglobulins. They are typically caused by enzymatic defects in the digestive system (e.g., lactose intolerance), although they might also result from pharmacological effects of vasoactive amines present in foods.[43] An example of a vasoactive amine is histamine, and when someone has a histamine intolerance, they have an imbalance between levels of released histamine and the ability of the body to metabolize it.[44] Many people have a lactose intolerance, which is usually caused by a reduction in lactase activity.[45] Lactase is the enzyme that breaks down lactose.

To better understand the difference between an allergy, sensitivity, and intolerance, let's use dairy as an example. Casein is a protein in dairy, and it is possible to have a casein allergy or a casein sensitivity. A casein allergy is IgE-mediated, and if someone has a casein allergy, they will usually experience overt symptoms within a few minutes or few hours of consuming dairy.

However, a casein sensitivity is IgG-mediated and can take a few hours or a few days to present with symptoms, and many times the person won't experience overt symptoms, which can make it even more challenging to diagnose. A lactose intolerance is different from a dairy allergy or sensitivity in that it doesn't involve the immune system, but instead involves a reduction of the enzyme lactase, which breaks down lactose.

Companies I have used for food allergen testing: Cyrex Labs Array #3, #4, #10, Alletess Comprehensive Food Panel, IgG, IgA.

Celiac panel. I discussed celiac disease in greater detail in section two. celiac disease is triggered by a combination of genetic and lifestyle factors. Regarding the genetics of celiac disease, more than 95% of patients with celiac disease share the major histocompatibility complex II class human leukocyte antigen (HLA) DQ2 or DQ8 haplotype.[46] If someone tests negative for these markers, there is a good chance they don't have celiac disease, although not having these markers doesn't completely rule this condition out.

In addition to testing for the genetic markers of celiac disease, one can also obtain a celiac panel. Although a negative celiac panel doesn't always rule out celiac disease, obtaining such a panel is usually a good place to start if someone suspects a gluten sensitivity issue. Some people only get the gliadin antibodies tested, but keep in mind that it's possible for these to be negative even if someone has celiac disease.

If a problem with gluten is suspected, you want to test the gliadin antibodies, the antibodies to tissue transglutaminase, and the anti-endomysial antibodies. It's also a good idea to test both immunoglobulin A (IgA) and immunoglobulin G (IgG) because if one of these immunoglobulins happens to be depressed, it can result in a false negative result, causing the person to think that their body doesn't react to gluten when the opposite is true.

TESTING FOR HYPERGLYCEMIA AND INSULIN RESISTANCE

One way to help determine if someone has high blood sugar levels is by doing a fasting blood glucose test. If someone has a glucose level of 100 mg/dl or greater, but less than 125 mg/dl, then this confirms that the person has hyperglycemia. However, from an "optimal" standpoint, you want this value to be between 70 and 90 mg/dl. Some sources will suggest a narrower range of between 70 and 85 mg/dl.

The glucose tolerance test is another test that can help determine if someone has blood sugar issues. With this test, the person fasts for a minimum of eight hours, and then a fasting blood glucose test is taken before they drink a glucose solution, and then their blood glucose levels are measured two hours later. If the levels are between 140 and 199 mg/dl then hyperglycemia is a factor, although some experts such as Dr. Mark Hyman recommend for the levels to be below 120 mg/dl after two hours.

There are variations of this test, as some doctors will test the blood glucose levels one, two, and three hours after drinking the glucose solution. It's also a good idea to test the fasting insulin levels, as well as testing insulin after doing the glucose challenge. If this value is high, then this is a sign of insulin resistance. Ideally, the fasting insulin levels should be less than 5 mg/dl, and less than 30 mg/dl after one or two hours of drinking the glucose solution.

C-peptide can also be a valuable test to help evaluate insulin production by the pancreatic beta cells. Elevated levels of C-peptide relates to high insulin production. A common reference range used by labs is 0.8-3.1 ng/ml.

Is It Necessary to Get a Thyroid Ultrasound?

An ultrasound uses sound waves to develop images, and it is the most sensitive imaging modality available for examining the thyroid gland. A thyroid ultrasound also has the benefit of being non-invasive, it doesn't use ionizing radiation, and it is less expensive than other imaging techniques such as an MRI and CT scan. However, does this mean that everyone with a suspected or confirmed case of Hashimoto's should consider getting a thyroid ultrasound?

Although having a thyroid ultrasound doesn't directly relate to finding or removing the triggers of Hashimoto's, I felt that this section on testing would be incomplete without briefly discussing this. While I'm sure many people reading this have already obtained a thyroid ultrasound, others haven't obtained one but might wonder if it is wise to obtain one.

Can a Thyroid Ultrasound Be Used to Diagnose Hashimoto's?

Although the diagnosis of Hashimoto's is usually confirmed by an elevated TSH combined with the presence of thyroid peroxidase and/or thyroglobulin antibodies, these antibodies are not always positive in those with Hashimoto's. When this is the case, getting a thyroid ultrasound can be beneficial, as, many times, this can confirm the presence of Hashimoto's.

Unfortunately, many medical doctors won't use an ultrasound for this purpose, as they will conclude that the person doesn't have Hashimoto's. If you fall under this category it is worth asking your doctor to order an ultrasound.

What's the Deal With Thyroid Nodules?

It is very common to have thyroid nodules. One journal article mentioned that while 4 to 7% of the population have palpable thyroid nodules, ultrasonography reveals that up to 67% of the population has them.[47] Another study mentioned that up to 35% of the population have thyroid nodules show up on an ultrasound.[48] While the statistics are conflicting, the good news is that most thyroid nodules are benign. As for why many people have thyroid nodules, one of the more common reasons relates to problems with estrogen metabolism. Estrogen not only can increase the risk of thyroid cancer, but it can also increase the risk of developing thyroid nodules.[49,50]

An iodine deficiency can also play a role, as thyroid nodules are four times more common in women than men, and their frequency increases with age and low iodine intake.[51] While iodine is controversial in the world of thyroid health (see Chapter 14), this mineral plays a role in estrogen metabolism. Thus, having an iodine deficiency can greatly increase one's risk of developing thyroid nodules.

When Is A Biopsy Necessary?

If you are considering having a biopsy done, read the article "Too Many Unnecessary Thyroid Biopsies Performed," which you can find if you do a Google search or visit **www.naturalendocrinesolutions.com/resources**. This is based on a report in JAMA internal Medicine[52] that involved 8806 patients, and three ultrasound nodule characteristics—microcalcifications, size greater than 2 cm, and an entirely solid composition—were the only findings associated with the risk of thyroid cancer. Based on these findings, the authors of the study suggested that rather than performing a biopsy of all thyroid nodules larger than 5 mm, one should instead require two abnormal nodule characteristics to determine if someone should require a biopsy. They mention how this would reduce unnecessary biopsies by 90% while maintaining a low risk of cancer.

In other words, if someone has a thyroid nodule and is concerned about it being malignant, it probably would be best to hold off on getting a biopsy unless if they had at least two of the following three characteristics:

1. A nodule size greater than 2 cm
2. An entirely solid composition
3. Microcalcifications of the thyroid nodule

OTHER TYPES OF TESTING

Although I listed some of the more common tests done by healthcare professionals, other tests can be beneficial to obtain in certain situations. For example, the organic acids test measures markers related to the mitochondria, and, while there isn't a perfect test for determining whether someone has mitochondrial dysfunction, the organic acids test can give an indication of this. Many people have problems with histamine, which is involved in allergies and inflammation, although it also acts as a neurotransmitter. Testing the histamine levels along with diamine oxidase (DAO) can provide some value in those who suspect a histamine intolerance. The company Dunwoody Labs offers an Advanced Intestinal Barrier Assessment, which measures histamine, DAO, and zonulin.

Which Tests Should YOU Choose to Do?

Now that I listed many different types of tests, you might be wondering which ones you should personally do. This depends on the person, as not everyone requires the same test. This also is where a comprehensive health history can be important, as this can determine whether someone needs more comprehensive testing. For example, while I recommend blood testing and adrenal saliva testing to just about all of my patients, I don't recommend a comprehensive stool panel to every patient. While it's true that a healthy gut is necessary in order to have a healthy immune system, I have helped many patients get into remission without having them do a stool panel.

Does this mean that those healthcare professionals who recommend stool testing to all of their patients are wrong? Of course not, as when it comes to testing, you can take one of two possible approaches:

Conservative vs. Comprehensive Testing

One approach is to be conservative with the testing and just start out with some basic tests (e.g., blood tests, a saliva panel), and then, if you aren't progressing as expected, you can always choose to do additional testing. I take this approach with most of my patients; although, at times I will recommend a comprehensive stool panel or other types of testing initially. The upside of being conservative with testing is that it can save the person money. The downside is that you might not detect the problem, and, as a result, the person will end up not progressing until more comprehensive testing is done.

Another approach is to do comprehensive testing on all patients from the start. The benefit of doing this is that you are more likely to find the cause of the problem. The downside is that not everyone needs comprehensive testing, and some people simply can't afford to spend a lot of money on tests. If you are experiencing severe symptoms, want to find answers quickly, and are able to afford more comprehensive testing, then this might be the best option. However, if your symptoms aren't too severe and/or you can't afford a lot of testing upfront, then it might make sense to take a more conservative approach.

Can Symptoms Be Used to Determine Which Tests Are Necessary?

Earlier in this chapter, I mentioned how you can't always go by symptoms when determining what tests you need. While knowing one's symptoms can be important, which is why I brought it up in Chapter 22, you can't always rely on symptoms. For example, the lack of digestive symptoms doesn't rule out gut problems. It's possible to have positive results on a comprehensive stool panel, even if you have no digestive symptoms. The reverse is true as well, as I've had patients with multiple digestive symptoms not show any significant findings on a comprehensive stool panel.

In many cases, it's a good idea to work with a competent natural healthcare professional, as they will give you guidance about what tests you should choose. They will conduct a thorough health history and try to use this information to determine which tests are necessary. Ultimately, the decision is yours to make, but it still can be helpful to receive some guidance.

Keep in mind that just about all healthcare professionals, including myself, have certain biases about testing. For example, while I like adrenal saliva testing, other practitioners don't do adrenal testing. Some healthcare professionals recommend a comprehensive stool panel to all of their patients, while others recommend it to some patients but not all of them, which is the approach I currently take.

I will add that while I commonly recommend basic tests initially, I'll usually give the patient an option to do some more comprehensive testing. In other words, after the initial consultation I'll recommend what I feel are the most important tests, but I'll also give some optional recommendations.

How Can You Order These Tests?

If you are currently working with a natural healthcare professional, they should be able to order one or more of these tests for you. If you aren't, then you can ask your primary care physician to order these. However, while medical doctors are increasingly open to ordering these "alternative" tests, many won't be willing to order them. If you are unable to order these tests on your own, please visit the website **www. naturalendocrinesolutions.com/testing**.

Detecting Triggers Through Testing Case Study

Glenda started working with me recently after being diagnosed with Hashimoto's. She did some initial testing, including blood tests and an adrenal saliva panel, and a few months after she started following my recommendations she noticed some positive changes in her symptoms. Many of her blood test markers improved, and she also did an updated adrenal panel that looked much better after initially revealing low cortisol levels and a depressed DHEA. However, her thyroid peroxidase and thyroglobulin antibodies remained elevated. At the time she didn't have any digestive symptoms, and she had regular bowel movements with well formed stools. However, I told her that something was missing, and we both decided that a comprehensive stool panel was a good next test to order.

She agreed to order a comprehensive stool panel, and sure enough, parasites were detected. To make a long story short, Glenda received treatment for the parasitic infection and her antibodies normalized shortly thereafter. There are a few lessons to learn from this case study. First, finding the trigger or triggers can be a challenge at times. But perhaps more importantly, you can't always rely on symptoms. While I can't say that I recommend a comprehensive stool panel to everyone, if someone isn't progressing then additional testing might be necessary, and you can't always rely on symptoms when determining what additional tests can be beneficial.

Chapter Highlights:

- There are flaws with relying on your symptoms in order to determine which tests are necessary.
- Adrenal testing can be accomplished through the blood, saliva, and urine.
- Other tests that can determine the health of the adrenals include the ACTH stimulation test, aldosterone, and Ragland's test.
- A comprehensive stool panel is one of the best, and perhaps the best test, for determining the health of the digestive system.
- An organic acids test evaluates for markers of yeast and bacterial overgrowth, although it also looks at other metabolites related to neurotransmitters, mitochondrial function, nutrients, and glutathione production.
- Testing for infections can be accomplished through the blood, stool, and urine.
- Sex hormone testing can be done through the blood, saliva, or urine.
- Some of the tests used for detecting environmental toxins include a provoked urine test, hair mineral analysis, blood testing, urine testing, and even stool testing.
- Nutrient deficiencies can be detected through the blood, hair, and urine.
- Unfortunately there isn't a perfect test for measuring all nutrient deficiencies.
- Food allergies are IgE-mediated, while food sensitivities are IgG-mediated and involve a delayed reaction.
- Some healthcare professionals are more conservative with their testing, while others recommend comprehensive testing to all of their patients.

Chapter Highlights, continued:

- As for which tests you should do, everyone is different, which is one reason why it's wise to work with a natural healthcare professional who can help determine which tests you will need.

• SECTION FOUR

REMOVING THE TRIGGERS

I N THIS SECTION, I will show you what you need to do in order to get into remission by removing your specific triggers. In Chapter 26, I start by talking about the foods you should eat and avoid, and then Chapter 27 discusses how you can balance your adrenals and sex hormones. Since having a healthy gut is essential to having a healthy immune system, I dedicated a separate chapter (Chapter 28) to healing the gut. In Chapter 29, I discuss how to eliminate harmful chemicals from your body, followed by how to correct nutrient deficiencies in Chapter 30. There are also chapters on overcoming infections (Chapter 31), getting a better night's sleep (Chapter 32), and how to deal with challenging cases (Chapter 33), which specifically focuses on Lyme disease, toxic mold, and SIBO.

Food Options vs. Supplements

Although you want to accomplish as much as you can through diet, I find that nutritional supplements are usually necessary to help someone achieve a state of remission. As mentioned in the opening paragraph, there is an entire chapter in section four dedicated to showing you which foods you should eat and which ones you should avoid (Chapter 26), but, in most of the other chapters, I also give supplement recommendations, including suggested doses. While I do recommend supplements to my patients, you need to keep in mind that taking a lot of nutritional supplements and herbs isn't always a good thing. This might seem like common sense, but it's common for people to be taking 20 to 30 different supplements prior to their first consultation with me.

And while many people do fine when taking multiple supplements and herbs simultaneously, you might want to consider starting with smaller doses and then gradually increase. In fact, one can argue that it might be best to start with one supplement at a time, and then you can add a new one every few days. This is especially true if you have a lot of known food and/or supplement sensitivities. The advantage of taking this approach is that if you happen to have a negative reaction, it will be much easier to pinpoint the specific supplement that is causing problems.

Note: For the food sources listed in this section, I commonly referenced the information provided on the World's Healthiest Foods website, which is whfoods.org. I found this to be a great resource, as it lists the foods that are highest in individual nutrients (e.g., magnesium, zinc, and iron).

Do I Give Specific Supplement Recommendations?

Although I do give suggested doses, please keep in mind that everyone is different, which is why I made sure to include the disclaimer you'll read next. In addition, I don't recommend specific supplement brands in this book (with a few exceptions) because I didn't want this section to focus on supplements. While I do recommend supplements to my patients and give supplement recommendations in this section, I also try to give plenty of food options as well. If you are interested in what specific brands of supplements I recommend, please visit **www.naturalendocrinesolutions. com/resources**.

DISCLAIMER: I just wanted to remind you that the information presented in this section is not a substitute for professional medical advice. Everyone is different, and, therefore, each person requires different supplements and doses, and some people do experience negative reactions with certain supplements and herbs. Please consult your healthcare practitioner before engaging in any treatments that are suggested in this section.

Work With A Competent Healthcare Professional

Since I'm a natural healthcare professional, I'm biased and feel like everyone with Hashimoto's should consult with a practitioner who has a lot of experience working with Hashimoto's patients. And while it might seem easy enough to self-treat your condition after reading section four, the truth is that Hashimoto's is a very complex condition. As a result, for optimal results, it is wise to work with an expert.

● CHAPTER 26 ●

ELIMINATING DIETARY TRIGGERS AND USING FOOD AS MEDICINE

I COMMONLY RECOMMEND THAT MY patients with Hashimoto's initially follow an autoimmune Paleo (AIP) diet because this diet eliminates the most common food triggers as well as foods that can cause a leaky gut. This doesn't mean that everyone with this condition needs to follow a strict AIP diet until they achieve a state of remission. Many people will only need to follow this diet for one to three months before reintroducing other foods.

Although some people with Hashimoto's do great when following an AIP diet, others struggle, and the stress associated with following an AIP diet can have a negative effect on one's recovery. In this chapter, I'll discuss the AIP diet and the different categories of foods, including those that are excluded from an AIP diet, and whether these foods can eventually be reintroduced, although I discussed the reintroduction of foods in greater detail in Chapter 23.

What I'd first like to do is discuss in greater detail the similarities and differences between a "standard" Paleo diet and an AIP diet. Here are the main **foods that are allowed** on a standard Paleo diet:

- Meat (beef, pork, chicken, lamb, etc.) and fish
- Eggs
- Fruits

- Vegetables (including the nightshades)
- Fermented foods (sauerkraut, kimchi, pickles, kombucha tea, unsweetened coconut yogurt)
- Nuts and seeds
- Herbal teas
- Coconut oil, olive oil, avocado oil

Foods that are excluded from a standard Paleo diet include all grains (including gluten-free grains), legumes, and dairy products. Of course, anything processed should also be avoided, which includes but isn't limited to refined foods and sugars, as well as fast food. A standard Paleo diet is restrictive with regards to what foods you can eat, although keep in mind that it is nutrient dense, and the goal isn't to restrict calories. Thus, while some people do struggle initially when following a standard Paleo diet, many of these people eventually thrive and wish they had followed this sooner.

Many people do better upon avoiding the grains, legumes, and dairy products. However, when someone also needs to avoid eating eggs, nuts and seeds, along with the nightshade vegetables, this makes it even more challenging. Not surprisingly, it's a greater challenge for a strict vegetarian or vegan to follow an AIP diet, as they won't be consuming any meat or fish.

Now that you know what foods are allowed and excluded on a standard Paleo diet, let's look at the foods that are allowed on an standard Paleo diet:

- Meat (beef, pork, chicken, lamb, etc.) and fish
- Fruits
- Vegetables (excluding the nightshades)
- Fermented foods (sauerkraut, kimchi, pickles, kombucha, unsweetened coconut yogurt)
- Herbal teas
- Coconut oil, olive oil, avocado oil
- Most coconut products (i.e., coconuts, coconut milk, coconut kefir)

You can see that the AIP diet is similar to a standard Paleo diet, but it excludes eggs, nightshade vegetables, nuts, and seeds.

Why Does An Autoimmune Paleo Diet Restrict so Many Foods?

Two main reasons why certain foods are excluded from an AIP diet are:

Reason #1: An AIP diet excludes common food allergens. Examples include gluten, dairy, eggs, soy, and corn. These foods can cause inflammation and, in some cases, can be autoimmune triggers, while other foods might not be a direct trigger but can still exacerbate an existing inflammatory condition. Gluten is the worse culprit. While not everyone has a problem with gluten from a symptomatic perspective, gluten can be a trigger of Hashimoto's. This is why I dedicated Chapter 5 to gluten in section two.

Reason #2: An AIP diet excludes foods that can cause an increase in intestinal permeability and/or can interfere with gut healing. For example, gluten isn't only a common allergen, but it can cause a leaky gut, which is a factor in many, if not all, cases of Hashimoto's. Other foods such as all grains, legumes, and the nightshade vegetables contain compounds that not only affect the absorption of nutrients but also, like gluten, can have a negative effect on the health of the gut. I'll discuss these and other excluded foods in greater detail in this chapter.

Keep in mind that, while not all of the foods excluded from an AIP diet are direct triggers of Hashimoto's, certain foods such as gluten, dairy, and corn can potentially be triggers through a molecular mimicry mechanism. Other foods such as eggs and the nightshades don't directly trigger Hashimoto's, but they have compounds that can increase intestinal permeability; thus they are potential "leaky gut triggers." This doesn't mean that everyone who eats eggs, tomatoes, or other excluded foods will develop a leaky gut, but when someone already has an increase in intestinal permeability it is a good idea to eliminate all of the potentially problematic foods in order to optimize gut healing.

The First Month

When someone with Hashimoto's consults with me for the very first time, I usually recommend that they follow a strict AIP diet for at least the first 30 days. While many people can benefit from following an AIP diet for a longer period, some people are ready to reintroduce foods after 30 days.

This doesn't mean that they can reintroduce any food, as, in most cases, the goal is to have the patient make the transition from an AIP diet to a standard Paleo diet. Some people do fine when reintroducing other "forbidden" foods such as gluten free grains and dairy, although I usually encourage my patients to try to avoid dairy and grains while trying to get into remission.

After the First Month

What do I recommend after the first 30 days? If the person is thriving on the AIP diet and is fine following this diet for a few additional months, then I'll encourage them to do so. If they are struggling with the diet, then I'm open to having them reintroduce some foods. I discussed reintroducing foods in great detail in Chapter 23.

Taking a Look at the Different Food Categories

In an attempt to make this easy to understand, I'll go through each category of food, discussing some of the main foods within each category that can be consumed and which ones should be avoided. Remember that everyone is different, and, while some people with Hashimoto's thrive when following a strict AIP diet, others struggle with this type of diet and do better when reintroducing certain foods.

Vegetables. Most people with Hashimoto's should eat a wide variety of vegetables each day, at least four to six servings of vegetables, although more than this would be even better. This includes vegetables such as artichokes, asparagus, broccoli, carrots, celery, kale, lettuce, onions, spinach, squash, sweet potatoes, and zucchini. As for whether they should be raw or cooked, if you can tolerate raw vegetables, then I would recommend eating a combination of both raw and cooked vegetables each day. Some people are only able to digest cooked vegetables while healing their gut.

It's important to eat a wide variety of vegetables. Not eating a wide variety of vegetable is one reason why many people find the AIP diet to be too restrictive. While this isn't the only reason, eating a wide variety of vegetables daily will make it easier for you to follow this diet.

Should You Avoid Cruciferous Vegetables?

Some people reading this are probably wondering if they should avoid cruciferous vegetables (e.g., broccoli, cabbage, kale, and cauliflower) due to their goitrogenic properties. Goitrogens consist of foods and other substances that can disrupt the production of thyroid hormone. A number of years ago, I did recommend that anyone with a hypothyroid condition completely avoid these foods, but when I finally did my own research, I found a lack of studies showing evidence of foods such as cruciferous vegetables having goitrogenic effects in humans. I'm not suggesting that people with hypothyroid conditions should eat large amounts of raw cruciferous veggies, but these are very healthy foods, and in most cases, eating a couple of servings per day won't cause any issues in those people with Hashimoto's.

While most people can eat a few servings of cruciferous vegetables each day, if someone has a moderate to severe iodine deficiency, then they might want to limit their consumption because the thiocyanates in cruciferous vegetables inhibit thyroid transport and the incorporation of iodide into thyroglobulin.[1] However, even in the presence of an iodine deficiency, eating one or two servings of cruciferous vegetables is fine for most people. If you are concerned, you can always choose to do a urinary iodine test to check your iodine status. Also, keep in mind that cooking cruciferous vegetables will help to reduce their goitrogenic properties, although this won't completely eliminate them.

Why Do the Nightshades Commonly Cause Problems?

Many people with Hashimoto's will want to be cautious about eating the nightshade vegetables, which include tomatoes, eggplant, white potatoes, and most types of peppers, because these foods contain compounds that can negatively affect the health of the gut. These compounds include lectins, alkaloids, and glycoalkaloids.

Lectins can potentially cause damage to the intestinal lining, which, in turn, can cause or exacerbate a leaky gut. Since a leaky gut is a factor in autoimmune conditions, it would make sense to avoid foods that have higher amounts of lectins while trying to restore your health back to normal. Legumes are another category of foods that are very high in lectins, which is why they're excluded from not only an AIP diet but also a AIP diet.

Sticking with the subject of nightshades, I'd like to discuss alkaloids and glycoalkaloids, and how they can have a negative impact on your health. I probably should warn you that the information included in these next few paragraphs will be somewhat advanced; thus, please feel free to skip this if you don't want to know about the compounds included in nightshades.

Capsaicin is an alkaloid found in spicy peppers. It's also the active ingredient in pepper spray and is responsible for the acute inflammation and burning feeling when sprayed, and might even cause bronchocon-striction.[2] Reports of pepper-spray-related injuries,[3,4] very well might be due to some people being highly sensitive to capsaicin.

This doesn't mean that everyone will have a negative reaction when consuming hot peppers, but it's something to keep in mind, and like toma-toes, eating these can prevent some people with Hashimoto's from going into remission. However, it's not just hot peppers that should be avoided; you will also want to avoid most other types of peppers. The exception might be small amounts of black pepper.

Solanine is a glycoalkaloid found in the nightshades, especially eggplant and potatoes, although it's also found in tomatoes and peppers. Solanine has fungicidal and pesticidal properties because these compounds are used as a form of protection by plants. The way it affects insects who feed on these plants is by the inhibition of acetylcholinesterase,[5] which breaks down acetylcholine.

Acetylcholine inhibitors can lead to problems with the nervous system, and can cause other health issues such as hypotension, bronchoconstric-tion, and hypermotility of the GI tract. This doesn't mean that everyone who eats these foods will have problems breaking down acetylcholine, but many people do react to the solanines and experience a significant improvement in their symptoms upon avoiding these foods.

Does Cooking Nightshades Reduce These Compounds?

Evidence shows that cooking can reduce the levels of some of these com-pounds found in the nightshades, such as solanine.[6] However, cooking won't complete degrade all of these compounds, and some people still have problems with cooked nightshades. Thus, it still is a good idea to initially avoid the nightshades, and, when eventually reintroducing these foods, it is a good idea to cook them.

Do the Vegetables You Eat Need to Be Organic?

Is it essential to eat only organic vegetables? Of course, this is ideal, but in some areas, it can be difficult to purchase organic food, and it is also more expensive. However, you do want to minimize your exposure to pesticides, and, while using a fruit and vegetable rinse can help to some extent, eating organic is best.

Over the years, I have referred my patients to the website of the Envi-ronmental Working Group (**www.ewg.org**) to obtain the Dirty Dozen and Clean Fifteen lists. The Dirty Dozen lists the twelve fruits and vegetables with the greatest concentration of pesticides, while the Clean Fifteen lists the fifteen fruits and vegetables with the least amount of pesticide residues.

Although I still find these lists to be beneficial and mention them to my patients, they are far from perfect. For example, while the foods on top of the Dirty Dozen might have the most pesticides, we need to keep in mind that some pesticides are more toxic than others. From what I understand, the Dirty Dozen list only considers the concentration of pesticides that a fruit or vegetable has, and not the type of pesticides. Thus, foods higher on the list have the greatest concentration of pesticides, but they might not have the most toxic pesticides.

While these lists aren't perfect, they still have some value, which is why I recommend them to my patients. This is yet another reason to try to eat mostly organic fruits and vegetables. While you won't completely eliminate your exposure to pesticides by eating organic produce, you will greatly minimize your exposure to these and other chemicals.

Sea Vegetables. Kelp and other sea vegetables have many health benefits, although they are also very high in iodine, which causes some health-care professionals to be concerned about their patients with Hashimoto's eating these types of foods. While I've worked with a few people with Hashimoto's who didn't tolerate eating iodine-rich foods, eating iodine-rich foods is different than taking iodine supplements, and many people do fine eating foods such as arame, dulse, kombu, and wakame.

Fruit. Most people with Hashimoto's can have at least a couple of servings of fruit per day, including avocados, blueberries, raspberries, blackberries, strawberries, apples, peaches, and pears. Certain fruits, including bananas, watermelon, and cantaloupe, are higher in sugar, but they also have healthy nutrients, and, in most cases, it's fine to eat these in moderation. There are exceptions, as, if someone has a Candida overgrowth, then it might be best to avoid fruits that are higher in sugar, and, at times, it might be wise to avoid fruit altogether while addressing this problem. Another situation when someone might need to restrict their consumption of fruit is having a fructose intolerance and/or problems with foods higher in FODMAPs, which include certain fruits such as apples, avocados, blueberries, peaches, and mangos.

Some healthcare professionals feel that eating fruit is similar to eating candy due to the fructose. While some studies show the harmful effects of pure fructose, there is a difference between consuming isolated forms of pure fructose and eating fruit (which also includes glucose and sucrose). Unlike eating candy or drinking sugary beverages such as soda, fruit consists of fiber, and studies show that the polyphenols included in fruit have anti-inflammatory properties.[7,8] In addition, a study involving type 2 diabetic patients showed that restricting fruit had no significant effects on hemoglobin A1C, weight loss, or weight circumference.[9]

However, I would recommend eating at least twice as many vegetables than fruit because I commonly see the opposite pattern, as it is common for people to eat four or five servings of fruit per day, and sometimes more than this, yet only eat a couple of servings of vegetables daily. One way you can sneak some more vegetables into your diet is by having a daily smoothie with one or two servings of vegetables. It's also a good idea to eat vegetables at each meal.

Eggs. Although eggs are very nutrient dense, and while I have some of my patients with Hashimoto's eat eggs, they can cause problems in some people for various reasons. First, regardless of whether someone has an autoimmune condition such as Hashimoto's, eggs are a common allergen. Some people have an IgE-mediated allergy, which involves an immediate reaction, while others have an IgG sensitivity, which involves a delayed reaction. Having a sensitivity to eggs is more common than having a true allergy.

In addition, compounds in egg whites can have a negative effect on gut health, specifically a protease called lysozyme. Thus, some people with Hashimoto's might have problems eating egg whites, yet do okay eating egg yolks. I recommend avoiding eggs altogether for at least one month, and if you are struggling with the diet and want to reintroduce eggs, it probably is best to first start out with eating egg yolks, and then, if all goes well, you can eventually reintroduce the egg whites.

Dairy. This is another food that is a common allergen. However, dairy has some good health benefits, especially raw dairy. Some people with Hashimoto's are able to tolerate certain forms of dairy without a problem once getting into remission. This includes raw dairy products, grass-fed butter, and ghee.

However, besides being a common allergen, casein (a protein in dairy) also cross reacts with gluten; thus, even if you don't have a dairy allergy or sensitivity, it still might pose a problem, which is why some healthcare professionals will recommend that all of their autoimmune patients permanently avoid dairy.

Fermented foods. Most people with Hashimoto's can benefit from eating some non-dairy fermented foods regularly. This includes kimchi, kombucha tea, sauerkraut, and pickles. Although fermented dairy products such as milk kefir and yogurt can also benefit one's health, since I typically have my patients avoid dairy, I recommend fermented dairy products be avoided while trying to restore their health. If someone has a condition such as small intestinal bacterial overgrowth (SIBO), or a histamine intolerance, they might not be able to tolerate any fermented foods until these imbalances have been addressed. If someone has a Candida overgrowth, eating fermented vegetables, such as sauerkraut, is usually fine, although kombucha and kefir can have a high yeast content and, thus, should be excluded.

Coconut products. Most people with Hashimoto's are able to consume coconut products, which include coconut butter, coconut milk, coconut oil, unsweetened coconut flakes, and unsweetened coconut yogurt. In addition, some evidence shows that coconut can help increase metabolism, which might offer yet another benefit to those with an underactive thyroid. Regarding coconut milk and coconut yogurt purchased at most health food stores, you need to be careful about other ingredients that you shouldn't consume. Thus, it probably is best to make your own coconut milk and yogurt. Similarly, some packaged coconut products (e.g., coconut water) are very high in sugar and should be avoided.

Meat. Most types of meats are fine to eat, including beef, chicken, turkey, lamb, and pork, although the quality of the meat is important. For example, if you plan to eat beef, then ideally, you should choose 100% grass-fed beef. If it's organic, that's even better. When eating poultry, organic pasture raised is preferred. Once again, perfection isn't necessary, as, if you have access to 100% grass-fed beef but it's not organic, then this is fine. If you eat organic poultry but it's not pasture raised, then this alone shouldn't prevent you from receiving great results.

Organ meats are very nutrient dense; thus, if you like organ meats such as liver and heart, then feel free to eat these. You also want to make sure the organ meats are from a good quality source. However, if you're like me and prefer not to eat organ meats, then that's not a problem, as you aren't required to eat organ meats to improve your health. However, there are some ways to sneak organ meats into your diet. For example, if having beef burgers, you can add liver or other organ meats to the ground beef.

With regards to eating liver, since this organ is involved in detoxification, some are concerned that it can be harmful to eat. I personally don't eat liver, but it's not out of fear that it will cause harm. While the liver is involved in eliminating toxins, keep in mind that the toxins aren't stored in the liver, and many healthcare professionals recommend eating liver because it has many healthy nutrients. Of course, quality is important, as it is best to eat liver from pasture-raised cows or bison.

How Much Meat Should You Eat?

Just as is the case with everything else related to diet, different people will have different opinions regarding how much meat should be eaten daily. Due to the lack of dietary choices, it is normal for people to eat more meat when following an AIP diet. This doesn't mean that it is a requirement to eat more meat per day, but don't feel guilty if you are eating more meat than usual while following an AIP diet, provided you are eating good quality meats.

The real question people want to know the answer to is, "How much meat and vegetables are necessary to eat for optimal health?" Another question you might have is, "How much meat is too much?" Some suggest looking at what hunter-gatherers ate in the past, but even this is up for debate. There is no consensus, and there probably will never be, but from all of the reading and research I've done, I recommend that the majority of foods you eat are vegetables, with a small amount of meat per meal. It's also fine to eat a few servings of fish per week, and you can also incorporate a small amount of fruit, some healthy oils, etc.

Seafood. This is yet another controversial food category, as some healthcare professionals will recommend that their patients minimize their consumption of seafood due to mercury and other environmental toxins, while others will say that it's fine to eat fish daily, providing they are wild and high in selenium because selenium binds to methylmercury, which is the mercury bound in fish.

However, while eating wild fish higher in selenium might sound like a good idea, I'm still not convinced that it's okay to eat fish daily. In addition, we also need to keep in mind that mercury isn't the only environmental toxin found in fish. For example, numerous studies show that PCBs in fish can cause adverse health issues.[10,11,12]

This doesn't necessarily mean you should avoid eating seafood, as, while I think it's fine to eat some wild fish, I usually tell my patients to limit their consumption of fish to two or three times per week. And I recommend they eat the smaller, wild fish that have less mercury and other environmental toxins. Regarding mercury in fish, the Natural Resources Defense Council has a pretty good guide that lists the fish with the least amount of mercury, those with a moderate amount of mercury, and those with a high amount of mercury. You can view this guide by visiting **http:// www.nrdc.org/health/effects/mercury/guide.asp**.

Nuts and Seeds. Although nuts and seeds are nutrient dense and are a good source of fiber, they are excluded from an AIP diet because they are difficult to digest, and there is a concern that they might interfere with gut healing. This might also depend on 1) the quantity of nuts and seeds eaten, and 2) how they are prepared, which I'll discuss shortly. There is also some concern about the phytates, as phytic acid is the major storage form of phosphorous in cereals, legumes, seeds, and nuts.[13] One of the main concerns with phytic acid is that it can inhibit the absorption of certain minerals such as iron, zinc, and calcium. There is also a concern that large amounts of phytic acid can be a factor in a leaky gut.

I always thought that lectins were the main reason why nuts and seeds were not included on an AIP diet, but, while nuts and seeds have lectins, they aren't as high in lectins as some other foods, such as legumes. This explains why legumes are excluded from a standard Paleo diet, while nuts and seeds are allowed. However, it's important to understand that some nuts and seeds have a higher lectin content than others. Unfortunately, I wasn't able to find a reliable list that includes the lectin content of the different nuts and seeds, but if I find such a list in the future I'll make sure to list it on the resources page of my website.

Although many people are aware that peanuts are a common allergen, many people also have tree nut allergies. I came across a study that showed that walnuts and cashews are the most allergenic tree nuts in the United States, whereas hazelnut is the most common nut allergy in Europe, and Brazil nuts, almonds and walnuts are the most common tree nut allergies in the United Kingdom.[14] Nuts and seeds are also high in oxalates, which are small molecules that have the ability to form crystals, which, in turn, can deposit in different areas of the body, including the thyroid gland. One of the main concerns is that having high levels of oxalates can lead to the development of kidney stones.

In any case, while I initially recommend that my patients with Hashimoto's avoid nuts and seeds, some people are able to reintroduce them after the first month or two without a problem. However, I will add that when I was dealing with Graves' disease, I didn't eliminate nuts and seeds for the first few months of following a natural treatment protocol, and I hit a roadblock in my gut healing. Upon eliminating the nuts and seeds from my diet, my gut health improved, and I eventually went into remission.

Gluten-Free Grains. Although some people do fine eating a small amount of gluten-free grains, such as rice, buckwheat, and quinoa (the latter is considered to be a pseudograin), these also have compounds that can have a negative effect on the health of the gut. Thus, it is a good idea for most people with Hashimoto's to go grain free, at least until their gut has been healed. I have had some patients with Hashimoto's reintroduce gluten free oats, rice, and/or quinoa and still receive good results, but other people don't do well unless if they exclude all grains from their diet.

Legumes. Legumes have some good health benefits, as they are a good source of protein, fiber, and certain nutrients such as folate, zinc, and calcium.[15] However, beans and legumes should ideally be avoided while trying to restore your health, since they can affect healing of the gut due to the high amount of lectins, saponins, and enzyme inhibitors.[16] In addition, for those with SIBO, it's important to know that legumes are considered to be high FODMAP foods due to the non-digestible galacto-oligosaccharides.[17] Legumes include beans, peas, lentils, peanuts, and other podded plants. The following are some of the more well-known legumes:

- Black beans
- Garbanzo beans (chickpeas)
- Green beans

- Kidney beans
- Lima beans
- Navy beans
- Pinto beans
- Soybeans
- Lentils
- Miso
- Dried peas
- Peanuts

Should Grains and Legumes Be Avoided Permanently?

Ultimately, my goal is to try to transition someone from an AIP Paleo diet to a standard Paleo diet. While a standard Paleo diet allows eggs, nightshades, nuts, and seeds, it excludes grains and legumes. Does this mean that grains and legumes should never be reintroduced?

I find that some people with Hashimoto's who get into remission can eat small amounts of these foods and do fine. To be honest, I can't say that I've known anyone who went into remission and relapsed because they were eating beans! However, since these foods have compounds that can increase gut permeability you should ideally wait until you are in a good state of health before reintroducing these foods, and if you do reintroduce grains, try to stick with gluten-free grains.

If you do choose to reintroduce legumes and/or grains you should consider soaking and fermenting them, which I'm about to discuss. I should also mention that some well known healthcare professionals recommend for everyone with Hashimoto's to avoid legumes and grains on a permanent basis, so without a doubt this is a controversial topic.

Although I'm focusing on grains and legumes here, I should add that some people aren't able to add back eggs and/or nightshades, even upon achieving a state of remission. You'll need to listen to your body carefully upon reintroducing these foods. The same is true with other foods as well.

What You Need to Know About Soaking, Sprouting, and Fermenting Nuts, Seeds, Grains, and Legumes

Soaking and sprouting nuts and seeds will help to reduce lectins and other compounds and make them easier to digest. And properly preparing other foods such as grains and legumes can also make them easier to digest. I must admit that when I was dealing with Graves' disease, I didn't soak and sprout the nuts and seeds prior to eating them. I'm not going to discuss in detail the "art" of soaking, sprouting, and fermentation, as there many books and YouTube videos that relate to this topic, along with information on the Internet. And you can visit my resources page at **www.naturalendocrinesolutions.com/resources**.

You might wonder why some of the excluded foods aren't allowed on an AIP diet if they are soaked, sprouted, and fermented? While properly preparing nuts, seeds, grains, and legumes can help to reduce these compounds, they won't completely eliminate them. Nevertheless, when someone decides to reintroduce any of these foods, it is a very good idea to properly prepare them. This doesn't mean that you will never be able to eat raw nuts and seeds again, but if you reintroduce any of these foods before your gut has fully healed and don't prepare them properly, then this might prevent you from getting into remission.

According to Dr. Steven Gundry, author of the book *The Plant Paradox*, pressure cooking can help to reduce the lectins in beans, tomatoes, potatoes, and quinoa. However, Dr. Gundry mentions that pressure cooking won't degrade the lectins in wheat, oats, rye, barley, or spelt. In other words, using a pressure cooker won't allow you to safely eat gluten-containing grains (oats don't inherently contain gluten but are often cross-contaminated), but it may allow you to safely eat other foods that are excluded from both an AIP and a standard Paleo diet.

Soy. This is yet another controversial food in the world of thyroid health. Soy is a common allergen, and most of the soy is genetically modified. Although a small amount of non-GMO fermented soy foods might be okay for some people to reintroduce, one's overall consumption of soy should be limited. I would definitely avoid processed soy products such as soy protein powder, soy burgers and chicken nuggets, soy milk, etc.

Sugar. Having a very small amount of natural sweeteners such as honey, pure maple syrup, or molasses is usually fine, although there are exceptions. For example, if someone has blood sugar imbalances, a Candida overgrowth, or a condition such as SIBO then certain natural sweeteners should be avoided. Other sweeteners such as agave, corn syrup, and high fructose corn syrup should be avoided by everyone due to the high amount of fructose.

Sugar alcohols are controversial, as while many people seem to do fine with them, others experience a lot of bloating and gas when consuming them. Most people with SIBO will experience a lot of gas when consuming sugar alcohols.

Can stevia be used a natural sweetener? While many healthcare professionals recommend stevia to their patients, others advise their patients to avoid it. One of the main concerns has to do with its effect on fertility, as a 1999 study showed that chronic administration of stevia on male rats may decrease fertility.[18] In addition, another study showed that stevia might inhibit the growth of Lactobacillus reuteri strains.[19] I'm not sure if we can conclude based on this single study that stevia can have harmful effects on the gut flora in humans; thus, more research is definitely needed.

If you do choose to add stevia to your tea or smoothies, make sure you avoid highly processed forms, such as Truvia, or consider adding a small amount of raw honey instead. I've always had a sweet tooth, and, while I used to add stevia to my green tea and herbal teas, I eventually stopped using it, and currently enjoy drinking both green and herbal tea without stevia, raw honey, etc.

Lou han guo, also known as monk fruit, seems safe to consume. Besides being a natural sweetener, a study I came across showed that it has antimicrobial properties, as it can inhibit the growth against Streptococcus mutans, Porphyromonas gingivalis, and Candida albicans.[20]

Herbs and spices. Spices can have a number of different health benefits, as some spices can help to decrease inflammation, others have antimicrobial properties, while others can help with blood sugar imbalances. However, not all spices are AIP-friendly. Towards the end of this chapter, I list some AIP-friendly spices you can consume.

Oils. For cooking, consider using coconut oil; although, if someone has problems with coconut oil, then they can use olive oil as an alternative. In the past, I thought that cooking with olive oil should be avoided due to it becoming easily oxidized and, therefore, causing more harm than good, but the research shows that extra virgin olive oil can resist oxidation fairly well.[21,22] I also love to use olive oil as a salad dressing.

However, you want to make sure you get good quality olive oil, as "olive oil fraud" is common, meaning that some unscrupulous companies use other unhealthy oils (i.e., soybean oil), and sell it as extra virgin olive oil.

You can learn more about this by reading the book *Extra Virginity: The Sublime and Scandalous World of Olive Oil*. Avocado oil is also fine to use, and while palm oil is allowed, the harvesting of palm trees for palm oil frequently results in the destruction of tropical forests, which, in turn, destroys the habitats of many animals.

Processed Foods. Obviously, these should be avoided while trying to restore your health. While some people are able to get away with eating a small amount of processed foods, for others it can have a negative effect on their recovery. After someone has restored their health, they should still try to eat mostly whole foods, although if someone has a healthy gut then eating some processed foods occasionally usually won't be a big deal. However, this depends on the person, as well as the type of food eaten.

Genetically modified foods. I would also try to avoid genetically modified foods while trying to get into remission. Because glyphosate can disrupt the gut flora and cause a leaky gut, as well as affect the phase one detoxification enzymes, it makes sense to do everything you can to avoid genetically modified foods. This is especially true while you are trying to get into remission, but even after you restore your health, you want to do try your very best to avoid or, at the very least, minimize your consumption of genetically modified foods.

What Can You Eat if You Are a Vegan or Vegetarian?

If you are a vegetarian or vegan, what is the best approach to take with your diet? Well, most of the same rules apply to those who eat meat, as vegetarians and vegans should eat whole foods while avoiding the refined foods and sugars. Keep in mind that I eat meat, as do many of my patients, but over the years, I have worked with many vegans and vegetarians. One of the big problems is that many vegans and vegetarians eat a lot of processed foods, although I'm sure that many reading this eat a healthy vegan or vegetarian diet.

If you are a vegan or vegetarian and insist on continuing to eat some of the excluded foods that can have an impact on gut healing (i.e., legumes, gluten free grains, nuts, and seeds) then these are the steps you should take to reverse the autoimmune process:

1) Consider testing for a leaky gut. Although I don't test most of my patients for a leaky gut, if someone is planning on eating foods regularly that can have a negative effect on gut healing, then it might be a good idea to do this type of testing for a couple of reasons. First, if you have a leaky gut, then it can be beneficial to determine the severity of it. Second, you can do retesting as one of the ways to monitor your progress.

For example, if you test positive for a leaky gut and choose to eat some properly prepared nuts, legumes, gluten-free grains, etc., you might choose to do another retest in three or four months to make sure your gut is healing. If it's not healing, then you probably will want to either reduce the amounts of "forbidden" foods that have lectins and other gut-disrupting compounds, or you might want to try eliminating these foods completely for a few months and then do another retest.

2) Try to follow a strict AIP diet for at least one month. I'm not suggesting that you should eat meat if you're a vegetarian, and if you're a strict vegetarian, you probably wouldn't listen to me even if I did suggest this! What I am recommending is avoiding all of the "excluded" foods for at least one month. In other words, avoid all of the foods that are common allergens, as well as those that have compounds that can increase the permeability of the gut…even if you did a leaky gut test and it came out negative.

After one month, if you don't feel any better and are struggling with the diet, then you can try adding small amounts of some of the foods that are normally excluded. If you choose to do this, I would reintroduce each food one at a time, every few days.

3) Properly prepare the excluded foods. If you choose to reintroduce legumes, gluten free grains, or nuts and seeds after the first month I would also make sure you properly prepare them. For example, soak and sprout any nuts and seeds you eat, and considering soaking and fermenting any grains and legumes you consume. As I discussed earlier, taking these steps will greatly decrease some of the compounds (e.g., lectins) that can prevent your gut from healing.

4) After the first month, minimize your consumption of the "excluded" foods. Although you might be fine eating some of the foods that normally aren't allowed on an AIP diet, you still want to minimize your consumption of these "forbidden foods." For example, if you are eating soaked nuts, seeds, and beans, along with gluten-free grains, don't eat large amounts of these foods. This is especially true if you ordered an intestinal permeability test and you tested positive for a leaky gut. But even if this test came out negative I still wouldn't load up on these foods, as I would try to eat at least six servings of fresh vegetables each day (although between nine and twelve would be even better), some fruit, and perhaps a small amount of these properly prepared "excluded" foods.

5) Eat and supplement with gut healing agents. Numerous studies show that L-glutamine can reduce intestinal permeability,[23,24,25] which is why many natural healthcare professionals recommend L-glutamine to their patients who have a leaky gut. Zinc and vitamin A can also help with the healing of the gut. Fermented foods such as sauerkraut can also help with gut healing by improving the health of the microbiome. Just as a reminder, many people with SIBO will experience digestive symptoms when eating fermented foods. Cabbage juice also has gut-healing properties.

6) Make sure you're getting all of the necessary nutrients. Although it is possible to eat a healthy vegetarian diet, many vegetarians and most vegans can greatly benefit from taking certain nutritional supplements regularly. For example, while vitamin B12 can be obtained from nutritional yeast, it probably will be necessary to take a vitamin B12 supplement such as methylcobalamin or hydroxocobalamin. Although fish oils aren't the only source of omega-3 fatty acids, keep in mind that most people have problems converting the alpha-linolenic acid from flax seeds, chia seeds, and walnuts into docosahexaenoic acid (DHA).

If you question whether or not you have one or more nutrient deficiencies then do some testing, which I discussed in the third section of this book. You can easily do a full iron panel, test for vitamin B12 and/or methylmalonic acid, do a fatty acid profile, etc.

A Summary of Foods Most People With Hashimoto's CAN EAT When Following a Strict AIP Diet

- **Most vegetables:** artichoke, arugula, asparagus, beets, broccoli, cabbage, carrots, cauliflower, celery, cucumber, kale, lettuce, mustard greens, onion, parsley, radish, spinach, squash, sweet potatoes, watercress, yams, zucchini

- **Fruits:** apples, apricots, avocados, bananas, blackberries, blueberries, cantaloupe, cherries, grapes, lemons, peaches, pears, plantains, raspberries, strawberries, watermelon
- **Fermented foods:** kimchi, kombucha, pickles, sauerkraut
- **Meats:** beef, chicken, lamb, pork, turkey, organ meats
- **Seafood:** Atlantic mackerel, clams, flounder, haddock, herring, mussels, salmon, sardines, shrimp, trout, whitefish
- **Coconut products:** coconut butter, coconut milk, coconut flakes (unsweetened), coconut oil, coconut yogurt (unsweetened)
- **Certain spices:** basal, cinnamon, coriander, cumin, garlic, ginger, lemongrass, mint, oregano, parsley, rosemary, sage, thyme, turmeric
- **Oils:** avocado oil, coconut oil, olive oil, palm oil

Note: while palm oil is allowed, the harvesting of palm trees for palm oil frequently results in the destruction of tropical forests, which, in turn, destroys the habitats of many animals. Indonesia might be a potential source of palm oil without the concern of deforestation.[26]

A Summary of Foods Most People With Hashimoto's SHOULD AVOID When Following a Strict AIP Diet

- **Dairy:** including but not limited to butter, cheeses, cow's milk, goat's milk, sheep's milk, whey, yogurt
- **Grains (even gluten-free):** including but not limited to amaranth, barley, buckwheat, corn, kamut, millet, oats, quinoa, rice, rye, spelt, wheat
- **Legumes:** including but not limited to black beans, lentils, peanuts, pinto beans, soybeans
- **Nightshade Vegetables:** including eggplant, paprika, peppers, tomatillos, tomatoes, white potatoes
- **Eggs**
- **Nuts and Seeds:** including but not limited to almonds, Brazil nuts, cashews, chia seeds, flax seeds, pecans, pistachios, sunflower seeds, pumpkin seeds, sesame seeds, walnuts
- **Alcohol:** Ideally all alcohol should be avoided while restoring your health. It's common for someone to ask if they can have an occasional glass of red wine. I would recommend to avoid all alcohol during the first 30 days of following an AIP diet. After the 30 days, some

people are able to reintroduce red wine without a problem, although in some people it can have a negative effect on their recovery.

Note: Many overlook the alcohol contained in herbal extracts. Ethanol is commonly used because it is a good solvent, and while I don't recommend liquid extracts to all of my patients, I find that most who need to take these progress fine.

- **Unhealthy Oils:** canola oil, peanut oil, soybean oil, safflower oil, cottonseed oil
- **All refined foods, fast food, etc.**

What AIP-Friendly Snacks Can You Eat?

One of the biggest challenges is to find snacks that are AIP-friendly. Thus, I'll list some snacks most people with Hashimoto's can safely consume. One thing to keep in mind is that while the snacks I have listed are AIP-friendly, this doesn't mean that it's okay to overindulge in these snacks. It's easy to eat too many servings of fruit, sweet potato chips, and other snacks.

- Plantain chips or crackers
- Sweet potato chips
- Kale chips
- Coconut chips or flakes
- Unsweetened coconut yogurt
- Tiger nuts
- AIP friendly beef jerky (e.g., Epic Bison Bacon & Cranberry bars)
- Sardines
- Baby carrots and other vegetables
- Fruit

Some question whether it is wise to snack at all. In other words, some healthcare professionals recommend that everyone eat every two to three hours to keep their blood sugar levels stable and, thus, recommend having snacks in between meals. In contrast, others will recommend only having two to three meals per day without snacks in between.

The truth is that it depends on the person. If someone has insulin resistance, then they might do better without having snacks between meals, and someone who has SIBO should also consider eating less frequently.

However, if someone has hypoglycemia, then eating snacks in between meals might be necessary until they address the cause of their blood sugar imbalances.

Remember That There Is No Single Diet That Perfectly Fits Everyone

Although I provided some guidance in this chapter, just keep in mind that everyone is different. Thus, there might be some people with Hashimoto's who are unable to eat one or more of the "allowed" foods due to food sensitivities, a Candida overgrowth, SIBO, etc. Others will choose to eat a few of the "excluded" foods, such as eggs, nightshades, nuts, seeds, and even properly prepared legumes and gluten free grains, yet still receive good results.

The problem is that it is impossible to predict who will do fine when straying from the diet, and who won't show a significant improvement in their health. While I realize the AIP diet is strict, if you choose to follow it for any length of time, try to be as strict as you can during this time in order to achieve optimal benefits. For example, if you choose to follow an AIP diet for 30 days before reintroducing certain foods, then during the 30 days, be strict.

The time of the year you begin this diet can be a very important factor in how successful you are. For example, if you plan on blocking out 30 days to follow a strict AIP diet you probably want to make sure you are not traveling during this time. Many people also have a difficult time following this diet during the holiday season (e.g., Thanksgiving, Christmas, Hanukkah). There is no "perfect" time to follow this diet, and you can always come up with an excuse to stray from the diet (e.g., birthdays, Valentine's day, and summer cookouts). However, certain times of the year do work better than others, and you want to do everything you can to set yourself up for success.

Should Gluten and Dairy Be Avoided Forever?

In a perfect world, those with Hashimoto's should avoid gluten and dairy permanently. Of course, we don't live in a perfect world, and, while some people will do everything they can to avoid gluten and dairy, some will either accidentally or intentionally be exposed to these foods.

Regarding dairy, besides it being a common allergen, it also can cross-react with gluten. Thus, even if you're gluten free, consuming dairy can lead to the production of gluten antibodies. However, some people are able to safely reintroduce dairy upon getting into remission. If this is the case with you, then it's best to consume healthier forms of dairy, such as ghee and raw dairy products.

As for gluten, there is no good reason to eat gluten, but unless if you eat home 100% of the time, then it can be very challenging to completely avoid gluten. This isn't to suggest that it can't be done, as, if someone has a condition such as celiac disease, then they need to strictly avoid gluten. Even if you don't have celiac disease, since gluten can cause a leaky gut in everyone, then this alone is a good argument to permanently avoid gluten.

Nevertheless, upon getting into remission, some people with Hashimoto's choose to reintroduce gluten, and, while some relapse, others seem to do fine. The problem is that it's impossible to predict who will do fine when reintroducing gluten and who will relapse; thus, if you do choose to reintroduce gluten please keep in mind that you are taking a risk.

AIP Diet Case Study

After being diagnosed with Hashimoto's, Christine did some browsing on the Internet and read where some people achieve significant improvement with a gluten and dairy free diet. As a result, she eliminated gluten and dairy for three months, ate mostly organic, and was hoping to see some good changes in both her symptoms and thyroid antibodies. While her symptoms did slightly improve after three months of avoiding gluten and dairy, her thyroid peroxidase and thyroglobulin antibodies remained elevated. She then came across my website and signed up for one of my free webinars, and after consulting with me I recommended for her to follow a strict AIP diet for a minimum of 30 days. After 30 days she felt better, and she decided to continue with the AIP diet for a few additional months. Not only did her symptoms further improve, but her antibodies greatly decreased. In fact, both antibodies were barely above the lab reference range after only three months of following the diet. Although I'm usually open to having people reintroduce foods sooner than later, Christine was so thrilled with the results that she wanted to continue with the AIP diet, and after a few months her thyroid antibodies had normalized, and she felt great from a symptomatic perspective. At this point she started reintroducing foods, and overall this went well, although unfortunately she experienced digestive symptoms upon reintroducing tomatoes. Because of this she cut out the tomatoes, but eventually she was able to make the transition to a standard Paleo diet. A few months later she did another thyroid panel with antibodies, and everything was still at optimal levels.

Action Steps You Can Take

While some will choose to make all of these changes at once, others will need to make gradual changes. If this describes you, then I would recommend taking the following action steps to modify your diet.

1. Incorporate more vegetables into your diet.
2. Reduce your intake of refined sugars.
3. Make sure you drink plenty of purified water.
4. If you eat a high carbohydrate breakfast, then replace this with a breakfast that is higher in protein and/or healthy fats.
5. Eat healthy fats including avocados, coconut oil, and olive oil.
6. Introduce a small amount of fermented foods.
7. Eliminate gluten from your diet.
8. Eliminate dairy from your diet.
9. Work on eliminating the other excluded foods from your diet.
10. Once you have eliminated all of the excluded foods, follow the elimination/AIP diet for at least 30 days
11. Please try your best to avoid genetically modified foods during this time.
12. Try to eat in a relaxed state, and make sure to thoroughly chew your food!

Notice that five of the first six action steps focused on adding foods, and not excluding foods because adding more healthy foods will make it easier to exclude other foods. One of the biggest complaints of following an elimination/AIP diet is that the person is hungry all of the time. However, in most cases, the reason for this is because they aren't eating a wide variety of vegetables and/or healthy fats.

Chapter Highlights:

- I commonly recommend for my patients with Hashimoto's to initially follow an autoimmune Paleo (AIP) diet for at least 30 days.
- An AIP diet is restrictive because 1) it excludes common food allergens, and 2) it excludes foods that can cause a leaky gut and/or can interfere with gut healing.
- I recommend eating at least five 1/2 cup servings of vegetables per day, and more than this would be even better.
- Make sure to eat a wide variety of vegetables.
- Most people with Hashimoto's can eat a few servings of cruciferous vegetables each day, although if someone has a moderate to severe iodine deficiency then they might want to limit their consumption.
- Many people with Hashimoto's will want to be cautious about eating the nightshades, which include tomatoes, eggplant, white potatoes, and most types of peppers.
- Sea vegetables have many health benefits, and while they are very high in iodine, many people with Hashimoto's seem to do fine eating these foods in moderation.
- Most people with Hashimoto's can have at least a couple of servings of fruit per day, although I would recommend eating at least twice as many vegetables than fruit.
- Some people with Hashimoto's might have problems eating egg whites, yet they might do okay eating egg yolks.
- Most people with Hashimoto's can benefit from eating some non-dairy fermented foods regularly, including sauerkraut, kimchi, kombucha, and pickles.
- Most types of meats are fine to eat, including beef, chicken, turkey, lamb, and pork, although the quality of the meat is important.

Chapter Highlights, continued:

- Legumes and grains are excluded from both a standard and an autoimmune Paleo diet, although some people with Hashimoto's chose to reintroduce these foods.
- Having a very small amount of natural sweeteners such as honey, pure maple syrup, and molasses is usually fine.
- Because glyphosate can disrupt the gut flora and cause or contribute to a leaky gut, as well as affect the phase one detoxification enzymes, it makes sense to do everything you can to avoid genetically modified foods.
- Remember that there is no single diet that perfectly fits everyone with Hashimoto's.
- Although following an autoimmune Paleo diet alone probably won't be enough to restore the health of most people, making these changes can lead to a huge improvement in your health, and, when combined with other factors, will greatly increase your chances of reversing your Hashimoto's condition.

CHAPTER 27

HOW TO BALANCE THE ADRENALS AND SEX HORMONES

WHILE IT CAN BE challenging to remove any of the triggers of Hashimoto's I discussed in section two, stress is, without question, one of the most challenging triggers to remove. You probably aren't going to remove all of your stressors; thus, the next best thing is to minimize the stressors while, at the same time, work on your stress-management skills and take other measures to improve the health of your adrenals.

I find that many of my patients with Hashimoto's focus on eating well and taking supplements, but most don't spend enough time on stress management. Some people just don't have the time to dedicate to this, while others feel that they do a good job of managing stress. Even if you think you have excellent stress-management skills, I still encourage you to block out time to work on stress management, which I'll discuss in this chapter.

I could have dedicated a separate chapter to balancing the sex hormones. However, I combined balancing the adrenals and the sex hormones into one chapter because, many times, improving the health of the adrenals will, in turn, help to balance the sex hormones. You almost always want to prioritize the adrenals, and this isn't just based on my clinical experience.

Most other healthcare professionals who practice functional medicine will also prioritize the health of the adrenals. Sure, there are integrative doctors who dispense bioidentical hormones to all of their patients without paying attention to the adrenals. While some people do need to take bioidentical hormones, you still want to improve the health of the adrenals first.

Understanding the Pregnenolone Steal

In order to help you better understand how problems with the adrenals can affect the sex hormones, I'll briefly discuss something called the pregnenolone steal. It's important to understand that all of the steroid and sex hormones are derived from cholesterol. Thus, if you have very low cholesterol levels, then this alone can result in low hormone levels. I need to emphasize this because many medical doctors commonly prescribe statins to their patients, which can result in very low cholesterol levels.

Thus, the hormone pathway starts with cholesterol, and the hormone pregnenolone is synthesized from cholesterol. This takes place in the mitochondria, and if someone has mitochondrial dysfunction, then this can affect the production of pregnenolone. However, if this isn't the case, pregnenolone can convert into either progesterone or DHEA, and these will convert into other hormones.

For example, DHEA can convert into androstenedione, which is a precursor of testosterone, and testosterone can convert into estradiol with the help of an enzyme called aromatase. Testosterone can also convert into dihydrotestosterone (DHT) via the enzyme 5α-reductase. Pregnenolone also converts into progesterone, which converts into 17-hydroxy progesterone, which ultimately is converted into cortisol.

The Body Prioritizes Cortisol Production Over the Sex Hormones

Out of all of the hormones I listed, the production of cortisol is a priority. If someone is in a stressed out state, cortisol will be produced at the expense of DHEA. Thus, with the hormone pathway I discussed, you'll recall that pregnenolone can be converted into both progesterone and DHEA, which, in turn, will convert into the other hormones I mentioned. If someone is stressed out, then this will inhibit the enzyme 17,20 lyase, which helps to convert 17-OH pregnenolone into DHEA, and 17-OH progesterone into androstenedione.

Consequently, if these enzymes are inhibited, DHEA and androstenedione will decrease. These hormones are precursors to testosterone, which converts into estradiol and DHT. Thus, the pregnenolone steal can result in decreased levels of DHEA, androstenedione, testosterone, estradiol, and

DHT. Keep in mind that not all of these hormones will become depleted simultaneously, as, initially, you might see some of these hormones depressed, while other hormones will look fine.

Thus, the pathway that converts pregnenolone into progesterone will predominate. However, cortisol is a priority over progesterone; thus, progesterone will also decrease in order to produce more cortisol. This is why this process is also referred to as the "cortisol steal" by some sources. You can halt and reverse this process by 1) reducing the stress in your life, and 2) improving your stress-management skills.

This doesn't mean that all sex hormone imbalances are caused by the pregnenolone steal, but this is where you want to focus initially. Thus, I'm going to focus on helping you improve your adrenal health first. Then, later in this chapter, I'll discuss other things you can do to balance your sex hormones.

Four Goals to Help You Achieve Optimal Adrenal Health

When trying to optimize the health of your adrenals, you have four main goals. Keep in mind that these goals aren't listed in the order of importance, although one can argue that the primary goal should be to eat well, followed by getting sufficient sleep, managing your stress-management skills, and then taking supplements and herbs to support the adrenals. However, you can argue that some people might not be able to get sufficient sleep without first improving their stress-management skills, and taking some supplements or herbs temporarily might be necessary to help some people to sleep better, do a better job of adapting to the stress, etc.

Goal #1: Eat well. Since I dedicated Chapter 26 to this, I'm not going to discuss this much here. You already know that you should eat a diet consisting of whole foods, while trying your best to avoid refined foods and sugars. While it's true that taking supplements temporarily might be required to correct nutritional deficiencies, you know that taking supplements isn't a substitute for eating a healthy diet.

Goal #2: Get sufficient sleep. Initially I was going to discuss sleep in this chapter, but I decided to dedicate Chapter 32 to overcoming sleeping difficulties and insomnia. Thus, if you have problems falling and/or staying asleep, I would read Chapter 32. Even if you sleep well, it's a good idea to read this chapter, as it might help you to get a better night's sleep.

Goal #3: Improve your stress-management skills. While some people reading this are doing a great job of managing their stress through meditation, yoga, or other mind-body medicine (MBM) techniques, many people aren't doing a good job in this area. In MBM, the body is the physical component that is able to experience physical sensations, such as pain and pleasure. The spirit can be thought of as the "life force" of the body. As for the mind, some consider this to be synonymous with the brain, while others consider both the mind and brain to be separate entities that work together.

Hippocrates described the connections between mental functions as being the mind, and the structure that produces these connections as being the brain. However, the British neurophysiologist Charles Scott Sherrington concluded that "The brain is the provider of the mind, and that the mental action lies buried in the brain…in that part most deeply recessed from the outside world, that is furthest from input and output."

Goal #4: Take certain nutritional supplements and herbs to support the adrenals. Although I commonly recommend nutritional supplements and herbs to support the adrenals, you really do need to focus on the previous three goals. In other words, if you take supplements but don't eat well, get sufficient sleep, and take measures for stress management, then you won't receive optimal results. Toward the end of this chapter, I'll discuss some of the nutritional supplements and herbs that can help support the adrenals.

Examples of Mind-Body Medicine Techniques

1. Meditation. This is probably the most well-known type of MBM. Many different types of meditation are practiced, and most involve four elements,[27] including a quiet location, a specific position, a focus of attention, and an open attitude. Many people practice meditation as a form of stress management, while others practice meditation for other reasons such as pain management. Mindfulness meditation is a type of meditation that helps us to pay more attention to our inner and outer experiences. In other words, it helps us to be aware of all of the surrounding physical and mental activities.

Many studies have shown the benefits of meditation. One randomized controlled trial showed that meditation may change brain and immune function in positive ways.[28] Another randomized controlled trial examined the effects of a one-month mindfulness meditation versus somatic relaxation training reporting distress.[29] The study showed that brief training in mindfulness meditation or somatic relaxation reduces distress and improves mood states. Another study showed that the practice of meditation reduced psychological stress responses and improved cognitive functions.[30]

How can you learn to meditate? You can read books on meditation or watch some videos on YouTube. Some areas have meditation groups or classes; thus, this is something to consider. Visit **www.meetup.com** or perform a search on Google or Bing for "meditation classes," followed by the name of your city.

2. Yoga. Yoga is another type of mind-body medicine, and many different yoga techniques exist. Hatha yoga is the most commonly practiced type in the United States and Europe, and some of the major styles of hatha yoga include Iyengar, Ashtanga, Vini, Kundalini, and Bikram yoga.[31] Certain yoga postures, such as a shoulder stand position known as sarvangasana, can help improve thyroid health.

While some people are able to learn how to do yoga by watching online videos, it probably is best to learn this in person from a certified yoga instructor. Visit Google or another search engine to find a nearby yoga studio you can join. Another option is to hire a yoga instructor one-on-one for a few sessions.

Many studies show how yoga can help with stress. A systematic review of the literature examined the mechanisms through which yoga reduces stress.[32] It showed seven mechanisms. Three of these are psychological mechanisms and include positive effect, mindfulness, and self-compassion.[32] Four of these mechanisms are biological and include the posterior hypothalamus, interleukin-6, C-reactive protein, and cortisol.[32]

Most people are aware that there are "psychological mechanisms" involved. However, the biological mechanisms prove that yoga can have a positive effect on the physiology of the body. Thus, when you hear someone discuss how yoga can help with stress, just remember that it does this by affecting the hypothalamus and decreasing cortisol. It can also reduce inflammation by modulating the proinflammatory cytokine interleukin-6 and by decreasing C-reactive protein (CRP).

While the specific psychological and biological mechanisms through which yoga reduces stress isn't important to memorize, it is necessary to realize that practicing yoga, along with other MBM techniques, can be just as important as eating well and/or taking supplements. I'm mentioning this because it's common for people with Hashimoto's (and other health conditions) to make dietary changes and take supplements, but they aren't blocking out time for stress management.

3. Biofeedback. Biofeedback is a MBM technique for modifying physiology to improve physical, mental, emotional, and spiritual health.[33] This intervention involves measuring a person's quantifiable bodily functions (e.g., blood pressure, heart rate, muscle tension) and, using this information, provide guidance and reinforcement for successful management of the physiological response to stress.[34] Some smaller studies have shown the effectiveness of biofeedback.

For example, one study assessed whether a self-directed, computer-guided meditation training program is useful for stress reduction in hospital nurses.[35] The results of the study showed that this program helped hospital nurses reduce their stress and anxiety. Another study showed that heart rate variability biofeedback decreases blood pressure in prehypertensive subjects.[36]

Although many types of biofeedback devices are utilized at clinician's offices, you can also purchase a device to use at home. Heart Math is a well-known company that has some wonderful technology, including the emwave2 and the Inner Balance. The emwave2 and Inner Balance programs measure something called heart rate variability (HRV). Heart rate variability involves a variation in the interval between heartbeats. It is a measure of the autonomic nervous system functioning and reflects an individual's ability to adaptively cope with stress.[37] Having a higher HRV is a sign of good adaptation and characterizes a person with efficient autonomic mechanisms, while having a lower HRV is usually an indicator of abnormal and insufficient adaptation of the autonomic nervous system.[38]

Why is it important to have a heart rate that is variable? Well, in the past, it was thought that the heart was supposed to have a regular, steady rhythm. However, even under resting conditions, there is supposed to be some degree of heart rate variability. HRV can be an important indicator of health and fitness. Having low HRV usually means that there is an imbalance of the autonomic nervous system, and evidence shows that reduced HRV can increase the risk of developing certain health issues.

One study showed that a reduced HRV could worsen the prognosis in people with myocardial infarction, chronic heart failure, unstable angina, and diabetes mellitus.[39] I personally use the Inner Balance from Heart Math as my main form of stress management. For more information, visit **www.heartmath.com**, as they have some videos and articles that discuss HRV in greater detail and how their programs can help.

Some of the factors that influence HRV include exercise, one's breathing patterns, and even your feelings and emotions. Having a negative attitude or being stressed out will most likely lead to a decrease in HRV. However, having a positive attitude and doing a good job of managing your stress can lead to increased HRV.

4. Hypnotherapy. Hypnotherapy is also considered to be a type of MBM. Hypnosis is a state of deep concentration, and can be used to help people with many different conditions. Hypnosis can be used not only for stress and anxiety,[40,41] but also might help with depression,[42] sleep disorders,[43] and irritable bowel syndrome.[44,45]

5. Other MBM Techniques. Some other MBM techniques include music therapy, visualization, tai chi, and qigong. When I recommend someone to choose one or more techniques to focus on stress management, any of these can greatly help. Although MBM can help greatly to manage your stress levels, remember that it can also help with other conditions, such as pain, high blood pressure, and depression. One way it helps with many conditions is by lowering the cortisol levels.

Mind-Body Medicine and Hashimoto's
Although most of the evidence for MBM relates to helping with stress, evidence also shows that MBM can help to modulate immune system function. In other chapters, I discussed how proinflammatory cytokines are a factor with autoimmune conditions such as Hashimoto's. I also discussed how certain nutrients could lead to a reduction in these cytokines. Also, certain MBM techniques can reduce proinflammatory cytokines.

One study found reduced TNF-α levels following 10 weeks of relaxation therapy among patients with tinnitus,[46] and other studies have reported reduced proinflammatory cytokine IL-1 following sessions of hypnosis and relaxation.[47,48] Yoga can modulate the immune system and lead to a lowering of proinflammatory cytokines and other inflammatory markers such as interleukin-6, interleukin-8, tumor necrosis factor alpha, and CRP.[49,50,51]

This doesn't mean that MBM techniques alone can reverse your Hashimoto's condition. I think it's safe to say that if someone eats poorly, then even if they practice MBM for a few hours each day, they will never achieve optimal health. Similarly, if someone has an environmental trigger such as infection or exposure to a heavy metal, then incorporating MBM techniques isn't going to remove the trigger. However, once the trigger has been detected and removed, combining a healthy diet with MBM can play a very important role in reversing the autoimmune process.

How to Incorporate Mind-Body Medicine Into Your Life

I trust you will agree that incorporating MBM is important; however, many people won't know where to start. This is what I recommend to do:

1. Choose one or more MBM techniques. If you already have experience incorporating a specific MBM technique (e.g., meditation), and if you enjoy this technique, then, of course, it makes sense to continue doing it.

2. Block out time each day to do it. I realize that it can be challenging to find the time to incorporate stress management. Even if you can only start with five minutes per day, that would still be beneficial. The key is to get into a routine. Then, hopefully, in the future, you can increase the duration of the MBM sessions.

3. Do it EVERY day. You should practice MBM every single day because, while doing MBM two to four times per week is certainly better than not doing anything, it's important to do something every day to help with the stress. This doesn't mean you need to incorporate the same MBM technique every day. For example, it's perfectly fine if you do yoga three days per week, and do a different MBM technique the other four days.

4. Learn how to appropriately use the techniques. This is also important, but the drawback is that it can take longer than five minutes per day, depending on what technique you choose. For example, if you choose yoga and are doing it for the first time then I would recommend being trained by a yoga instructor and not to try learning it on your own by watching online videos. However, if you are incorporating deep breathing or meditation, there are plenty of "guided trainings" that you can use. If you are able to join a local group or attend classes then this probably

is the best option, although if you visit **www.naturalendocrinesolutions.
com/resources**, I'll list some of the online programs and phone apps I
recommend.

Supporting the Adrenals Through Diet

In order to support the adrenals through diet, you want to do the
following:

Eat plenty of healthy fats. This includes avocados, coconut oil, and olive
oil. Proteins such as meat and fish can be consumed, as can organ meats.
Those who successfully make the transition from an autoimmune Paleo
(AIP) diet to a standard Paleo diet can also eat eggs, nuts, and seeds

Consider adding sea salt. Those who have low cortisol levels should consider adding sea salt to their food. In Chapter 6, I mentioned some studies
that showed a relationship between salt and autoimmunity, although these
involved consuming excessive amounts of salt. Adding a small amount
of sea salt to your diet, shouldn't trigger or exacerbate an autoimmune
response.

Minimize your consumption of sugar. Ideally, you want to avoid eating all
refined sugars, and, while most people with Hashimoto's can eat a few
servings of fruit per day, those with conditions such as insulin resistance
or a Candida overgrowth will want to limit their intake to one or two
servings of low glycemic index fruits per day. Also, please make sure you
eat at least twice as many servings of vegetables than fruits.

Stop drinking coffee (at least for now). Although there are some health
benefits to drinking coffee, caffeine can have a negative effect on the health
of the adrenals. This is especially true for those who are slow metabolizers of caffeine. But regardless of whether someone is a slow or fast
metabolizer of caffeine, while restoring your health, I usually advise my
patients to take a break from highly caffeinated beverages such as coffee
and black tea. While green tea has some wonderful health benefits, those
with adrenal issues probably should stick with an organic decaffeinated
green tea.

Supporting the Adrenals Through Nutritional Supplements and Herbs

Nutrients and Herbs for Low Cortisol Levels. Let's take a look at some nutrients and herbs that can benefit those with low cortisol levels. Keep in mind that those with low cortisol levels won't need to take everything I list here. It's also important to remember that while taking supplements and herbs can help, it's even more important to focus on lifestyle factors, such as stress management. I discussed how to test for cortisol levels in Chapter 25.

Vitamin C. The adrenal gland has one of the highest concentrations of vitamin C in the body.[52] Certain studies show that vitamin C plays a crucial role in the health of both the adrenal cortex and adrenal medulla.[52] Another small study showed that taking high doses of ascorbic acid was associated with reduced stress reactivity of systolic blood pressure, diastolic blood pressure, and subjective stress, and with greater salivary cortisol recovery.[53]

Although ascorbic acid is only one component of vitamin C (the antioxidant wrapper), just about all studies relating to vitamin C involve ascorbic acid. Nevertheless, when I recommend vitamin C in supplement form I prefer for my patients to take a food-based vitamin C complex, as this also includes the necessary cofactors.

Note: Vitamin C can be taken regardless of what the adrenal saliva test looks like, as anyone who is dealing with a good amount of stress can benefit from taking vitamin C. However, it is especially useful for those who have depressed cortisol levels.

Suggested Dosage: 500 to 2,000 mg per day

Food Sources: papaya, broccoli, Brussels sprouts, strawberries, pineapple, oranges, cauliflower, kale, cabbage

Pantothenic acid (vitamin B5). Pantothenic acid is one of the more important B vitamins for those with depressed cortisol levels, as it is a component of coenzyme A, which is required to generate energy from fats, protein, and carbohydrates. Taking pantothenic acid can help to stimulate the production of cortisol and progesterone.[54] While you can take a separate pantothenic acid supplement, in most cases It's better to take this as part of a B vitamin complex.

Note: Although pantothenic acid can be safely taken by most people, since it can help to enhance the production of cortisol, it is especially helpful to take for those who have low or depressed cortisol levels.

Suggested Dosage: 250 to 500 mg per day
Food Sources: shiitake mushrooms, cauliflower, broccoli, sweet potatoes, asparagus, turnip greens, celery, avocados

Other B Vitamins. Although vitamin B5 is well known for supporting the adrenals, some of the other B vitamins can also be beneficial in those with low cortisol levels. Both vitamin B6 and folate can affect cortisol secretion.[55] Vitamins B1, B2, and B3 can also benefit the adrenals and improve cortisol secretion.[56]

If you deal with a high amount of stress, then taking a B complex supplement for extra support might be a good idea. However, you can also do some testing to determine your levels of the B vitamins. Getting a standard blood test at a local lab won't accurately determine whether you have a deficiency of all of the B vitamins.

One option is micronutrient testing through a company such as Spectracell. Genova Diagnostics has a test called the NutrEval, which measures not only the B vitamins, but other nutrients as well. Yet another option is organic acids testing, as the organic acids test by Great Plains Laboratory measures the metabolites associated with vitamin B2, B6, B12, along with biotin. The Organix from Genova Diagnostics also looks at the metabolic intermediates of the B vitamins.

Licorice. Licorice is an herb that is commonly used by many natural healthcare professionals. Glycyrrhizic acid, or glycyrrhizin, is the main compound in licorice root. Licorice can help to increase cortisol levels, as it inhibits 11 beta-dehydrogenase 2 (11 beta-HSD2), which is an enzyme responsible for the conversion of cortisol to cortisone. Thus, this herb essentially decreases cortisol metabolism, prolonging the life of cortisol.

If you choose to take a licorice supplement, you need to be careful about taking high doses, or even smaller doses over a prolonged period. Although I commonly recommend this herb to my patients with depressed cortisol levels, taking high doses of licorice root, or even smaller doses for a prolonged period, can lead to hypokalemia (potassium deficiency) and/or high blood pressure.[57]

Suggested Dosage: 250 to 500 mg with breakfast and/or lunch
Note: I recommend taking licorice around each low cortisol reading. For example, if you get a salivary cortisol test and have depressed cortisol

levels in the morning and early afternoon, then I would take licorice root first thing in the morning, and then right around lunchtime.

Eleuthero (Siberian ginseng). This is an adaptogenic herb that can help support the hypothalamic pituitary adrenal (HPA) axis, and help people to better adapt to stress.

Suggested Dosage: 250 to 500 mg with breakfast and/or lunch

Rhodiola. Rhodiola rosea is a popular plant in traditional medical systems in Eastern Europe and Asia with a reputation for stimulating the nervous system, decreasing depression, enhancing work performance, eliminating fatigue, and preventing high altitude sickness.[58] Like eleuthero, rhodiola can help people to better adapt to the stress.

Suggested Dosage: 125 mg to 500 mg with breakfast and/or lunch

Cordyceps. Cordyceps sinensis is a fungi that acts as an adaptogen and, therefore, can help support the HPA axis, and it has other health benefits. One study showed that an extract of cordyceps caused an increase in cortisol.[59]

Suggested Dosage: 250 to 500 mg with breakfast and/or lunch

Glandulars for adrenals, pituitary, and hypothalamus. Although there are times when I use glandulars in my patients to support the adrenals, pituitary gland, and/or hypothalamus, no scientific evidence shows that these glandulars provide any health benefits. However, this doesn't mean that glandulars can't be beneficial, as there also aren't any studies I'm aware of that show they aren't effective.

In other words, the lack of clinical trials conducted on these glandulars, as well as on other supplements and herbs, doesn't mean that they can't benefit some people. Far more studies are conducted on drugs not because drugs are more effective than nutritional supplements and herbs but because the pharmaceutical companies have plenty of money to spend on these studies. This isn't true when it comes to studies on herbs and other supplements.

Note: Usually, adrenal glandulars are given when someone has depressed cortisol levels. I don't recommend taking adrenal glandulars for longer than two consecutive months so that the body doesn't become dependent on them.

Nutrients and Herbs for Elevated Cortisol Levels. Let's take a look at some nutrients and herbs that can benefit those with high cortisol levels. Just as is the case with depressed cortisol levels, when someone has elevated cortisol levels, you don't want to rely on taking supplements but, instead, want to use them for additional support while you focus on improving lifestyle factors, including stress management and getting sufficient sleep.

Phosphatidylserine. Phosphatidylserine is produced naturally by the body and is important in maintaining cellular function. If someone has elevated cortisol levels, then taking phosphatidylserine can help to lower these levels.[60,61]

Suggested Dosage: 100 to 500 mg/day before each high cortisol episode

Food Sources: organ meats such as liver, kidneys, and heart have the highest amount of phosphatidylserine.[62] Certain legumes such as white beans and soybeans contain phosphatidylserine, although these, of course, are excluded from both a standard and AIP diet.

Phellodendron bark (Relora). A few studies show that the herb Relora can help to reduce cortisol levels.[63,64] Thus, taking this herb before each high cortisol episode can be helpful.

Suggested Dosage: 250 to 500mg before each high cortisol episode

Ashwagandha (Withania somnifera). This herb has both tonic and adaptogenic properties; thus, it can be used as a general tonic to increase energy; improve overall health and longevity; and prevent disease in athletes, the elderly, and pregnant women.[65] Ashwagandha is also an adaptogenic herb, which means that it helps the body adapt to stress. However, ashwagandha is a member of the nightshade family, and while many people with Hashimoto's do fine when taking this herb, those who are following a strict AIP diet should avoid taking this herb.

Suggested Dosage: 250 to 500mg before each high cortisol episode

How to Have Healthy Sex Hormone Levels

The pregnenolone steal is responsible for many sex hormone imbalances. However, when it comes to a "true" estrogen dominant state (i.e., elevated estradiol levels), addressing the pregnenolone steal and improving the health of the adrenals usually isn't sufficient. When someone has elevated estrogen levels, that person needs to do two things. First, they need to reduce their exposure to exogenous estrogens. Second, they need to support detoxification and estrogen metabolism.

This is assuming they have a case of "true" estrogen dominance. After all, if someone has a progesterone deficiency and normal levels of estrogen, then this is also considered to be a state of estrogen dominance. In this situation, the low progesterone levels very well could be the result of the pregnenolone steal. However, if someone has elevated levels of estradiol, then they need to make sure they reduce their exposure to exogenous estrogens while at the same time increasing the clearance of estrogen from their body.

Here is a list of specific things to keep in mind about minimizing one's exposure to exogenous estrogens:

1. Be cautious about taking bioidentical hormones...especially hormone creams. My goal here isn't to be critical of hormone creams. Although taking bioidentical hormones can be necessary at times, if you're not careful, they can cause problems. Even if you are careful, they can still cause problems.

I've had a number of patients who were taking small doses of hormone creams, yet had very high levels of estrogen show up on a hormone panel. And even though the focus here is on estrogen dominance, I also should say that I've seen elevated levels of progesterone and testosterone due to bioidentical hormones. I don't recommend bioidentical hormones too frequently, but when I do, I advise my patients to take them sublingually.

Another thing to keep in mind is that cross-contamination can happen with hormone creams. For example, if you aren't taking bioidentical hormones, but your significant other is taking bioidentical testosterone in the form of a cream, you can be exposed to the testosterone during intercourse. If your spouse doesn't wash his or her hands after applying the hormone cream then cross-contamination can occur this way as well. While the focus here has been on bioidentical hormones, there are also potential risks with taking synthetic estrogen or progesterone, such as Premarin and Provera.

2. Be aware of the side effects of oral contraceptives. Not all oral contraceptives include estrogen, as some only include progestin. Others include a combination of estrogen and progestin, and these can affect estrogen metabolism. One effect of oral contraceptives is that they can increase the incidence of gallbladder disease,[66] and one factor could be the effect that estrogen has on bile metabolism.

Oral contraceptives can also result in nutrient deficiencies. Some of the potential nutrient deficiencies caused by oral contraceptives include vitamins B2, B6, B12, C, and E and the minerals magnesium, selenium, and zinc.[67] My goal isn't to convince women who are currently taking oral contraceptives to abruptly stop, but many aren't aware of the potential side effects I mentioned here.

3. Minimize your exposure to xenoestrogens. Natural products play an important role in this, as I discussed in Chapter 8. While there are numerous sources of xenoestrogens, drinking water out of plastic bottles is probably the biggest culprit. While drinking bottled water every now and then isn't a big deal for most people, drinking water out of plastic bottles frequently is likely to cause problems with your health. Also, in the long run, it's less expensive to get your own water purification system, along with your own water bottle. I personally use a glass water bottle with an outside padding from the company Lifefactory.

Xenoestrogens are also found in pesticides, herbicides, food storage containers, thermal paper receipts, many household products and cosmetics, and many other sources. While it's impossible to completely avoid exposure to xenoestrogens, most people can take measures to reduce their exposure to them.

4. Eat a healthy diet. You, of course, want to avoid eating foods with xenohormones. Hormones are frequently fed to livestock to increase their size, and most non-organic fruits and vegetables are sprayed with pesticides that contain xenohormones. The best way to minimize your exposure to xenohormones through diet is by eating organic food.

Understanding the Basics of Estrogen Metabolism

In addition to minimizing your exposure to exogenous estrogens, you also want to make sure you have healthy estrogen metabolism. It probably is a good idea to briefly discuss some of the basic facts regarding estrogen. There are three main types of estrogen, which includes estradiol, estrone, and estriol. Estradiol is considered to be the dominant estrogen, and it can be converted into estrone. Estrone, in turn, can convert into estradiol. Both of these hormones can convert into estriol, which is primarily produced during pregnancy by the placenta.

During premenopause, most estrogens are produced in the ovaries. In postmenopause, estrogen production from the ovaries greatly decreases, and most of the estrogen is produced through the aromatization of androgens (i.e., testosterone) in the fat cells, although this conversion can also take place in other tissues such as the skin and bone. Testosterone is converted into estradiol, while androstenedione is converted into estrone.

Estrogens bind to certain receptors, and there are two main types of estrogen receptors: estrogen alpha and estrogen beta. Estradiol and estrone both lead to the formation of estrogen metabolites, which I discussed in Chapter 25. These include 2-hydroxyestrone (2-OH), 4-hydroxyestrone (4-OH), and 16α-hydroxyestrone (16α -OH).

The enzyme catechol-o-methyltransferase (COMT) is involved in the detoxification and excretion of estrogens. Thus, supporting detoxification/methylation can help with the elimination of estrogens. Not surprisingly, if someone has a genetic polymorphism of the COMT gene, this can affect the methylation of estrogens. In addition, certain cofactors are necessary to support the methylation of estrogen, including S-adenosylmethionine (SAMe) and magnesium.

A process called glucuronidation is also involved in the detoxification of estrogen, and an enzyme called beta-glucuronidase can prevent the excretion of estrogen and allow it to re-enter the circulation. Some stool panels test for this enzyme, and if someone has elevated levels of beta-glucuronidase, they will want to support the gut flora and increase their fiber intake. Calcium D-glucarate can also reduce beta-glucuronidase activity.

Since this information on estrogen metabolism might have been a little bit advanced for some people, I'll briefly summarize the important points:

- There are three main types of estrogens, and estradiol is considered to be the dominant estrogen.
- The 2-OH metabolite has weak estrogenic activity, and is labeled as being the "good" estrogen.
- The 4-OH and 16α-OH metabolites have a greater amount of estrogenic activity, and higher levels of these metabolites might increase the risk of developing certain types of cancers.
- Thus, you want to have high levels of the 2-OH metabolite and low levels of the 4-OH and 16α-OH metabolites.
- The enzyme catechol-o-methyltransferase (COMT) is involved in the detoxification and excretion of estrogens; thus having a genetic defect of the COMT gene can affect the detoxification of estrogens.

• An enzyme called beta-glucuronidase can prevent the excretion of estrogen and allow it to re-enter the circulation. Someone with elevated levels of beta-glucuronidase will want to support the gut flora and increase their fiber intake.

What can you do to improve estrogen metabolism? Eating a healthy diet is of course important, and at times, taking nutritional supplements and herbs can be beneficial. Thus, let's take a look at both of these:

Supporting Estrogen Metabolism Through Diet
In order to support estrogen metabolism, you want to do the following:

• **Eat plenty of vegetables to help support detoxification.** Eating plenty of vegetables, especially cruciferous vegetables, can help to increase glutathione levels, which helps to support the detoxification pathways.
• **Eat plenty of vegetables to help support methylation.** Methylation is necessary when it comes to protein synthesis, detoxification, the formation of neurotransmitters, and the regulation of hormones, and it has many other functions. Methylenetetrahydrofolate reductase (MTHFR) is an enzyme that is vital for re-methylation of homocysteine to methionine. Folate is one of the more important nutrients, as it is necessary not only for the breakdown of homocysteine, but also for the synthesis of neurotransmitters such as serotonin, epinephrine, and dopamine. Green leafy vegetables are an excellent source of folate, along with asparagus and broccoli.
• **Eat foods that support glucuronidation.** Earlier I mentioned that glucuronidation is involved in the detoxification of estrogens. Some foods that support glucuronidation include apples, kale, broccoli, and watercress.
• **Eat plenty of fiber.** Many people think of fiber as playing a role in regular bowel movements, which is true. However, having sufficient fiber is also important for the health of your microbiome, which, in turn, can help lower beta glucuronidase.
• **Consume ground flaxseeds.** Much controversy surrounds phytoestrogens, which are compounds that have weak estrogenic or antiestrogenic activity. Flax and soy are two of the more well-known foods among others that have phytoestrogens. Phytoestrogens have the ability to bind to the estrogen receptors and are thus classified by

some sources as being endocrine disruptors. However, it appears that phytoestrogens mostly bind to the estrogen receptor beta (ERβ), which is the "good" estrogen receptor.

If you eat soy then you want to make sure it's organic and fermented, but even if this is the case, I think it's a good idea to minimize your consumption of soy. If you are following a strict AIP diet, then you would be avoiding not only soy but flaxseeds as well, along with other nuts and seeds. However, I find that many people with Hashimoto's are able to reintroduce a small amount (e.g., one tablespoon) of ground flaxseeds per day. I recommend buying the flaxseeds whole and grinding them on your own (I use a coffee grinder I purchased on Amazon) because ground flaxseeds and flaxseed oil turn rancid faster than whole flaxseeds.

- **Exercise regularly.** Numerous studies demonstrate that regular exercise can have a positive effect on estrogen metabolism, and can even reduce the risk of estrogen-dependent cancer.[68,69]

Supporting Estrogen Metabolism Through Nutritional Supplements and Herbs

Although you want to do as much as you can through diet, sometimes, supplementation is necessary. Here are some of the supplements that can help support estrogen metabolism:

Diindolylmethane (DIM). 3,3'-diindolylmethane (DIM) is derived from indole-3-carbinol, which is found in cruciferous vegetables. Studies show that DIM can positively affect estrogen metabolism.[70,71] While you can take a supplement that has DIM, I recommend getting most of the DIM from eating cruciferous vegetables.

Suggested Dosage: 100 to 500mg/day

Calcium D-glucarate. This has been extensively studies by researchers, and one of its main health benefits is in the inhibition of beta-glucuronidase, which is an enzyme produced by bacteria in the gut. Inhibiting beta-glucuronidase can help support the body's ability to detoxify estrogens.

Suggested Dosage: 500 to 1,000 mg/day

N-Acetylcysteine (NAC). This is a source of the amino acid cysteine and is a precursor to glutathione, which helps to support detoxification.

Suggested Dosage: 600 to 1,800 mg/day between meals

Support glucuronidation. While supporting the gut flora and taking calcium D-glucarate can help to reduce beta-glucuronidase activity, some of the other nutrients that can help to support glucuronidation include quercitin, curcumin, resveratrol, milk thistle, omega 3 fatty acids, and magnesium.

Supplement Recommendations for Progesterone Production:

Although I'm going to list a few nutritional supplements that can increase progesterone production, please keep in mind that the best way to increase progesterone levels is by improving the health of the adrenals.

Chaste Berry Extract (Vitex agnus-castus). Extracts of the fruits of chaste tree are commonly used to treat premenstrual symptoms. One way it seems to accomplish this is by increasing progesterone levels.

Suggested Dosage: 100 to 500 mg/day

Maca (Lepidium meyenii). Maca root is an adaptogenic herb that can balance hormone levels by supporting the hypothalamic pituitary gonadal (HPG) axis. This in turn can support progesterone production in some women.

Suggested Dosage: 500 to 1,000 mg/day

How Can Hyperprolactinemia Be Corrected?

In Chapter 16, I discussed the correlation between hyperprolactemia and autoimmunity. Although prolactin isn't a sex hormone, I figured I'd briefly discuss how to address high prolactin levels in this chapter.

As for how to correct hyperprolactinemia, conventional medical treatment usually involves the patient taking dopamine agonists because dopamine can inhibit the secretion of prolactin by the anterior pituitary cells. As for a natural approach, I just mentioned how the herb chaste tree (also known as Vitex) is known for helping to increase progesterone levels, and evidence suggests that it can successfully lower high prolactin levels in many women.[72,73]

If someone is pregnant or has just given birth, it's normal for these levels to be high, and if a woman is breastfeeding, then giving a dopamine agonist will affect the production of breast milk. Other factors can cause elevated prolactin levels such as a tumor (referred to as a prolactinoma). Taking a dopamine antagonist (which are used to treat schizophrenia) will also cause hyperprolactinemia.

Also, keep in mind that even if the high prolactin levels can trigger an autoimmune response, using medication or an herb such as chaste tree to lower the prolactin levels won't necessarily suppress the autoimmune response. In other words, removing the trigger is important, but other actions are usually necessary to suppress the autoimmune component of the condition. I pointed this out in section one when discussing the importance of downregulating NF-kappaB and increasing regulatory T cells.

Chapter Highlights:

- The hormone pathway starts with cholesterol, and the hormone pregnenolone is synthesized from cholesterol.
- The pregnenolone steal explains how chronic stress can lead to low levels of the sex hormones.
- The body prioritizes the production of cortisol over the sex hormones.
- Four goals to help you achieve optimal adrenal health are 1) eat well, 2) get sufficient sleep, 3) improve your stress-management skills, and 4) take certain nutritional supplements and herbs.
- Some examples of mind-body medicine techniques include meditation, yoga, biofeedback, and hypnotherapy
- Yoga can modulate the immune system and lead to a decrease in proinflammatory cytokines and other inflammatory markers.
- In order to support the adrenals through diet, you want to eat plenty of healthy fats, consider adding sea salt, minimize your consumption of sugar, and stop drinking coffee.
- Some nutrients and herbs that can benefit people with low cortisol include vitamin C, vitamin B5, licorice root, glandulars, and adaptogenic herbs such as eleuthero and rhodiola.
- Some nutrients and herbs that can benefit people with elevated cortisol levels include phosphatidylserine, relora, ashwagandha, and cordyceps.
- Having healthy adrenals is essential in order to have balanced sex hormones, although you also want to minimize your exposure to exogenous estrogens, and, at times, will need to support estrogen metabolism.

Chapter Highlights, continued:

- In order to support estrogen metabolism through diet you want to eat plenty of vegetables, eat foods that support glucuronidation, eat plenty of fiber, consume ground flax-seeds, and exercise regularly.
- Some supplements that can support estrogen metabolism include DIM, calcium d-glucarate, and NAC.
- Supplements that can support progesterone production include chaste tree and maca root.
- Evidence shows that chaste tree can successfully lower high prolactin levels in many women.

CHAPTER 28

HEALING YOUR GUT THROUGH THE 5-R PROTOCOL

THE 5-R PROTOCOL RELATES to the healing of the gut, which is part of the triad of autoimmunity. Many sources refer to this as a "4-R Protocol," but the Institute for Functional Medicine updated it and added a fifth "R." So let's go ahead and discuss each of the five components, which will give you the information you need to heal your gut.

1. Remove

As you know, in order for someone to develop Hashimoto's, they must be exposed to an environmental trigger. Thus, in order to reverse the auto-immune component, you need to find and remove the trigger. The same is true for healing a leaky gut. While many will take supplements, such as L-glutamine, and eat gut-healing foods, such as bone broth, to heal their gut, it's important to first detect and remove the leaky gut trigger.

Here are some of the more common leaky gut triggers:

Food allergens. I dedicated two chapters to food allergens, one on gluten (Chapter 5), and another on dairy and other food allergens (Chapter 6). Gluten is the main culprit, as it can cause a leaky gut in everyone. Also, gluten can be a direct environmental trigger through a molecular mimicry mechanism.

Infections. The literature describes numerous infections that can cause an increase in intestinal permeability. These include H. pylori,[74] Blastocystis hominis,[75] and giardia.[76] A Candida overgrowth can also cause a leaky gut,[77,78] and evidence shows that small intestinal bacterial overgrowth (SIBO) can cause an increase in intestinal permeability.[79] Just as a reminder, an increase in intestinal permeability is synonymous with a leaky gut, and so I'll use these interchangeably throughout this chapter.

Environmental toxins. Some of the environmental toxins that have been shown to increase the permeability of the gut include PCBs,[80] mercury,[81] and arsenic.[82]

Drugs. Besides the stress that many drugs put on the liver, some medications can also cause an increase in intestinal permeability. These includes NSAIDs and antibiotics.[83,84] For example, while taking an antibiotic won't directly trigger Hashimoto's, a history of taking antibiotics can make you more susceptible by causing an increase in intestinal permeability.

Proton pump inhibitors (PPIs), also known as acid blockers, inhibit the secretion of gastric acid in the stomach, along with the colonic proton pumps. Evidence shows that PPIs such as omeprazole and lansoprazole can affect intestinal barrier function.[85] Even in situations when these drugs don't directly cause a leaky gut, PPIs have a negative effect on the gut microbiome, which can cause SIBO and Clostridium difficile,[86,87,88] and these can cause an increase in intestinal permeability.

Stress. Evidence indicates that both acute and chronic psychological stress can cause an increase in intestinal permeability.[89,90]

Systemic Inflammation. Proinflammatory cytokines can result in an increase in intestinal permeability.[91]

Detecting the triggers is the most difficult component of the 5-R protocol. However, this book gives you copious information to help find and remove your triggers. Let's look at the other four components of the 5-R Protocol:

2. Replace

This component involves replacing certain factors that play a role in digestion. I'm going to focus on digestive enzymes, betaine HCL, bile salts, and dietary fiber.

Digestive Enzymes. These include enzymes to break down protein (proteases), carbohydrates (amylase), and fat (lipase).

What causes a deficiency of digestive enzymes? Some of the different factors that can cause a deficiency of digestive enzymes include damage to the microvilli, stress, nutrient deficiencies, and environmental toxins.

Signs of a digestive enzyme deficiency: indigestion or a sense of fullness and bloating or flatulence two to four hours after eating a meal.

Plant vs. Animal Sources

Both plant and animal sources of digestive enzymes can be effective. For vegetarian sources, bromelain and papain are two of the more well-known plant-based enzymes, and digestive enzymes can also be derived from microbial sources, such as fungal organisms (e.g., Aspergillus). Pancreatin is an example of a digestive enzyme derived from an animal source (e.g., a porcine or bovine pancreas).

Should You Take Proteolytic Enzymes?

Proteolytic enzymes have three main purposes. One is to break down protein, and I commonly recommend digestive enzymes to my patients to assist with this. Usually, I don't recommend a separate proteolytic enzyme for just protein, but, instead, a supplement that includes enzymes that break down proteins, fats, and carbohydrates.

While taking proteolytic enzymes with meals can help to break down protein, taking proteolytic enzymes in between meals can help to reduce inflammation. One rat study, looking at the role of chymotrypsin, trypsin, and serratiopeptidase on edema, found that chymotrypsin and serratiopeptidase were more effective than aspirin in a subacute model of inflammation.[92] Certain proteolytic enzymes such as serratiopeptidase can also act as biofilm disruptors.[93] I'll discuss biofilm disruptors in Chapter 31.

Food-Based Digestive Enzymes

Although many people with Hashimoto's can benefit from taking a digestive enzyme supplement, some can rely on their body's production of digestive enzyme. In addition, food-based sources of digestive enzymes include bromelain in pineapple, papain in papaya, and amylase in mangos.

What You Need to Know About Hydrochloric Acid (HCL)

Many people with Hashimoto's have low gastric acid (stomach acid), and can benefit from taking betaine HCL with meals. Gastric acid consists mostly of hydrochloric acid, which is released from the parietal cells of the stomach. It plays a role in activating pepsinogen into the active enzyme pepsin, which, in turn, breaks down proteins. In addition, gastric acid has antimicrobial properties that can prevent the development of certain gut infections as well as SIBO.

What causes hypochlorydria (low stomach acid)? Some of the different factors that can cause low stomach acid include nutrient deficiencies, hypothyroidism, and intestinal dysbiosis, including SIBO.

Signs of a HCL deficiency: sense of fullness during or after eating, bloating or belching immediately after eating, undigested food in the stool, one or more nutrient deficiencies (especially iron and vitamin B12), and brittle fingernails

Recommended dosage of betaine HCL: 350 to 3,500 mg/day

Note: If taking betaine HCL, please make sure you do so with meals high in protein (at least 15 grams). You also want to start with a low dosage (i.e., one capsule with each meal), and if you experience heartburn or any other type of burning sensation, this is a sign that you are taking too much and should decrease the dosage. For example, if you were taking three capsules of betaine HCL with meals and were doing fine, but upon increasing the dosage to four capsules, you experienced burning, then you should decrease the dosage back to three capsules per meal and stick with this dosage.

Foods That Promote the Production of Gastric Acid

Some of the foods that can increase gastric acid production include fermented vegetables (e.g., sauerkraut, kimchi, and pickles), apple cider vinegar, and Swedish bitters. It also is a good idea to minimize the amount of water you drink with your meals, and, since stress can reduce stomach acid levels, you might also want to consider doing some deep breathing for a few minutes before your meals.

Bile Salts. Some people can also benefit from supplementing with bile salts, which are involved in fat emulsification. This is especially true for those who have had their gallbladder removed, as getting gallbladder surgery doesn't address the bile metabolism issues commonly associated with these conditions. Some other people can also benefit from taking bile salts, such as those who have problems emulsifying fats. Bile also plays an important role in estrogen metabolism, and, like gastric acid, also has antimicrobial properties.

Signs of bile insufficiency: the incomplete absorption of fats, which presents as steatorrhea (the excretion of abnormal quantities of fat with the feces); diarrhea is also common

Suggested Dosage of bile salts: 500 to 1,000 mg/day in the form of ox bile

Foods that Promote Bile Production

Some of the foods that can help with the formation of bile include beets, ginger, radishes, and artichoke.

Dietary Fiber. Although dietary fiber doesn't fall under the same category as digestive enzymes, betaine HCL, and bile salts, many people don't consume enough dietary fiber, which is important for many reasons. First, fiber helps to feed the good bacteria in your gut. Having sufficient dietary fiber is also important for having regular bowel movements, which is important for eliminating harmful chemicals from the body.

How Much Dietary Fiber Should You Consume?

The recommended fiber intake for children and adults is 14 grams of fiber per 1,000 calories.[94] For example, if you consume an average of 2,000 calories per day then you should be eating 28 grams of fiber per day. If you average 2,500 calories per day then you should aim for 35 grams of fiber per day. If you aren't sure how many calories you consume daily you can use a free program such as **www.myfitnesspal.com**, where you can enter your food diary and it will tell you approximately how many calories you consume daily. You can also use this program to keep track of how much fiber you are consuming.

Some sources suggest that we should be eating even more fiber daily. Evidence suggests that our ancestors ate up to 100 grams of fiber each day![95] I don't expect you to eat this much fiber, but you might want to aim for at least 50 grams of fiber consumption daily.

Fiber can be soluble and insoluble, and most people eat mostly insoluble fiber. Soluble fiber is found in foods such as oat bran, barley, nuts, seeds, beans, lentils, peas, and some fruits and vegetables, while some common sources of insoluble fiber include vegetables and whole grains. Many of these foods are excluded from both an AIP and a standard Paleo diet. Thus, many people with Hashimoto's will rely heavily on vegetables as their source of fiber. However, it's important to understand that while some foods can be classified as being strictly "soluble" or "insoluble," many foods will have a combination of different types of fiber.

Resistant starch can also be a good source of insoluble fiber in those with Hashimoto's. Resistant starch isn't broken down by digestive enzymes, and thus reaches the large intestine and is fermented by bacteria, which classifies it as a type of fermentable fiber. Some AIP-friendly sources of resistant starch include plantains, green bananas, and cassava.

The Role of Butyrate

Eating a good amount of fiber can lead to higher butyrate levels. Butyrate is a short-chain fatty acid (SCFA) that is produced by the bacterial fermentation of fiber in the colon. Acetate and propionate are two other abundant SCFAs, although butyrate is the preferred energy source for epithelial cells located in the colon. SCFAs have a number of different functions, but one important function is to lower colonic pH, which can inhibit the growth of potential pathogens, while at the same time promote the growth of beneficial bacteria, including bifidobacteria and lactobacilli.[96]

SCFAs also have anti-inflammatory effects and play a role in the regulation of immune system function. For example, evidence shows that butyrate can help increase regulatory T cells (Tregs), while decreasing Th17 cells.[97] In section one, I discussed how increasing Tregs and decreasing Th17 cells could help to suppress autoimmunity.

Fiber and the Autoimmune Paleo Diet

Many of the best food sources of fiber are excluded from an autoimmune Paleo (AIP) diet. These include nuts, seeds, legumes, and grains. Thus, if you are following a strict AIP diet, it can be very challenging to get sufficient fiber from your diet. Where should people with Hashimoto's get their fiber from if they are following this type of diet? Vegetables and fruits are the main sources, which is why you want to make sure you eat plenty of these foods daily.

Based on the food diaries of my patients, many people with Hashimoto's don't eat enough servings of vegetables per day. It's also important to understand that the type of vegetables you eat, as well as fruit can make a difference. For example, one ½ cup serving of broccoli will provide more fiber than one cup of spinach. With fruit, a medium apple or pear will have a lot more fiber than one cup of grapes. You can also get fiber by eating starches such as plantains and sweet potatoes.

Here are some of the top high-fiber foods that can be eaten by those who are following an AIP diet:

AIP-friendly foods highest in fiber:
- Apples
- Artichokes
- Avocados
- Blackberries
- Broccoli
- Coconut
- Brussels Sprouts
- Figs (dried)
- Pears
- Plantains
- Raspberries
- Sweet potatoes

3. Reinoculate

Although I commonly recommend probiotic supplements to my patients, it's important to understand that the bacteria in probiotic supplements don't seem to colonize the intestine themselves or modify the overall diversity of the intestinal microbiota.[98] However, studies have shown that taking probiotic supplements can significantly change the types of bacteria and, as a result, can have a significant capacity to remodel the microbiome.[98] In addition, our diet has a direct effect on our microbiome, which is why you want to eat plenty of prebiotic and probiotics sources of foods.

While much research has been done involving the use of probiotics supplements, the approach we take now very likely won't be the approach we take in the future. When recommending probiotic supplements, some healthcare professionals will recommend formulations with specific, well-researched probiotic strains, while other doctors won't pay as much attention to the specific strains included, but instead will focus more on the diversity.

Food Sources of Prebiotics and Probiotics: While it can be beneficial to take a probiotic supplement, you should also eat food sources of probiotics, such as sauerkraut, kimchi, and pickles. Some examples of prebiotic foods include Jerusalem artichokes, asparagus, onions, chicory, bananas, and other fruit; even green tea is considered to be a source of prebiotics.[99,100] Prebiotic foods are important because they feed the good bacteria, such as bifidobacteria and lactobacilli, and they're good sources of short-chain fatty acids.

Which Strains of Probiotics Should You Take?

I can't say that I'm an expert on the different probiotic strains. However, when I recommend a probiotic supplement to my patients, I try to recommend probiotics that include well-researched strains, which greatly improve the chances of taking a supplement with therapeutic actions because specific strains have specific functions. I will briefly mention the benefits of some of the strains I commonly recommend to my patients:

Lactobacillus acidophilus. This is probably the most well-known species, and it is resistant to gastric acid and bile salts, along with pepsin and pancreatin. The strains Lactobacillus acidophilus LA-5 and LA-14 have been shown to inhibit certain pathogens.[101,102]

Bifidobacterium lactis. This species produces large amounts of antimicrobial substances. It also modulates the immune system response to help against pathogens. The strains Bifidobacterium lactis BB-12 and HN019 are known for their antipathogenic and immune enhancement effects.[103,104,105]

Lactobacillus casei. This probiotic also improves the health of the immune system, and can be effective against certain pathogens such as H. pylori[106] and Candida albicans.[107] Evidence indicates that the strain Lactobacillus casei CRL 431 (along with Lactobacillus rhamnosus CRL 1224) can be effective against Aspergillus flavus,[108] which is a fungi.

Lactobacillus plantarum. A few strains of lactobacillus plantarum have proven to be beneficial. Lactobacillus plantarum 299v has been shown to provide effective symptom relief, particularly of abdominal pain and bloating, in patients with irritable bowel syndrome.[109,110] Lactobacillus plantarum Lp-115 also can benefit people with gastrointestinal disorders.[111]

Lactobacillus rhamnosus. Numerous studies have shown the benefits of Lactobacillus rhamnosus GG in reducing the incidence of ear infections and upper respiratory infections in children[112] and antibiotic-associated diarrhea.[113] One study showed that Lactobacillus rhamnosus HN001 (along with Bifidobacterium longum BB536) can modulate the gut microbiota, which in turn can cause a significant reduction of potentially harmful bacteria and an increase of beneficial ones.[114] Another study I came across showed that taking Lactobacillus rhamnosus HN001 in early pregnancy may reduce the prevalence of gestational diabetes mellitus.[115]

Saccharomyces boulardii. Saccharomyces boulardii is another well-researched strain with many different health benefits. It is well known for helping people who have a Candida overgrowth.[116,117] It also can be useful in the maintenance treatment of Crohn's disease.[118] It can help to improve intestinal permeability,[119] and help reduce inflammation and dysfunction of the gastrointestinal tract in intestinal mucositis.[120]

Other probiotic strains. Some other beneficial probiotic strains include Bifidobacterium lactis Bl-04, Bifidobacterium longum Bl-05, Bifidobacterium bifidum Bb-06, and Lactobacillus casei Lc-11.

What About Soil-Based Probiotics and Fecal Transplants?

Two examples of soil-based probiotics include bacillus subtilis and bacillus coagulans. These are also known as spore-based probiotics. These bacterial spores offer the advantage of a higher survival rate during the acidic stomach passage and better stability during the processing and storage of the product.[121] One study involving a spore-based probiotic called Megasporebiotic showed that it could help decrease proinflammatory cytokines and reduce the symptoms associated with a leaky gut.[122] Over the last few years, many healthcare professionals have started recommending spore-based probiotics to their patients with good results.

I'm not asked as much about fecal microbiota transplants, but I figured it was worth mentioning this here because this can potentially help with certain health conditions. This essentially involves the transmission of fecal microorganisms from a healthy donor into the gastrointestinal tract of a patient, and the primary goal of this procedure is to restore a normal microbiome in patients with conditions associated with dysbiosis.[123] It seems to be very effective in helping people with clostridium difficile, along with Crohn's disease and ulcerative colitis.[123,124,125] While I haven't come across any evidence of fecal microbiota transplants benefiting those with Hashimoto's, case reports have shown favorable outcomes in Parkinson's disease, multiple sclerosis, myoclonus dystonia, chronic fatigue syndrome, and idiopathic thrombocytopenic purpura.[126]

4. Repair

A leaky gut occurs when the intestinal barrier is compromised. Epithelial tight junctions form a selective permeable seal between the cells of the small intestine. In other words, these tight junctions of the small intestine allow some smaller molecules to pass through, but not other larger molecules. However, certain factors can disrupt these tight junctions, allowing larger proteins and other molecules to pass into the bloodstream, where they normally shouldn't be. Thus, the immune system sees them as being foreign and mounts an immune system response.

For example, the way gluten can cause a leaky gut is by causing a release of zonulin, a molecule that regulates the tight junctions of the small intestine, opening up the tight junctions between cells and allowing larger molecules to pass through into the bloodstream. Infections can also have a similar effect. Because of this, zonulin can be a marker of impaired gut barrier function.

As for how to repair the gut, a lot can be accomplished through diet, and in Chapter 26, I discussed how the AIP diet can help with gut healing by eliminating foods that can cause gut inflammation, along with an increase in permeability. In addition to avoiding foods that can have a negative effect on gut healing, certain foods can aid in healing the gut, which I'm about to discuss.

Note: Please remember that in order to heal your gut, you need to remove the leaky gut trigger, which is the first component of the 5-R protocol. While this might sound obvious, many people who follow a strict diet and take gut-healing supplements don't receive optimal results because they haven't addressed those factors that compromised the gut in the first place.

Foods That Can Help With Gut Healing

Some of the foods that can help heal the gut include bone broth, fermented foods, and cabbage juice. I'd like to focus on bone broth, as many people are aware of the healing benefits of bone broth. Not only are more and more people drinking bone broth these days, but now people are adding bone broth protein powders to their smoothies. Is this a case of "bone broth fever," or is there justification to drinking bone broth regularly?

I can't say that drinking bone broth is required to heal a leaky gut, but it can help because it has multiple gut healing agents, including collagen, glutamine, glycine, and proline. While making your own bone broth is probably the best option, doing this is admittedly time consuming. For those who don't have the time to make their own bone broth, some companies, such as Wise Choice Market, sell premade organic beef bone broth from grass-fed cows.

Nutritional Supplements and Herbs That Can Help With Gut Healing

L-glutamine. One of the most common nutrients used to help heal a leaky gut by natural healthcare professionals is L-glutamine. Glutamine is an amino acid, and is considered to be the most abundant free amino acid in the blood.[127] In helping to heal a leaky gut, glutamine is the primary energy source for enterocytes, which are the cells of the small intestine.[128] A number of different studies show that taking glutamine can help reduce intestinal permeability.[129,130,131]

Suggested Dosage: Between 4,000 and 12,000 mg/day taken in between meals

Is Glutamine an Excitotoxin?

Some are concerned that glutamine is an excitotoxin, but this isn't true. However, glutamine can convert into glutamate, which can cause excitotoxicity in some people. If someone has a defective glutamine-glutamate-GABA cycle, then this can lead to the buildup of glutamate. However, if this is working properly, then glutamine is converted into glutamate, but this, in turn, is converted into GABA. Thus, taking L-glutamine can lead to excessive amounts of glutamate in a small percentage of people. If you are concerned about this, you can start with very small doses of L-glutamine, and, assuming you don't experience any negative symptoms, you can then gradually increase it.

Demulcent Herbs. Demulcents help to soften and soothe dry and irritated mucous membranes, and this allows new intestinal cells to grow. Three of the most commonly used demulcents are deglycyrrhizinated licorice (DGL), slippery elm, and marshmallow root.

Suggested Dosage of deglycyrrhizinated licorice: 250 to 500 mg/day
Suggested Dosage of slippery elm: 250 to 500 mg/day
Suggested Dosage of marshmallow root: 250 to 500 mg mg/day

Zinc. Zinc supplementation has been shown to have a protective effect on the epithelial barrier.[132] Another study showed that impaired intestinal barrier function improved following supplementation of zinc, along with vitamin A.[133] Some healthcare professionals specifically recommend zinc carnosine for gut healing because of a study showing that zinc carnosine can offer protection against an increase in intestinal permeability.[134]
Suggested Dosage of zinc carnosine: 50 to 75mg/day

Vitamin A. Zinc and vitamin A supplementation can improve impaired intestinal barrier function[133] because Vitamin A and its derivatives have been shown to regulate the growth and differentiation of intestinal cells.[135]
Suggested Dosage: I'm cautious about listing a dosage here, as there are risks in taking too high of a dosage of vitamin A. However, I will say that with some patients, I'll recommend 10,000 IU/day of active vitamin A, and I know some healthcare professionals who will recommend higher doses than this. Nevertheless, vitamin A toxicity is a concern.

5. Rebalance

I'm not going to discuss this component in detail here, as I've explained some of these factors in other chapters. However, I did want to briefly discuss the parasympathetic nervous system, as this plays a big role in having optimal digestive health.

The parasympathetic nervous system is one of two branches of the autonomic nervous system, with the other branch being the sympathetic nervous system. The parasympathetic nervous system consists of the vagus nerve, which, in turn, innervates most of the tissues involved in nutrient metabolism, including the stomach, pancreas, and liver.[136] Thus, activation of the parasympathetic nervous system will lead to activation of vagal efferent activity, which can influence how nutrients are absorbed and metabolized.[136] In other words, activation of the parasympathetic nervous system can increase the absorption of the nutrients you consume.

How do you activate the parasympathetic nervous system? One of the best ways is by practicing mind-body medicine, which I discussed in Chapter 27. This includes meditation, yoga, and biofeedback. For example, evidence shows that yoga can directly stimulate the vagus nerve and enhance parasympathetic output.[137] In the same chapter, I also discussed how heart rate variability could help achieve a state of coherence, which is associated with a relative increase in parasympathetic activity.

Can You Focus on Multiple Components Simultaneously?

You might wonder if you can address more than one component of the 5-R protocol simultaneously. For example, if someone has an H. pylori infection, is it acceptable to take digestive enzymes and probiotics at the same time the infection is being eradicated, and perhaps even taking some gut healing agents? You can address multiple components simultaneously, and most healthcare professionals do so, including myself.

However, there is nothing wrong with focusing on one "R" at a time. For example, it's perfectly fine to first focus on removing the factor that is causing the leaky gut. After all, you can't fully heal your gut until you address the first "R." Then, once this has been accomplished, you can focus on the other components.

I will add that if you focus on the "remove" component first, after you remove the factor that caused the leaky gut you then might want to focus on the other components simultaneously. In other words, you might want to initially focus on removing the factor that caused the leaky gut, and then take measures to replace, reinoculate, repair, and rebalance the body.

Chapter Highlights:

- The first component of the 5-R protocol is remove, as you want to remove the factors that caused the leaky gut.
- Some of the more common leaky gut triggers include food allergens, gut infections, environmental toxins, drugs, stress, and systemic inflammation.
- The second component of the 5-R protocol is replace.
- Some of the things you want to consider replacing include digestive enzymes, hydrochloric acid, bile salts, and dietary fiber.
- The third component of the 5-R protocol is reinoculate.
- While it can be beneficial to take a probiotic supplement, you should also eat food sources of probiotics.
- Spore-based probiotics offer the advantage of a higher survival rate during the acidic stomach passage and better stability during the processing and storage of the product.
- The fourth component of the 5-R protocol is repair.
- Some of the foods that can help heal the gut include bone broth, fermented foods, and cabbage juice.
- Supplements that can help with gut healing include L-glutamine, demulcent herbs, zinc, and vitamin A.
- The fifth component of the 5-R protocol is to rebalance your body through sleep, stress management, and other lifestyle factors.
- One of the best ways of activating the parasympathetic nervous system is by practicing mind-body medicine.
- While some people will incorporate all of the components of the 5-R protocol simultaneously, others will choose to focus on removing the factor that caused the leaky gut, and then, once this has been accomplished, they will focus on the other four components of the 5-R protocol.

CHAPTER 29

HOW TO REDUCE YOUR TOXIC LOAD

IN CHAPTER 8, YOU learned about many of the different sources of environmental toxins you're frequently exposed to. In this chapter, I'll discuss what you can do to reduce your toxic load and support your detoxification pathways. Keep in mind that I'm not suggesting that everyone needs to follow all of the detoxification strategies I'll be discussing, and towards the end of the chapter, I'll discuss some action steps you can take.

I'd like to begin by discussing the detoxification pathways. There are two primary phases of detoxification. In the phase one detoxification system, which is known as "biotransformation," certain toxins are converted into intermediate metabolites that can be more harmful than the original compound.

In the phase two detoxification system, also known as the conjugation process, these intermediate metabolites are combined with certain molecules and become less toxic and water soluble. These metabolites are eventually excreted, which is considered to be phase three detoxification. In phase one, these toxins can be more harmful, as these intermediate metabolites can cause damage to the proteins, DNA, and RNA if they don't go through phase two detoxification. Thus, this can have harmful effects if someone has compromised phase two activity.

The Role of Cytochrome P450 Enzymes in Detoxification

Cytochrome P450 (CYP450) enzymes are produced by the liver, although they are also found in other areas, including the kidney, small intestine, lung, adrenals, and most other tissues. These enzymes are utilized in phase one detoxification. There are 58 different CYP450 enzymes, and different enzymes will play different roles in the metabolism of environmental toxins, which include medications. The CYP450 enzymes can be inhibited or induced by certain drugs, as well as by certain nutrients and herbs. An inducing agent can increase the rate of another drug's metabolism, whereas an inhibiting agent can decrease or inhibit the drug's metabolism.

CYP450 enzymes are also essential in the metabolism of certain nutrients, such as vitamin E,[138] and hormones such as estrogen, as the first step in the metabolism of estrogens is the hydroxylation catalyzed by CYP450.[139] The CYP450 enzymes are also necessary for the metabolism of vitamin D.[140]

Genetic Polymorphisms Can Affect Detoxification

I'd like to briefly discuss some of the genetic factors that can play a role in detoxification. I realize that the next few paragraphs will be advanced for many people, and while the environment plays a huge role in toxic overload, we can't overlook the importance of genetic factors. While you can't change your genes, you can take measures to better support your detoxification pathways and improve methylation despite the presence of certain genetic polymorphisms.

Polymorphisms are common genetic defects that can occur in the CYP450 family, which, in turn, can affect the detoxification process. This is especially true for the phase one metabolism of drugs, since almost 80% of drugs are metabolized by these enzymes.[141] For example, if someone has a polymorphism of CYP2D6, then they would be considered to be a "poor metabolizer".[141] Polymorphisms of other CYP genes are also common, including CYP1A1, 2A6, A13, 2C8, 3A4, and 3A5.

What is the significance of these genetic polymorphisms? Having certain polymorphisms of the CYP450 enzymes can reduce the person's ability to detoxify. Some of these polymorphisms have been linked to chronic health conditions. Of course, most people aren't tested for these polymorphisms; thus, when prescribing a specific medication, the medical doctor will simply recommend what he or she thinks is the appropriate dosage. In the future, more and more people are going to be tested for these genetic polymorphisms, which, in turn, will impact the drug recommendations given by medical doctors.

Reminder: Glyphosate Inhibits the Cytochrome P450 Enzymes

In section two, I dedicated an entire chapter to glyphosate (Chapter 20), and mentioned that glyphosate can inhibit the CYP450 enzymes. This is yet another reason to try to eat organic whenever possible, as this will decrease your exposure to this chemical. Some non-GMO crops are sprayed with glyphosate right before they are harvested, which is why purchasing non-organic, non-GMO foods alone isn't sufficient. Glyphosate can also be found in the water supply, which is yet another reason to drink purified water.

How Do Nutrient Deficiencies Affect Detoxification?

Nutrients are necessary for the proper functioning of the detoxification pathways. Some of the more important nutrients required for phase one detoxification include vitamins B2, B3, B6, B12, folate, magnesium, zinc, copper, iron, and molybdenum. Glutathione is an antioxidant that plays an important role in both phase one and phase two detoxification. The amino acids glycine, cysteine, and glutamine are precursors of glutathione, although other amino acids such as taurine and methionine are important for phase two detoxification.

When looking at phase one detoxification, remember that intermediary metabolites are produced, and these metabolites can lead to the formation of free radicals. Thus, it is important to have sufficient antioxidants to help neutralize these free radical reactions. This not only includes glutathione, but others such vitamin C and vitamin E. This doesn't mean that you need to take all of these as supplements, as you ideally want to get most of your antioxidants from food, specifically vegetables and fruits.

The Complexity of Phase Two Detoxification

Phase two involves the conjugation of the intermediate metabolite with another molecule to make it less toxic and water soluble. This process can be quite complex, as many pathways are required in this phase. These includes glucuronidation, sulfate conjugation, methylation, amino acid conjugation, glutathione conjugation, and acetylation. Having problems with any one of these pathways can affect phase two detoxification.

Several factors can cause these pathways to become less efficient. Having a genetic defect such as an MTHFR polymorphism can be a major factor in some cases. Having certain nutrient deficiencies can also be problematic.

For example, acetylation involves attaching acetyl Co-A to environmental toxins to help eliminate them from the body. Nutrients that play a role in acetylation include pantothenic acid (vitamin B5), vitamin C, vitamin B1, vitamin B2, and magnesium. If any of these nutrients are deficient, then this can have a negative effect on acetylation. When it comes to methylation, which involves conjugating toxins with methyl groups, three of the most important nutrients include folate, vitamin B6, and vitamin B12.

Glutathione synthesis depends on nutrients as well, including magnesium. Other important nutrients and amino acids are required (I mentioned glycine, cysteine, and glutamine earlier), but if someone has a severe magnesium deficiency, yet they take N-acetylcysteine to help increase glutathione levels, they won't be able to accomplish this if the magnesium deficiency isn't addressed. In addition, sulfur can be used to increase the synthesis of glutathione, which is why sulfur-rich vegetables contribute to over 50% of dietary glutathione.

Thyroid Hormones and Detoxification

Thyroid hormones play an important role in detoxification. One study with mice showed that hypothyroidism could affect the metabolism of xenobiotics by suppressing the CYP3A enzyme, while inducing the CYP2B enzyme.[142] Studies also show that a thyroid hormone imbalance can affect the CYP450 enzymes.[143,144,145]

This means that having hypothyroidism due to Hashimoto's thyroiditis can have a negative effect on detoxification. While Hashimoto's is an immune system condition, for optimal detoxification, it is necessary to correct any thyroid hormone imbalance.

How to Minimize Your Exposure to Environmental Toxins

Next, I'd like to discuss some things you can do to minimize your exposure to environmental toxins. After all, while it's important to take measures to eliminate these chemicals from your body, it's even more important to take precautions to minimize your exposure to them. Of course, you won't be able to completely avoid exposure to these chemicals, but you want to do everything you can to reduce your exposure to them.

Eat well. Everyone reading this book knows that it is important to eat mostly whole foods, while minimizing the refined foods and sugars. If you eat mostly whole foods, then you won't have to be concerned about the ingredients added to refined foods, as many of these ingredients are harmful to your health. These chemicals include artificial flavors and colorings, as well as preservatives, GMOs, and other harmful ingredients.

Regarding whole foods, certified organic is best in order to minimize your exposure to toxic ingredients. This is especially true with meat, fruits, and vegetables, although it can apply to other types of foods as well. Concerning fruits and vegetables, if you are unable to purchase organic produce then you might want to check out the Dirty Dozen and Clean Fifteen lists from the Environmental Working Group (**www.ewg.org**). The Dirty Dozen lists the top twelve fruits and vegetables with the greatest amount of pesticides, while the Clean Fifteen list includes the top fifteen fruits and vegetables with the least amount of pesticides. These lists are updated each year.

You want to eat a good variety of fruits and vegetables every day, as this will help to ensure that you get the nutrients necessary to support the detoxification pathways. This is especially true for vegetables, so try to eat at least four to six servings of fresh vegetables per day, and more than this would be even better. I usually recommend eating both raw and cooked vegetables, although some people might not be able to tolerate raw vegetables initially; thus, you might have no choice but to only eat cooked vegetables, at least until you improve the health of your digestive system.

I realize that some people with hypothyroid conditions are cautious about eating cruciferous vegetables, although eating one or two servings of these foods each day usually won't pose a problem for most people with Hashimoto's. Cruciferous vegetables are the primary source of isothiocyanates and other glucosinolate derivatives that are known to induce phase II detoxifying enzymes, including glutathione S-transferases.[146]

What Type of Water Should You Drink?

Much controversy exists over the different types of water to drink. I would recommend that you avoid drinking tap water due to the chlorine and fluoride added, and other environmental toxins, including heavy metals, solvents, and pharmaceuticals. If you have well water, it might not have chlorine and fluoride, but it can include other environmental toxins, such as arsenic.[147,148,149]

Although testing your water is an option, there isn't a test I know of that will measure all of the possible environmental toxins that might be contaminating your water. In addition to not drinking tap water, and possibly well water, you also might want to consider investing in a filtration system that allows you to bathe in cleaner water. At the very least, consider purchasing a filter to put on your showerhead that reduces chlorine and some other chemicals. For specific recommendations, please visit **www.naturalendocrinesolutions.com/resources**.

Concerning drinking water, I personally drink both reverse osmosis water and a good quality spring water out of a glass bottle. The downside of reverse osmosis is that that this type of filtration not only removes all of the minerals but can also waste a lot of water. However, it removes most of the harmful chemicals from the water, which is a great benefit. While tap water can be a good source of calcium, magnesium, and potassium, most of the minerals you obtain come from the food you eat. Supplementation is also an option for those who are concerned about the "risks" of drinking reverse osmosis water.

Spring water out of glass bottle is also a good option to consider, as this will have minerals, and thus is alkaline in nature. Mountain Valley Springs has an excellent quality spring water out of a glass bottle, although it can become quite expensive drinking a few glass bottles of spring water per day, especially if you are purchasing this water for a large family. One solution is to drink a combination of reverse osmosis water and spring water out of a glass bottle. For example, I drink two cups of Mountain Valley Springs water every morning, but otherwise I drink reverse osmosis water.

Purchase natural household products. In addition to eating well, you want to try purchasing mostly natural products. If you can switch to all organic products, that would be great, but if you are unable to do this, then prioritize the household cleaners and cosmetics you purchase. At the very least, make sure any household products that you use regularly are natural or organic. For specific brand recommendations on household cleaners and cosmetics, please visit **www.naturalendocrinesolutions.com/resources**.

It would be great if you can switch to all natural and organic products, but I realize this can be expensive. While I can argue that in the long run, it will be less expensive when you consider the negative impact these chemicals can have on your health, I realize that many people still won't switch out all of their products, and if you can't truly afford to buy every-thing natural, then you need to prioritize. You can also visit the Environ-mental Working Group's Skin Deep website (**www.ewg.org/skindeep**) to find out which household products are the most toxic. Many people are using body creams they think are natural, but actually include chemicals that either have been proven to be unsafe or haven't been tested.

You can also make your own household products. Essential oils can be great for this, as there is a lot of research on the different health benefits of essential oils, and you can use them to make toothpaste, soap, shampoo, deodorant, etc.

Use a natural dry cleaning company. Dry cleaning involves a few different chemicals that can be harmful to your health. Tetrachloroethylene, also known as perchloroethylene, has been the dominant solvent used in dry cleaning worldwide,[150] and can be carcinogenic.[151] Perchloroethylene is toxic to the liver, kidneys, and central nervous system, and may be a human carcinogen.[152] According to the EPA, approximately 28,000 dry cleaners use perchlorethylene.[153] Some dry cleaners are using alternative solvents, butylal and high-flashpoint hydrocarbons.[154] However, there currently seems to be insufficient toxicological and health information to determine their safety, especially for butylal.[154]

Can't you use an organic dry cleaners? Even if you have an organic dry cleaners nearby, you do need to be careful, as some advertise as being "organic cleaners" or "eco-friendly," when this isn't the case. You might want to see if one of the local dry cleaners offers "wet cleaning," which is a nontoxic alter-native to conventional dry cleaning.[155] If you choose to use a conventional dry cleaners, I wouldn't put the dry cleaned clothes in your bedroom closet for at least 48 hours after they are cleaned. Instead, remove the plastic bag and place the dry-cleaned clothes outside to air out.

Consider replacing your carpeting. If you are renting, then this prob-ably isn't an option. And even if you own your own home, replacing the carpet with hardwood floors can be very expensive. However, if the chemicals from your carpeting are having a negative impact on your health, then this is something to strongly consider. Besides these chemicals potentially being a factor in your Hashimoto's condition,[156] if you have children, studies show that formaldehyde used in carpeting and furniture might increase the risk of childhood asthma.[157] Also, if you get hardwood floors installed, you want to make sure that they are low-VOC.

Use low or no-VOC paints. These days, it's easy to purchase paint that is low in VOCs. However, keep in mind that some low-VOC paints may still have significant emissions of some individual VOCs.[158] Thus, it probably is best to get a "zero" VOC paint.

Be careful when buying new furniture. When you buy new furniture, try your best to avoid those that have flame retardants. You might want to try to get furniture made from polyester, wool, or cotton fillings. Since most people spend anywhere from one quarter to one third of their day in bed, it makes sense to consider investing in a "natural" mattress. Although I'm not suggesting that the chemicals from your mattress are responsible for your Hashimoto's condition, this doesn't mean that these chemicals can't have a negative impact on your current and future health.

I came across a study that looked at the effects of mattress emissions in mice.[159] The study showed that all mattresses caused pulmonary irritation, and the authors concluded that some mattresses emitted mixtures of volatile chemicals that have the potential to cause respiratory-tract irritation and can decrease airflow velocity. They also mentioned that organic cotton padding caused very different effects, increases in both respiratory rate and tidal volume.

Use safe cookware. Aluminum cookware should be avoided due to leaching of aluminum.[160] Stainless steel is a safer option, and is what I use, although it can be an overlooked source of nickel and chromium.[161] Cast iron is another option to consider, and using this cookware might benefit those with an iron deficiency.[162]

Invest in a quality air purification system. One of the best things you can do is invest in a quality air-purification system. A HEPA filtration system is recommended. Please visit the resources page on my website for some brand suggestions.

How to Reduce Your Exposure to Electronic Pollution

Let's not forget about electronic pollution, as this also can have a negative effect on your health. The reason for this has to do with EMFs, which are electromagnetic fields we are constantly exposed to. Some of the products that emit electromagnetic fields include televisions, refrigerators, cell phones, computers, vacuum cleaners, hair dryers, and fluorescent lights. Although you probably won't be able to eliminate your exposure to EMFs, here are eight things you can do to minimize your exposure to electronic pollution:

1. Focus on your bedroom. Try to spend your resting hours away from EMFs. Consider getting rid of all of the electronics in your bedroom. If you insist on having a television in your bedroom, and perhaps a DVD player and/ or a DVR, unplug these devices at night.

Don't use an electric alarm clock, as these are high in EMFs. So are electric blankets. If you absolutely refuse to use a battery-operated alarm clock then make sure that your electric alarm clock or cell phone is at least six feet away from your bed. Turn your cell phone on airplane mode at night. Electric fans also emit EMFS.

2. Position your refrigerator carefully. Your refrigerator will emit a good amount of EMFs, and keep in mind that EMFs emit through walls. So for example, if your living room couch is located on the other side of the wall where your refrigerator is, then whenever you or anyone else sits on the couch they will be exposed to EMFs from the refrigerator. The same concept applies to other devices. If you have a big screen television in your living room, and on the other side of the wall is a bed, then, assuming this television is plugged in all of the time, that person on the other side will be exposed to EMFs while sleeping. However, if the television is unplugged at night then this will help to reduce their EMF exposure.

3. Don't carry around your cell phone. I realize that, at times, you might need to have your cell phone. I don't bring my cell phone everywhere I go when I'm in my home, although I'm usually guilty of carrying my cell phone with me when I leave my house. Also, when talking on your cell phone, don't hold the phone up against your head. Cell phones are great pieces of technology, but people really do need to cut down on their usage.

4. Reduce your exposure to other electronic devices. In addition to minimizing your cell phone use, also try to cut down on your usage of other electronic devices that emit EMFs such as computers, televisions, e-readers, handheld video games, hairdryers, and electric blankets. You especially want to be cautious about using wireless devices, including cordless phones, Bluetooth headsets, and other Bluetooth devices.

5. Turn off the Wi-Fi each night. While it would be great if you can hardwire your house, I realize that most people who have Wi-Fi are unlikely to get rid of their Wi-Fi router, including myself. While you might be exposed to the Wi-Fi from your neighbors, it still will benefit your health if you turn your Wi-Fi off each night when you go to bed.

6. Incorporate earthing. This is also known as grounding, and it involves an exchange of electrons from the earth to your body. Some research shows how this transfer of electrons can help to improve the health of people by neutralizing free radicals. In some people, this can cause a reduction in pain, improved sleep, and other health benefits.

Earthing can be done by placing your bare feet outside on the ground (e.g., the grass, dirt, or sand if you live near a beach). However, there are ways to engage in earthing while inside your home or at work, as you can buy "earthing mats" and "earthing sheets" to use on your bed or in your office so that you can receive the benefits of earthing if working a desk job, and while sleeping. If you don't want to purchase any "earthing equipment," taking 15 to 30 minutes each day to walk barefoot outside can offer some good benefits.

A few studies have been done on the benefits of earthing. One study looked at the role of earthing in neuromodulation, and it found that earthing could help to restore natural, electrical status of the electrical environment of the organism and, thus, the nervous system.[163] Another study involving 40 adult participants looked to see if earthing improves mood, and it was concluded that a one hour contact with the earth improved mood more than expected than by relaxation alone.[164]

7. Consider investing in a gauss meter. I have a Cornet gauss meter, which seems to do a pretty good job of measuring EMFs. For more information on this, I would visit the website **www.electricsense.com**, which discusses the different gauss meters. Some apps you can download on your smartphone to help with the detection of EMFs, although they don't seem to be as reliable as a gauss meter.

8. Consider moving if necessary. I realize that this is an extreme measure that most people won't take, and, fortunately, most people don't need to do this. However, you need to consider the long-term effect of electronic pollution on your health. For example, if you live near a cell phone tower, then over the years, this can have a negative effect on your health. While living near a cell phone tower doesn't guarantee that you will develop cancer or another chronic health condition, why take the chance?

Supporting Detoxification Through Diet

Now that I've explained in detail how to minimize your exposure to environmental toxins, I'd like to discuss how to support your detoxification pathways through eating well. In order to support the liver through diet, you want to do the following:

Enhance phase one detoxification. You can accomplish this by eating plenty of cruciferous vegetables, flax lignans, and omega-3 fatty acids.

Use diet for the protection against phase one metabolites. You can accomplish this by eating antioxidant-rich foods, especially a wide variety of fruits and vegetables.

Promote methylation. Eat foods rich in folate, such as dark green leafy vegetables. Eat foods rich in vitamin B6, including turkey, beef, chicken, salmon, sweet potatoes, and spinach. Eat foods rich in vitamin B12, including liver, beef, chicken, fish, and eggs.

Stimulate bile production. Eating foods such as dark green leafy vegetables, celery, watercress, dandelion, and garlic will help with this.

Eat cilantro. A few studies show that cilantro, also known as Chinese parsley, can help with the binding and excretion of heavy metals, including mercury[165] and lead.[166] Some people find cilantro to have a foul taste, while others enjoy eating it, and this "cilantro preference" has a genetic component.[167] If you do like cilantro, consider consuming one-quarter cup per day to help support detoxification.

Drink plenty of water daily. Drink 40 to 50% of your body weight in ounces. For example, if you weigh 140 pounds, drink 56 to 70 ounces of water per day. Avoid drinking tap water and water out of plastic bottles frequently, and either drink purified water, or spring water out of a glass bottle. Drinking green tea has some great health benefits and can help with the elimination of environmental toxins. The caffeine can be an issue with some people, although you can drink an organic decaffeinated green tea. Drinking herbal teas can also offer some health benefits.

Enhance bowel movements. Constipation is common with those who have an underactive thyroid, which can affect your ability to eliminate toxins. Some of the most common causes of chronic constipation include a) not drinking enough fluids, b) not eating enough foods rich in fiber, c) having intestinal dysbiosis, d) having certain nutrient deficiencies (e.g., magnesium), e) some medications, and f) having bile metabolism problems. People with small intestinal bacterial overgrowth who have high methane levels will also commonly have chronic constipation

Supporting Detoxification Through Nutritional Supplements and Herbs

Although you can do a great job of supporting your detoxification pathways through diet, taking certain nutritional supplements and herbs can also be beneficial. While I will give suggested doses, everyone is different, and keep in mind that it is always possible to have a negative reaction when taking any type of supplement. Thus, it is always best to work with a competent natural healthcare professional.

Milk Thistle. This is a well-known herb that can protect the liver from oxidative stress by increasing the endogenous production of glutathione, and this herb has demonstrated anti-inflammatory and T cell-modulating effects.[168] Milk thistle can also promote protein synthesis, regenerate liver tissue, enhance glucuronidation, and protect against glutathione depletion.[169] Evidence shows that milk thistle might offer protection from the toxic effects of heavy metals.[170,171]
  Suggested Dosage: 250 to 500 mg/day

N-acetylcysteine. This is a precursor to glutathione, an antioxidant that supports the detoxification pathways. NAC can also act as a heavy metal chelator. It seems to be most effective in the chelation of mercury,[172] and it can be effective with arsenic poisoning.[173,174,175]
  Suggested Dosage: 600 to 1,800 mg/day between meals

Alpha lipoic acid. Alpha-lipoic acid is a naturally occurring compound synthesized in the mitochondria. It can assist in detoxification by scavenging free radicals, chelating heavy metals, and it can also restore intracellular glutathione levels.[176] The research shows that alpha lipoic acid is an effective chelator of heavy metals, including mercury and lead.[177,178] Alpha lipoic acid seems to work better for lead toxicity when used in combination with another chelating agent.[178,179] Alpha-lipoic acid consists of two forms: R-lipoic acid and S-lipoic acid. Many healthcare professionals prefer R-lipoic acid since this is the naturally occurring form and, thus, seems to be better utilized by the body.

You need to exercise caution if you have mercury amalgams, as there is the potential risk of the redistribution of metals if alpha lipoic acid isn't used carefully.[180] Thus, if you have mercury amalgams, then it is wise to take lower doses of alpha lipoic acid, and to be cautious about taking other chelating agents as well. To play it safe, it probably would be best to work with a competent healthcare professional.

Suggested Dosage: 200 to 600 mg/day

Acetylated or Liposomal glutathione. You can also choose not to take the glutathione precursors and, instead, take a liposomal or an acetylated form of glutathione. Regarding the effects glutathione has on toxic metals, one study demonstrated three specific roles glutathione has in protecting the body from mercury toxicity.[181] Another study showed that intracellular glutathione could help to protect against cadmium toxicity.[182] Glutathione also offers protection against lead.[183] Selenium is a cofactor for glutathione production. Thus, someone with a selenium deficiency will most likely have low glutathione levels.

Suggested Dosage of Acetylated glutathione: 200 to 600 mg/day
Suggested Dosage of Liposomal glutathione: 250 to 500 mg/day

Trimethylglycine (TMG), also known as anhydrous betaine. TMG plays a role in metabolizing homocysteine into methionine. TMG has been shown to protect the liver and raise S-adenosylmethionine (SAMe) levels. SAMe is important because it is the primary methyl donor in the body, and methyl groups are necessary for optimal health and well-being, as they play a critical role in the expression of genes.

Suggested Dosage: 500 to 1,000 mg/day

Schisandra. You don't hear about this herb as much as some of the others I mentioned, although schisandra can support the lungs, adrenals, and liver.
Suggested Dosage: 250 to 1,000 mg/day

Dandelion root. Enhances liver and gallbladder function by supporting bile production, and assists the liver in the filtration of accumulated environmental toxins.
Suggested Dosage: 250 to 500 mg/day

What's the Deal With Chlorella?

Chlorella is a fresh water green alga rich in proteins, vitamins, and minerals. Daily dietary supplementation with chlorella may reduce high blood pressure, lower serum cholesterol levels, accelerate wound healing, and enhance immune functions.[184] Chlorella also can help to counteract heavy metal toxicity, especially that of mercury[185] and cadmium.[186]

However, evidence suggests that chlorella can stimulate the immune system by increasing the Th1 response.[187,188] Because of this, some healthcare professionals are concerned that taking chlorella can exacerbate the autoimmune response in some people with Hashimoto's. Although I don't commonly recommend chlorella to my patients, over the years, I have had some patients with Hashimoto's take chlorella without any adverse effects. However, you still want to exercise caution, and if you do choose to take chlorella, you want to make sure it's a clean source.

Other Tips to Help Eliminate Harmful Chemicals From Your Body

Invest in an infrared sauna. Many natural healthcare professionals, including myself, recommend using infrared sauna therapy to help with the elimination of toxins. Infrared (also known as thermal radiation) is a band of energy in the complete electromagnetic spectrum and it has been used effectively to treat certain maladies.[189] At the cellular level, electromagnetic radiation alters cell membrane potentials and affects mitochondrial metabolism.[189,190] Visit **www.naturalendocrinesolutions.com/resources** for some infrared sauna recommendations.

Which Environmental Toxins Are Eliminated Through Sweating?

Research shows that numerous environmental toxins are eliminated through sweat. This includes heavy metals,[191,192] bisphenol A (BPA),[193] and phthalates.[194] Just keep in mind that in addition to eliminating toxins, you will also lose some of the minerals through sweat, which is why it's a good idea to add electrolytes to water, or you can drink some coconut water, which is a good source of electrolytes.[195]

Although I wasn't able to find any studies related to Hashimoto's and sauna therapy, I did find a study that looked at the effects of infrared sauna in people with the autoimmune conditions rheumatoid arthritis and ankylosing spondylitis.[196] The study involved 17 patients with rheumatoid arthritis and 17 with ankylosing spondylitis, and showed that infrared sauna was well tolerated and didn't lead to any adverse effects or exacerbation of disease. In addition, pain and stiffness decreased, and even fatigue decreased.

Infrared Sauna Protocol:
1. Drink at least 8 to 16 ounces of water prior to going into the sauna
2. Pre-heat sauna for 15 to 30 minutes
3. Place a towel on the chair you'll be sitting on
4. Begin your session when the sauna reaches 100 degrees Fahrenheit
5. Initially, start with 10 to 15 minutes in the sauna at 100 degrees Fahrenheit every other day
6. Gradually increase the time until you reach a duration 25 to 40 minute sessions at a temperature between 100 and 130 degrees Fahrenheit
7. After the sauna, drink 16 to 24 ounces of water with electrolytes
8. Use your sauna at least two to three times per week

Coffee Enemas. While I can't say I have most of my patients do coffee enemas, over the years, I have consulted with patients who had done regular coffee enemas prior to consulting with me, and most of the feedback has been positive. Obviously, it wasn't enough to restore their health or else they wouldn't have consulted with me in the first place, but many reported that they experienced significant improvement upon doing coffee enemas. So, it's something to consider incorporating.

Colon hydrotherapy. Before going through my masters in nutrition degree, I wasn't a big fan of colonics. However, after completing a class dedicated to biotransformation and detoxification, I realized the benefits of colon hydrotherapy and colonic irrigation. Dr. Walter Crinnion, a naturopathic doctor who focuses on biotransformation and detoxification, taught this class. He would commonly say that if he could choose only one method of detoxification, it would be colon hydrotherapy.

However, colon hydrotherapy usually isn't the first treatment option I recommend to my patients to eliminate environmental toxins. I find that using food, supplements, and infrared sauna therapy are excellent methods to help support detoxification in most patients. Nevertheless, in some people, environmental toxins are a big issue, and going through multiple sessions of colon hydrotherapy can cause a significant improvement in their condition.

Is Chelation Therapy a Safe Option?

Chelation is a process that uses synthetic or natural agents to bind to heavy metals, although some chelating agents can also bind to minerals, resulting in their excretion from the body. Chelation therapy can help with the excretion of certain heavy metals.[197] I don't recommend intravenous chelation therapy as the primary treatment method for heavy metals, although I know some healthcare professionals will recommend this to anyone who has high levels of toxic metals. I'm not opposed to using oral chelating agents if someone has higher levels of heavy metals, although these also come with some risks if someone isn't careful.

Some examples of chelating agents include DMSA, DMPS, and EDTA. Although EDTA seems to be more effective in chelating lead than DMSA or DMPS, there is evidence that using EDTA to mobilize lead causes redistribution of lead and cadmium into the soft tissues.[198] It has been suggested that using DMSA helps to increase the excretion of lead if DMSA was given after using EDTA.[198] DMPS increases urinary excretion of arsenic, cadmium, lead, methylmercury, and inorganic mercury.[199] Whenever using any type of chelating agent, you also want to increase glutathione levels through diet and/or supplementation, which will help with the clearance of these toxins.

Another thing to keep in mind is that using these chelating agents can result in the loss of minerals from the body. For example, in a study involving a DMPS challenge test there was significantly increased excretion of copper, selenium, zinc, and magnesium.[200] DMSA can also result in the loss of essential minerals, including potassium and chromium.[201]

Exercise Caution if You Have Mercury Amalgams

There is the potential risk of the redistribution of metals when using chelating agents, especially DMSA, DMPS, and EDTA. Some natural chelating agents, such as alpha lipoic acid, can also cause the redistribution of metals if you don't take the proper precautions. I'm not too concerned about eating foods that have chelating properties, such as cilantro, but if you have mercury amalgams, you do need to be cautious if you take any supplements or synthetic agents that have the ability to chelate heavy metals.

Action Steps You Can Take for Optimal Detoxification

To make it easier to understand what steps you should take, I'll prioritize the detoxification strategies:

1. Minimize your exposure to environmental toxins. Please try to do your best to minimize your exposure to environmental toxins. Probably the best place to start is in your own home, as you want to try to use as many natural cleaning products and cosmetics as you can, whenever possible purchase natural furniture and carpeting, and minimize your exposure to EMFs.

2. Support the detoxification pathways through diet. It's important to eat well in order to heal your gut and to support the detoxification pathways. If you don't know where to start, try eating at least four to six servings of vegetables per day, although more than this would be even better. Also, eat a good variety of different vegetables. I mentioned how adequate selenium levels are important for glutathione production. While Brazil nuts can be a good source of selenium, their selenium content is variable, and they are excluded from an AIP diet. Sardines are an excellent source of dietary selenium, and have much lower levels of mercury than most other fish.[202]

3. Drink plenty of water. I recommend either reverse osmosis water and/or a good quality spring water out of a glass bottle. This doesn't mean that there aren't other good options, but either way, I would try to avoid drinking tap water regularly as well as water out of plastic bottles.

4. Consider nutritional supplements and herbs to support detoxification. If you just followed the first three action steps, this would help greatly, although, sometimes, taking certain nutritional supplements and herbs can be beneficial. Examples include milk thistle, NAC, or a liposomal or an acetylated form of glutathione.

5. Utilize infrared sauna therapy. I realize that not everyone will be able to afford an infrared sauna, although depending on where you live you might be able to find a local spa, salon, or fitness club that offers infrared sauna therapy.

Chapter Highlights:

- Cytochrome P450 enzymes are produced by the liver, and they are utilized in phase one detoxification.
- These cytochrome P450 enzymes not only play a role in detoxification, as they are also essential in the metabolism of certain nutrients.
- Polymorphisms are common genetic defects that can occur in the cytochrome P450 family, which, in turn, can affect the detoxification process.
- Thyroid hormones play an important role in detoxification, and numerous studies also show that a thyroid imbalance can affect the cytochrome P450 enzymes.
- Some of the things you can do to minimize your exposure to environmental toxins include 1) eating well, 2) drinking purified water, 3) purchasing natural household products, 4) using a natural dry cleaning company, 5) replacing your carpeting, 6) using low or no-VOC paints, 7) buying natural furniture, 8) using safe cookware, and 9) investing in a quality air-purification system.
- Some of the products that emit electromagnetic fields include televisions, refrigerators, cell phones, computers, vacuum cleaners, hair dryers, and fluorescent lights.
- You can support detoxification through diet by eating plenty of vegetables, including cruciferous and dark green leafy vegetables, foods rich in vitamin B6 and B12, and cilantro; drinking plenty of purified or spring water; and eating sufficient fiber.
- Some of the supplements and herbs that can support detoxification include milk thistle, NAC, alpha lipoic acid, an acetylated or liposomal glutathione, TMG, schisandra, and dandelion root.
- Some other methods of eliminating toxins include infrared sauna therapy, coffee enemas, and colon hydrotherapy.

CHAPTER 30

CORRECTING YOUR NUTRIENT DEFICIENCIES

MANY PEOPLE UNDERESTIMATE THE impact of nutrient deficiencies, but being deficient in one or more nutrients can have a dramatic effect on your health. As discussed in section two, nutrient deficiencies can set the stage for the development of Hashimoto's and other chronic health conditions. For those who already have Hashimoto's, which describes those reading this book, having one or more nutrient deficiencies will make it more challenging to achieve a state a remission. While eating well is essential for anyone who has Hashimoto's, or any other health condition, eating a nutrient-dense diet alone usually won't correct nutritional deficiencies.

What's the Difference Between Macronutrients and Micronutrients?

When discussing nutrient deficiencies, I'm not just referring to vitamins and minerals. You need to consider both macronutrients and micronutrients. The macronutrients include protein, fats, and carbohydrates. However, examples of micronutrients include vitamins, minerals, and antioxidants. I'm not going to get into detail about the different macronutrients and micronutrients here, as that's beyond the scope of this book; although, in Chapter 13, I did focus on seven specific nutrients.

Of course, with any diet, the goal is to obtain balance. For example, while some people consider the autoimmune Paleo (AIP) diet to be too restrictive, most people can get sufficient protein (e.g., meat and fish), healthy fats (e.g., avocados and healthy oils), and carbohydrates (fruits and vegetables) when following this diet. As for getting enough of the micronutrients, this is also possible, as eating a wide variety of vegetables will greatly help with this. Some people make the mistake of thinking that both an AIP and standard Paleo diet are mostly "meat-based" diets, but, ideally, you want to fill your plate with plenty of vegetables. Although some people eat meat with each major meal, others choose to eat a small portion of meat or fish once or twice per day.

The problem is that there is so much conflicting information, as one source will tell you to eat a very high protein diet, while others will recommend more of a ketogenic diet, which isn't meant to be a long-term diet. The truth is that everyone is different, and, sometimes, you need to listen to your own body. For example, if you feel better eating a larger serving of meat with each meal, then go ahead and continue doing this while trying to get into remission; although, I would still make sure you are eating plenty of vegetables. However, if you only want to eat a small serving of meat once or twice per day, this is also fine. Even though meat is nutrient dense, this doesn't mean that you are required to eat a lot of meat.

What's the Difference Between the RDA, RDI, and DRI?

Many decades ago, the Recommended Daily Allowance (RDA) was created by the United States government. The RDA was an estimate of the nutrients most people required in order to prevent nutritional deficiencies from developing. Over the years, it became clear that these guidelines weren't ideal, as many people who met the RDA requirements still had nutritional deficiencies. Thus, while it's important to obtain a sufficient amount of vitamins and minerals from diet and nutritional supplements, most people need to get more than what the RDA suggests. In the 1990s, the RDI (Reference Daily Intake) was introduced. The Dietary Reference Intake (DRI) was introduced in 1997 to broaden the guidelines of the RDA. Then, to make matters even more confusing, on supplement labels, you'll see the "Daily Value (DV)," which is the recommended intakes for nutrients.

Without question, in order to prevent nutrient deficiencies from developing, it is important to eat a nutrient-dense diet. However, when correcting nutrient deficiencies, I find that supplementation is almost always required. When I make a supplement recommendation to one of my patients, it's common for them to look at the label on the bottle and question why the dosage I'm recommending is well above the DV.

For example, the DV for selenium is 55 mcg, but many people with Hashimoto's need to take a much higher dosage of selenium than the DV. Studies show that taking 200 mcg of selenium is necessary to have a therapeutic effect,[203,204] which is why many natural healthcare professionals recommend higher doses of selenium to their patients. The same concept applies to most other micronutrients.

How Much Protein, Carbohydrates, and Fats Are Required?

Let's switch gears to the macronutrients, as a common question I am asked is, "How many grams of protein, carbohydrates, and fats should I eat?" This can get confusing, as different sources provide different recommendations. The truth is that most people aren't going to keep track of the amount of protein, fats, and carbohydrates they eat every day. And while free computer programs and apps can help with this, in most cases, you don't have to keep track of everything you eat.

For example, if you eat many vegetables, some fruit, and eat minimal refined foods and sugars, then you should be fine with the amount of carbohydrates. As for fats, make sure to have at least one or two servings of healthy fats per day in the form of avocados, olives, and healthy oils (i.e., coconut oil, olive oil, avocado oil). Many people who initially follow an AIP diet will eventually be able to reintroduce a small amount of nuts and seeds each day, which are another good source of fat. And if you eat meat, then this also will provide some fat along with protein.

As for how much protein you should eat, the Dietary Reference Intake is 0.8 grams of protein per kilogram of body weight, or 0.36 grams per pound. For example, according to the DRI, someone who weighs 150 lbs. should eat approximately 54 grams (2 ounces) of protein per day. However, many healthcare professionals feel that this is too low and is the bare minimum needed to prevent muscle loss. As a result, some will recommend for their patients to eat up to 2.0 grams of protein per kilogram. I personally think that eating between 1.0 and 1.5 grams of protein per kilogram of body weight is fine for most people. One kilogram equals approximately 2.2 pounds, and so for example, if someone weighs 150 pounds (68 kilograms), then they should eat between 68 and 102 grams (2.4 and 3.6 ounces) of protein per day.

7 Steps to Correct Nutrient Deficiencies

Hopefully, you have a better understanding of the difference between macronutrients and micronutrients. What I'd like to do next is discuss seven different things you need to do to correct nutrient deficiencies.

Step #1: Consider testing for nutrient deficiencies. This is probably the least important of the seven steps because there isn't a perfect test that accurately determines all of the different nutrients. For more information on testing for nutrients, please read Chapter 25.

It's also worth mentioning that besides doing testing for nutritional deficiencies, certain physical signs can indicate a deficiency. For example, ridges on fingernails can indicate an iron deficiency, whereas transverse depressions in the nail plate (known as Beau's lines) are frequently caused by a severe zinc deficiency. Burning of the tongue is commonly caused by a vitamin B12 deficiency. A sore tongue can also be related to a vitamin B12 deficiency, although other nutrient deficiencies can be factors, including folate, zinc, or iron. Dry skin can be caused by nutrient deficiencies as well, including fatty acids, vitamin A, and vitamin E. While a thyroid hormone imbalance can lead to hair loss and/or dryness, the same is true with certain nutrient deficiencies, including iron and essential fatty acids.

Step #2: Eat a nutrient-dense diet. As mentioned in Chapter 26, I recommend for most people with Hashimoto's to start out by following an elimination/AIP diet, and to eventually make the transition to a standard Paleo diet. Although both of these are restrictive (especially the AIP diet), they are nutrient-dense. However, one of the biggest problems is that many people don't eat enough vegetables.

Although I recommend eating a minimum of four to six servings of vegetables daily, I would strive to eat between 9 and 12 servings per day. In other words, while it's common for people to eat a lot of meat and a few vegetables while following either an AIP diet or a standard Paleo diet, you want to eat more vegetables than meat. While grass-fed beef, pasture-raised poultry, organ meats, and wild fish are very nutrient dense, eating a wide variety of vegetables every day is just as important as and perhaps even more important than eating meat. I'm not suggesting for everyone to follow a vegetarian diet, as while I do have patients who are vegetarians and vegans, most of my patients eat meat, and I personally eat meat as well.

My point is that if you eat a good amount of vegetables per day, then you won't need to eat as much meat to get the necessary nutrients.

Step #3: Try to eat mostly organic foods. Although it would be great if everything you eat is organic, if you must prioritize then make sure that any meat, vegetables, and fruit you eat is organic. If you initially follow an AIP diet and eventually reintroduce eggs, then these should be organic as well. The obvious reason for this is to minimize your exposure to the chemicals that are in these conventional foods. For example, non-organic meat is commonly filled with hormones and antibiotics.

Remember that you also need to consider what the animal eats. This is why, ideally, you want to eat 100% grass-fed beef, as most conventional cows are fed grains, which will affect the nutrient density of the meat. Similarly, most organic chickens are also fed grains, which is why you want to try to eat pasture-raised chickens. I know this isn't always possible, and I admit that, at times, I eat organic chicken and not pasture-raised. The same is true with eggs, as, while I frequently purchase pasture-raised eggs, at times, I will purchase organic eggs that aren't pasture-raised.

As for fruits and vegetables, you ideally want these to be organic in order to minimize your exposure to the conventional pesticides and herbicides used. I discussed the effects of these chemicals in section two.

What if You Can't Eat Mostly Organic Foods?
I realize that everyone is in a different situation, and, therefore, some people won't be able to eat mostly organic foods. If you eat mostly conventional meat, fruit, and vegetables, will this prevent you from achieving a state of remission? Not necessarily, as I've had patients with Hashimoto's restore their health even when eating whole foods that were not organic. However, it is best for your overall health to try to eat as many organic foods as you can.

Besides the potentially harmful effects of the chemicals in certain foods, remember from section two that glyphosate causes the chelation of minerals. Thus, if you eat foods that have glyphosate then this not only will make it difficult to correct any existing nutrient deficiencies but also can lead to a worsening of current nutrient deficiencies.

Step #4: Heal the gut. While eating nutrient dense foods and avoiding refined foods is important to correct nutrient deficiencies, it is equally important to heal the gut. It makes sense that having optimal digestion and absorption is essential for correcting nutrient deficiencies. For more information on how to heal the gut, please read Chapter 28.

One thing I didn't mention so far is that healthy intestinal bacteria play a role in the synthesis of certain nutrients, including the B vitamins and vitamin K2.[205] Thus, while diet and nutritional supplementation can help to correct nutrient deficiencies, having a healthy microbiome is also essential.

Step #5: Take nutritional supplements. While it would be great to be able to correct nutritional deficiencies through diet alone, moderate to severe nutrient deficiencies usually require supplementation. One of the main reasons for this is because the crops are not as rich in vitamins and minerals as they were many years ago. Unfortunately, modern agricultural methods are responsible for this, as improper farming practices, along with the use of pesticides and herbicides, have caused the depletion of the soil of essential nutrients. We also need to keep in mind that the animals that eat these plants are also malnourished, which means that any meat you eat also isn't as nutrient-dense as it was in the past.

When Choosing Supplements, Don't Forget That Quality Matters
Everyone reading this understands that there is a difference between eating good quality food and poor quality food. The same concept applies when taking nutritional supplements and herbs. Choosing good quality supplements can be challenging for someone who doesn't know what high quality ingredients to look for. What I usually do is first look at the company's multivitamin, assuming they have one. You can find out a lot about a supplement company simply by looking at their multivitamin.

For example, magnesium oxide is poorly absorbed, yet because it is cheap, it is commonly used by supplement manufacturers. Cyanocobalamin is a lower quality form of vitamin B12 that is commonly used. This doesn't mean that these nutrients won't get absorbed at all, but better quality forms of magnesium include magnesium glycinate, magnesium malate, and magnesium citrate. Methylcobalamin and hydroxocobalamin are higher quality forms of vitamin B12. Synthetic folic acid is also of low quality, as you want the supplement to include natural folate (i.e., L-5-methyltetrahydrofolate). These are just a few examples, but if you look at the multivitamin from your favorite supplement company and it includes magnesium oxide, cyanocobalamin, and/or folic acid, then this is usually a good indication that this company doesn't use high quality ingredients.

The supplements you take should also have minimal fillers. Fillers are commonly added by supplement manufacturers, and while many of them are harmless, others are more controversial. In most cases, I'm not too concerned about a supplement having a couple of fillers, but it depends on what these are. If this is a topic that interests you, please visit **www.naturalendocrinesolutions.com/resources** for more information. Obviously, you want to avoid supplements that have artificial ingredients.

Should the Supplements Be Third-Party Tested?

In 2007, the FDA published something called "Current Good Manufacturing Practices" (cGMPs) for nutritional supplements and herbs. In addition, a few third-party companies test the quality of supplements. NSF International is one of these third-party organizations, as they test thousands of supplements and herbs to make sure the supplements contain the ingredients listed on the label, and they also conduct a toxicology and contaminant review.

Australia's Therapeutic Goods Administration (TGA) is the pharmaceutical regulatory agency of the Government of Australia, and it's supposed to be one of the toughest regulatory agencies in the world. While many supplement companies are NSF certified, fewer companies are TGA certified. Once again, this doesn't mean that supplement companies that aren't certified by third-party agencies don't sell good quality supplements, and I admit that I use a few supplement companies that aren't certified by a third party. But if you are choosing a supplement company on your own and are concerned about the supplements not including ingredients that are on the label and/or having a high level of contaminants, then it might be best to choose a supplement company that has been tested by a third party.

Should You Take a High-Potency Multivitamin/Mineral Formulation?

Some healthcare professionals recommend for their patients to address specific nutrient deficiencies by taking individual nutritional supplements, while others recommend for all of their patients to take a high potency multivitamin with minerals. Just for simplicity sake, I'm going to refer to it as a multivitamin, but just know that I'm referring to a multivitamin with minerals. In the past, I have been in favor of using individual supplements to correct specific nutrient deficiencies.

However, there are few advantages of taking a high potency multivitamin. First, it can be challenging to detect certain deficient nutrients through testing. For example, if you were to order a micronutrient panel that tests for all of the vitamins and minerals and it only shows one or two nutrient deficiencies, can you completely rely on this data? Of course, you can do other types of testing, and although I do some testing for nutrients, there is no perfect method of detecting all of the nutrient deficiencies; thus, one can make a good argument that taking a high potency multivitamin is a way to ensure that you correct any existing deficiencies.

Another advantage of taking a high potency multivitamin is that, in a perfect world, the person would only have one bottle to keep track of compared to taking individual supplements. For example, if someone does some testing and it's determined that they are low or deficient in magnesium, zinc, iron, and vitamin B12, they can either purchase four separate bottles (one for each nutrient deficiency), or they can purchase a single high potency multivitamin. However, this doesn't necessarily mean that they would need to take fewer pills, as a serving size of a good quality multivitamin will almost always include multiple capsules.

There are also some downsides of having everyone take a high potency multivitamin. First, there might be some ingredients in the multivitamin that you don't need or want to take. For example, most multivitamins include iodine, and while I find that most people with Hashimoto's do okay with smaller doses of iodine (i.e., 200 mcg or less), some people still prefer not to supplement with any iodine.

Another thing to consider is that some people who take a high potency multivitamin will still have to take individual supplements. For example, most high potency multivitamins have vitamin D, but if you have a moderate to severe vitamin D deficiency, then there might not be enough vitamin D in the multivitamin; therefore, you would have to take a separate vitamin D3 supplement. Also, depending on the multivitamin you choose to take, there is a chance you might have to supplement separately with one or more other nutritional supplements.

So what's the final verdict? Different healthcare professionals will have different opinions, as some give a high potency multivitamin to all of their patients, while others never give one to their patients. I don't recommend a high potency multivitamin to all of my patients with Hashimoto's, although I do recommend such a supplement at times.

For those who do take a high potency multivitamin, just remember that the goal isn't to be on this for a prolonged period. Thus, while some people choose to continue taking a multivitamin after restoring their health, others rely on getting their nutrients from the foods they eat. Of course, either way, you want to continue eating a nutrient-dense diet.

Step #6: Be aware of medications that deplete nutrients. You also want to try your best to avoid medications that can deplete nutrients such as oral contraceptives,[206] acid blockers,[207] statins,[208] and Metformin.[209] If, for any reason, you need to take these medications, you should take nutritional supplements in order to help prevent nutrient deficiencies from developing.

For example, if you are taking an acid blocker, it would be a good idea to take a high-potency multivitamin, and the same is probably true for those taking oral contraceptives. However, if you are taking a statin then the main concern is having a deficiency in CoQ10; thus, taking a CoQ10 supplement would be a good idea. If you take higher doses of Metformin and/or take it for a prolonged period, then the main concern is a vitamin B12 deficiency; thus, you might want to consider doing a serum B12 and a urinary methylmalonic acid, and, if necessary, take a vitamin B12 supplement.

Step #7: Consider the impact of certain genetic polymorphisms. Everyone has genetic polymorphisms, but some of these can have a greater impact on the nutrients than others. For example, the MTHFR gene plays a role in folate metabolism, and if someone is homozygous (has two genes) for MTHFR C677T, then this decreases the activity of the enzyme by up to 70%, whereas if someone is heterozygous (has one gene) for MTHFR C677T then this will decrease the activity of the enzyme by 35%.[210] In other words, those who have a homozygous polymorphism for MTHFR C677T are more likely to have a reduced ability to break down folic acid.

Correcting Nutrient Deficiencies Through Supplementation

It's challenging to recommend supplement doses in general, and this is especially true with regards to vitamins, minerals, and other nutrients because some people not only are more deficient in certain nutrients than others, but also don't eat as many nutrient dense foods as others eat. Thus, it really is best to work with a competent healthcare professional.

In addition, I gave specific nutrient recommendations in some of the other chapters in this section. For example, in Chapter 27, I gave suggested doses for vitamin C and vitamin B5, while in Chapter 28, I gave suggested doses for L-glutamine, zinc, and vitamin A. In Chapter 32, I will give suggested doses for magnesium and chromium. Below, I list some suggested doses for a few nutrients I haven't covered, along with some food sources. Keep in mind that with some of the nutrients listed, higher doses are indicated at times.

Selenium. I discuss selenium in detail in Chapter 13.
Suggested Dosage: between 100 and 250 mcg/day
Food sources. As mentioned in section two, seafood and organ meats are considered to be the richest food sources of selenium. Other good sources include shrimp, sardines, salmon, turkey, chicken, lamb, and beef.

Calcium. Although calcium is important (just like every other mineral), most people don't need to take calcium supplements. This is true even if you don't consume dairy. However, I'll still list a suggested dosage below for those situations when calcium supplementation is required.
Suggested Dosage: between 200 and 500 mg/day
Food sources. Some non-dairy food sources of calcium include sardines, collard greens, turnip greens, mustard greens, broccoli, and kale.

Boron. Boron is a trace mineral that is important for bone health, as it affects the metabolism of calcium, magnesium, and phosphorus. It also impacts the body's use of estrogen, testosterone, and vitamin D, reduces inflammatory markers, and increases antioxidant enzymes including glutathione peroxidase.[211]
Suggested Dosage: 3 mg/day
Food sources: Some of the best food sources of boron include avocados, red wine, and pecans.

Vitamin D. I discuss vitamin D in detail in Chapter 13. Before supplementing with vitamin D, I recommend being tested, which I discussed in section three.
Suggested Dosage: 2,000 IU to 10,000 IU/day
Food Sources: Salmon, sardines, dairy, eggs, shiitake mushrooms

Vitamin K2. There are two main types of vitamin K2, which include menaquinone-4 (MK-4), and menaquinone-7 (MK-7). MK-4 is what's mostly found in animal foods, while natto is a source of MK-7. Both of these can be excellent sources of vitamin K2. Regarding vitamin K2 supplements, both MK-4 and MK-7 seem to raise vitamin K2 levels in an experimental setting, but lower doses of MK-7 typically are required when compared to MK-4.

Suggested Dosage: 50 to 500 mcg/day of MK-4 or 45 mcg/day of MK-7

Food Sources: Vitamin K2 is mostly found in animal foods such as eggs, cheese, butter, beef, and is also found in natto

Vitamin B1. Also known as thiamine, this is a water-soluble essential vitamin that is required for glucose production. The persistent fatigue that commonly accompanies Hashimoto's may very well be linked to a thiamine deficiency in some cases.

Suggested Dosage: 50 to 200 mg/day

Food Sources: Legumes and beans are excellent sources of thiamine. However, legumes are excluded from both a standard Paleo and an AIP diet. Many fish are also high in thiamine. Trout and tuna have some of the highest sources, while beef and pork also contain higher amounts. Eggs are also a good source of thiamine.

Vitamin B2. Also known as riboflavin, it's worth mentioning that thyroid hormone regulates the enzymatic conversion of riboflavin to its active coenzyme forms in the human adult.[212]

Suggested Dosage: 10 to 50mg/day

Food Sources: Meat and fish are good sources of riboflavin, and certain fruit and vegetables, especially dark-green vegetables, contain higher concentrations.

Vitamin B12. There are a few different types of vitamin B12, and I usually recommend either methylcobalamin or hydroxocobalamin, and occasionally will recommend adenosylcobalamin.

Suggested Dosage: 500 to 2,000 mcg/day

Food Sources: Some of the best food sources of vitamin B12 include fish (sardines, salmon, and cod), lamb, shrimp, and beef.

Folate. Although many supplements include synthetic folic acid, when I recommend a folate supplement, I usually recommend methylfolate. Folinic acid is also an active form of folate, although it is a non-methylated form.

Suggested Dosage: 500 to 2,000 mcg/day

Food Sources: Some of the best food sources of folate include spinach, romaine lettuce, broccoli, cauliflower, and asparagus.

Vitamin B6. Pyridoxal 5'-phosphate (P-5-P) and pyridoxine hydrochloride are the two common forms of vitamin B6 seen in supplements. Vitamin B6 is an essential coenzyme that is involved in the metabolism of amino acids, carbohydrates, and lipids.

Suggested Dosage: 25 to 50 mg/day

Food sources: Some good food sources of vitamin B6 include turkey, beef, chicken, salmon, sweet potatoes, cabbage, cauliflower, sunflower seeds, spinach, and bananas

EPA and DHA. I discuss omega 3 fatty acids in detail in Chapter 13.

Suggested Dosage: 1,000 to 2,000 mg/day of EPA and 500 to 1,000 mg/day of DHA

Food Sources: Fish is the best food source of omega 3 fatty acids, with sardines and salmon having a high omega 3 fatty acid content. Other good sources include grass-fed beef, walnuts, and flaxseeds

Chapter Highlights:

- Macronutrients include protein, fats, and carbohydrates, while micronutrients include vitamins, minerals, and antioxidants.
- The Recommended Daily Allowance (RDA) was replaced by the RDI (Reference Daily Intake), although many people who meet these requirements still have nutritional deficiencies.
- In order to prevent nutrient deficiencies from developing, it is important to eat a nutrient-dense diet; although, supplementation is usually necessary to correct existing nutritional deficiencies.
- When choosing nutritional supplements, the quality of the supplement can make a big difference.
- Some healthcare professionals recommend for their patients to address specific nutrient deficiencies by taking individual nutritional supplements, while others recommend that all their patients take a high potency multivitamin with minerals.
- Seven steps to correct nutrient deficiencies include 1) confirming nutrient deficiencies through testing, 2) eating a nutrient-dense diet, 3) eating mostly organic foods, 4) healing the gut, 5) taking nutritional supplements, 6) being aware of medications that deplete nutrients, 7) considering the impact of certain genetic polymorphisms

CHAPTER 31

OVERCOMING INFECTIONS

THE FIRST "R" OF the 5-R protocol involves removing certain factors that can have a negative impact on the health of the gut. One of those factors is infections. Different types of pathogens can potentially trigger Hashimoto's. These include bacterial, viral, fungal, and parasitic infections. While I discussed many of these pathogens in Chapter 9, in this chapter, I'm going to discuss the treatment options for these different types of infections.

While I will be listing specific nutritional supplements and herbs that can help to eradicate infections, it's important to remember that you need to do more than take supplements in order to receive optimal results. While taking natural antimicrobials can be an important part of eradicating infections, doing other things to improve the health of your immune system is equally important. Having a healthy immune system not only can help make the antimicrobial agents more effective but will also prevent these infections from coming back. In addition, some infections, such as viruses, can't be completely eradicated; therefore, having a healthy immune system will help to keep these viruses in check.

Before you can heal your gut and, thus, have a healthy immune system, you do need to remove those factors that are causing intestinal dysbiosis and a leaky gut. In Chapter 28, I mentioned that you can address all of the components simultaneously, but removing your triggers is the most important factor. Some people choose to focus on detecting and removing their triggers first, and then, once this has been accomplished, they focus on the other aspects of the 5-R protocol (replace, reinoculate, repair, and rebalance).

When Should Conventional Methods Be Considered?

Although the focus of this chapter will be on using natural agents to eradicate infections, there is a time and a place for prescription drugs. Prescription antibiotics, antivirals, and antifungals can be necessary at times. This is when it is wise to work with a healthcare professional who can give you the different options, and then you can decide which option is best for you. For example, if a patient of mine tests positive for H. pylori, I will explain to them the benefits and risks of both natural and conventional treatment options. While, in most cases, I prefer the natural treatment approach, ultimately, it is the patient's decision.

You might be wondering what the risks and benefits are of both types of treatment. Well, it does depend on the infection. Sticking with the example of H. pylori, the risk of taking the conventional treatment approach, which usually includes taking two different antibiotics, is that the drugs not only will have antimicrobial effects against H. pylori, but they will also harm a lot of the good bacteria in your gut. The benefit is that prescription antibiotics work faster than taking natural agents. The benefit of a natural treatment approach for H. pylori is that it won't be as harsh on the gut flora as antibiotics. The downside is that it will usually take longer to eradicate H. pylori when using natural antimicrobials.

However, if someone has acute Lyme disease, then taking the conventional medical approach might be the best option. Of course, this is just my opinion, as some natural healthcare professionals treat acute Lyme disease naturally, but everything comes down to risks vs. benefits. While I prefer to try to avoid antibiotics and other prescription drugs whenever possible, in my opinion, the risk of failing to appropriately address an acute case of Lyme disease is greater than taking antibiotics because acute Lyme disease can progress to chronic Lyme disease, which is even more difficult to eradicate. Many people with chronic Lyme disease have unbearable pain, neuropathy, chronic fatigue, and other symptoms.

Should All Infections Be Eradicated?

Some controversy exists over whether certain microorganisms should be eradicated. For example, while H. pylori can be a potential trigger for Hashimoto's and increase the risk of peptic ulcers and gastric cancer in certain people, some sources claim that H. pylori can be beneficial to our health. For example, evidence shows that the eradication of H. pylori can increase the risk of developing gastroesophageal reflux disease.[213,214,215]

Thus, if someone with Hashimoto's tests positive for H. pylori, should they receive treatment to eradicate this bacteria? After all, the only way to prove that H. pylori is the autoimmune trigger is to eradicate it and see if the person goes into remission. There is always the possibility that someone can have H. pylori, but another factor can be the autoimmune trigger. Or perhaps they have multiple triggers, with H. pylori being one of them. Either way, when one of my Hashimoto's patients tests positive for H. pylori, I will recommend for them to receive treatment to eradicate the bacteria.

Another controversial example involves Blastocystis hominis, as some sources consider this to be a commensal organism. One older study concluded that Blastocystis hominis "is a commensal germ of the intestinal tract, even in subjects free of gastro-intestinal manifestations, and does not usually require prescription of an antibiotic."[216] Another study showed that 8% of stool samples harbored Blastocystis, but also mentioned that it was a commensal organism.[217]

Eventually, it was suspected that Blastocystis hominis might be a possible cause of intestinal diseases.[218,219] One of these studies concludes that "Blastocystis hominis is a potential pathogen that may or may not require drug therapy depending on the overall clinical circumstances, the severity of symptoms, and the presence of other pathogenic organisms".[219] Another more recent study mentioned how this species isn't commensal, and is now being regarded as a parasitic organism.[220]

If Blastocystis hominis were indeed pathogenic, then it would make sense to eradicate it if present on a stool test, right? Well, since it might be a potential trigger of Hashimoto's, if someone with this condition tests positive for this parasite, then it probably is wise to eradicate it. Similarly, if someone doesn't have Hashimoto's but has digestive symptoms, then it also would be wise to kill off this parasite. Some recommend for those who test positive for Blastocystis hominis but are asymptomatic to not receive treatment.[221] However, if this is a potential trigger for autoimmunity, it might make sense to eradicate it even if gastrointestinal symptoms aren't present. This is the approach I take in my practice.

Natural Agents to Eradicate Infections

Although most medical doctors will recommend prescription drugs to eradicate infections, what can be done from a natural perspective? The specific treatment depends on the type of infection. For example, if someone has a parasitic infection, conventional medical treatment usually involves prescription drugs such as metronidazole, while natural treatment methods commonly involve herbs such as oregano oil, wormwood, black walnut, and clove oil.

Most medical doctors will treat a Candida overgrowth using prescription antifungals such as nystatin or fluconazole, while a natural healthcare professional might try using oregano oil, caprylic acid, monolaurin, Saccharomyces boulardii, and/or other natural antifungal agents. I'll now list some of the natural agents used for different pathogenic infections, and discuss what they are commonly used for. Then, at the end of the chapter, I'll list some basic treatment protocols for bacterial, viral, fungal, and parasitic infections.

Garlic. Studies show that garlic can help with H. pylori,[222,223] and it is effective against other types of bacteria, including those strains that have become resistant to antibiotics.[223] Garlic can be effective against both gram-negative and gram-positive bacteria.[224]

Garlic can also has antimicrobial properties against yeast and parasites, and a few studies even demonstrate that garlic has antiviral activity.[225,226] I commonly recommend garlic to help with the eradication of all different types of infections. While consuming whole garlic can be beneficial, when taking it in a form of a supplement, I usually recommend Allicin supplements. Allicin is the major active component of garlic.

Oregano oil. Oregano oil can also eradicate certain pathogens, including bacteria, as well as fungi such as Candida.[227,228] Oregano oil can also be effective in treating parasites.[229] This is also something I commonly use for bacterial and parasitic infections, along with a Candida overgrowth.

Goldenseal. This herb helps with inflammation and infection. Its antibacterial activity has been attributed to its alkaloids, the most abundant of which is berberine.[230] Several studies demonstrate how effective berberine is when it comes to certain microorganisms, including Streptococcus mutans, Staphylococcus aureus, and Chlamydia pneumoniae.[231,232] I can't say that I use goldenseal frequently, but I do commonly use berberine to help with certain types of infections, especially bacterial infections.

Mastic Gum. A few studies have shown that mastic gum can help to eradicate H. pylori.[233,234] If a patient of mine has H. pylori, I will almost always recommend mastic gum, along with a few other natural antimicrobials.

Cat's Claw (Uncariatomentosa). Cat's Claw has immunomodulating, antimicrobial, and antiviral properties.[235,236] Some consider this herb to be a contraindication for certain autoimmune conditions such as Hashimoto's, although I have given it to some of my patients without any issues. However, just as is the case with all of these antimicrobials I'm listing in this chapter, to be on the safe side, it probably would be best to work with a natural healthcare professional before taking Cat's Claw.

Yerba Mansa extract. Yerba mansa has antimicrobial properties against certain bacterial pathogens, including Staphylococcus aureus, Streptococcus pneumoniae, and Geotrichimcandidum.[237]

Caprylic Acid. Caprylic Acid has antimicrobial properties,[238] especially against Streptococcus agalactiae, Streptococcus dysgalactiae, and Streptococcus uberis.[239] However, this can also be effective against other microorganisms,[240] and can especially be effective in someone who has a Candida overgrowth.

Pau D' Arco (Tabebuia avellanedae). For many decades, preparations made with this plant were used in South and North America as antineoplasic, antifungal, antiviral, antimicrobial, antiparasitic, and anti-inflammatory treatment.[241]

Colloidal Silver. Colloidal silver is commonly used as an antimicrobial. One study showed evidence that colloidal silver is a broad-spectrum antimicrobial agent against aerobic and anaerobic bacteria,[242] although another study showed that colloidal silver didn't have any antimicrobial effect in vitro on certain microorganisms.[243] While colloidal silver can help with chronic infections, its best use might be with more acute infections.

Although I personally have seen some good results with colloidal silver, some have expressed concerns about its safety. This includes the National Center for Complementary and Integrative Health at the National Institutes of Health (NIH), as if you visit their website you'll see that they discuss colloidal silver potentially causing serious side effects, such as argyria, which is a bluish-gray discoloration of the skin. This is probably based on a few case reports that showed the onset of argyria following the use of supplements that included colloidal silver.[244,245] This admittedly is rare, but it's still something to keep in mind, especially for those who consume large doses of colloidal silver, or smaller amounts over a prolonged period.

The NIH also mentions that colloidal silver might interfere with the absorption of certain medications, including levothyroxine. I personally haven't seen this in the research, although if you take thyroid hormone replacement and choose to take colloidal silver, you might want to play it safe and take the colloidal silver two to four hours after taking the medication.

Wormwood (Artemisia absinthium). Wormwood is commonly used by natural healthcare professionals for the treatment of parasites.[246,247] I commonly recommend wormwood for my patients with parasitic infections.

Black Walnut (Juglans nigra). Although many natural healthcare professionals (including yours truly) use black walnut for parasitic infections, I couldn't find evidence in the literature that it can eradicate parasites. However, I did find evidence that it can help to eradicate pathogenic bacteria and Candida.[248]

Uva ursi. This is also known as bearberry, which is commonly given for urinary tract infections,[249] although it can also help with other types of bacterial and yeast infections.

Licorice root. A few studies have shown that glycyrrhizic acid, which is a component of licorice root, can prevent Epstein-Barr virus (EBV) replication.[250,251] Apparently, glycyrrhizic acid interferes with an early step of the EBV replication cycle.[251]

Lysine. Many people take lysine as a preventative measure for herpes outbreaks. A few different studies show that supplementing with lysine might help to prevent the reactivation of herpes simplex viruses.[252,253]

Quercetin. Quercetin is a naturally occurring flavonoid, and evidence indicates that quercetin has antiviral activity against EBV.[254]

Probiotics. Lactobacillus and bifidobacteria are the most common probiotics, but Saccharomyces boulardii is a nonpathogenic yeast that can help to eradicate certain infections, such as Clostridium difficile[255] and Candida albicans.[256,257] Also, evidence shows that S. boulardii can help to eradicate certain parasitic infections, such as Blastocystis hominis.[258]

One study involving symptomatic children with Blastocystis hominis showed that this was more effective than metronidazole.[258] Spore-based probiotics might also have some antimicrobial activity, as one study showed that Bacillus subtilis and Bacillus pumilus exhibited antimicrobial activity against a number of different pathogens, including Escherichia coli, Salmonella typhimurium, Shigella dysenteriae, Yersinia enterocolitica, and Aspergillus ochraceus.[259]

Are There Risks Associated With Natural Antimicrobials?

While natural antimicrobials are less harsh on the gut flora than prescription antibiotics, this doesn't mean that they are completely harmless. For example, evidence shows that grapefruit-seed extract can be effective against more than 800 bacterial and viral strains, 100 strains of fungus, and a large number of parasites.[260] While on the surface, this may sound positive, keep in mind that many strains of these microbes are beneficial to the body. Besides grapefruit-seed extract, other natural agents can also eradicate some of the beneficial microorganisms, such as oregano oil.

Of course everything comes down to risks vs. benefits, and in most cases, when someone has a pathogenic infection or a Candida overgrowth, using natural antimicrobials will be less harsh on the body than prescription drugs. However, I just want to let you know that you need to be cautious about randomly taking large doses of natural antimicrobials, especially for a prolonged period. Keep in mind that not every natural antimicrobial has a negative effect on the gut flora. Garlic is one natural agent that has antimicrobial effects against pathogenic bacteria, yeast, viruses, and parasites, yet doesn't seem to have a negative effect on our gut flora.

If you are taking either natural antimicrobials or prescription antibiotics, and are also taking a probiotic supplement, it is a good idea to take the probiotic supplement two hours before or after the antimicrobial agents because if you take a prescription antibiotic, or even some natural antimicrobials at the same time as taking a probiotic supplement, you will kill some of the probiotics strains included in the supplement.

When Should Biofilm Disruptors Be Used?

A biofilm is a group of microorganisms (e.g., bacteria, yeast) that form a protective layer. Bacterial biofilms can be resistant to both prescription antibiotics[261] and natural antimicrobials. Candida albicans can also form biofilms, which makes them resistant to certain antifungal medications such as Fluconazole,[262] as well as natural antimicrobials. Since many people with Hashimoto's have these types of infections, it can be beneficial to understand how to disrupt these biofilms.

If someone has an infection, how can you tell if the bacteria or yeast have biofilms? Unfortunately, most labs that test for infections don't test for the presence of biofilms; thus, when treating these infections you are faced with a couple of different options.

One option is to take the necessary treatment without any biofilm disruptors, and hope that biofilms aren't present. The second option is to take biofilm disruptors when treating any bacterial or yeast infection. Evidence shows that biofilm-related infections account for at least 65% of all human infections.[263] Thus, it might be a good idea to play it safe and take some type of biofilm disruptor when combating any type of infection.

Which Microorganisms Are Known to Have Biofilms?

Many different microorganisms have biofilms. I'm not going to list all of them here, but some of the more common ones include H. pylori,[264,265,266] Borrelia burgdorferi,[267] Yersinia enterocolitica,[268] Escherichia coli,[269,270] Klebsiella pneumoniae,[271] Mycoplasma,[272,273,274] and Candida albicans.[275,276,277,278] You'll notice that some of these were mentioned earlier as being associated with Hashimoto's.

Natural Agents That Can Disrupt Biofilm

A few different natural agents have been shown to dissolve the biofilm matrix. This includes N-acetylcysteine (NAC), which not only can increase glutathione, but can also reduce and prevent biofilm formation.[279,280,281,282] Some studies specifically show that NAC can inhibit biofilm formation by H. pylori[283] and Candida albicans.[284]

Proteolytic enzymes, which break down proteins, can help to degrade biofilm when taken on an empty stomach.[285,286,287] Examples of proteolytic enzymes include serratiopeptidase, endopeptidase, and exopeptidase. I mentioned colloidal silver earlier, and a number of different studies showed that colloidal silver can be effective against the biofilm of Candida albicans.[288,289,290] A few studies also showed that colloidal silver has antibiofilm activity in Staphylococcus aureus.[291,292]

Lactoferrin is an iron-binding glycoprotein present in milk, and also has antimicrobial activities by withholding iron from iron-requiring bacteria.[293] Numerous studies show that lactoferrin can inhibit biofilm formation.[294,295,296] It's worth mentioning that colostrum is rich in lactoferrin. Iodine also is a biofilm disruptor, at least when used topically, which is why it is commonly used externally for wounds.[297,298]

Natural Treatment Protocols for Different Types of Infections

I'm going to give a few different general protocols for bacterial, viral, fungal, and parasitic infections. Please keep in mind that whereas prescription medication can usually eradicate infections rapidly, in most cases, it will take at least one to four months to eradicate infections taking a natural treatment approach. In addition, doses will vary depending on certain factors (e.g., person's body weight). Also, while I realize it can be tempting to self-treat your condition, if you are dealing with an acute or chronic infection, it is best to work with a competent healthcare professional.

Natural Treatment Protocol for Bacterial Infections:

Allicin: 250 to 500 mg 3x/day
Berberine: 500 mg 2x/day
Oregano oil: 200 mg 3x/day
Optional: Biofilm disruptor such as NAC or Klaire Labs Interfase
Note: If someone has H. pylori, I would add mastic gum to the protocol (1,000 mg 2x/day)

Natural Treatment Protocols for Active Viral Infections:

Licorice root: 250 to 500 mg 2x/day
Note: Licorice root is contraindicated in those with hypertension. De-glycyrrhizinated licorice (DGL) has been manufactured to avoid the side effects of licorice by removing the active compound glycyrrhizin, but this form is not effective in combating viruses.

Quercetin: 250 to 500 mg 2x/day
Note: While doing research for this book, I discovered that kimchi is a good source of quercetin,[299] which is another reason to eat fermented foods regularly. Other good sources of quercetin include asparagus, red leaf lettuce, broccoli, and apples.[300]
Monolaurin: 500 to 3,000 mg 2x/day
Olive Leaf: 250 to 500 mg 3x/day

Natural Treatment Protocol for a Candida Overgrowth:

Oregano oil: 200 mg 3x/day
Caprylic acid: 250 to 500 mg 3x/day
Olive leaf: 250 to 500 mg 3x/day
Uva Ursi: 200 mg 3x/day
Saccharomyces boulardii: 500 mg 2x/day
Biofilm disruptor (i.e., Klaire Labs InterFase): start with one capsule 30 minutes prior to taking the antifungal herbs; after a few days, increase to 2 capsules
Note: In addition to taking the natural antimicrobials, when dealing with a Candida overgrowth, you will also want to eliminate fruit juice, refined sugars, kombucha, kefir, alcohol, and minimize your consumption of fruit and starchy vegetables. If the Candida overgrowth is severe, then complete elimination of fruit and starchy vegetables may be required. It is also is essential to improve the overall health of your immune system in order to fully address a Candida overgrowth and prevent a recurrence.

Natural Treatment Protocol for Parasites:

Oregano oil: 150 to 200 mg 3x/day
Wormwood: 250 to 500 mg 2x/day (take for 10 days, followed by a 10 day break, then take for another 10 days)
Black Walnut: 50 to 250 mg 3x/day
Clove oil: 1-2 drops 3x/day
Saccharomyces boulardii: 500 mg 2x/day

How to Minimize Die-Off Reactions

Die-off reactions, also known as Herxheimer reactions, are common when following an antimicrobial protocol. Although you can get die-off symptoms when following any type of antimicrobial protocol, these symptoms seem to be worse when following an anti-Candida protocol. Some of the common die-off symptoms include headaches, fatigue, bloating, gas, nausea, and, in some cases chills, itchiness, muscle pain, and/or rashes.

One way to minimize die-off symptoms is to support the liver prior to starting the antimicrobial protocol. You also might want to consider starting slowly with any antimicrobial protocol. In other words, start with a smaller dosage and gradually increase it. Although it might take longer to eradicate the infection taking this approach, you are less likely to experience extreme die-off symptoms. In addition, please make sure you are well hydrated, as this will help to flush out the bacteria and yeast toxins. Taking 1,000 to 2,000 mg of vitamin C per day might also help.

If the die-off symptoms are extreme, then taking 10 to 30 grams of activated charcoal per day in divided doses might help by binding to the toxins released by the yeast or bacteria. However, before doing this, it is wise to contact the natural healthcare professional you're working with who gave the recommendations for the antimicrobial protocol. Molybdenum might also help with yeast die off by converting the acetaldehyde (a byproduct of yeast) into acetic acid.

Why Are Some Infections More Difficult to Eradicate?

It can be quite frustrating to take natural antimicrobials for a few weeks or a few months, only to do a retest and discover that the infection is still present. Here are some reasons why natural antimicrobials might not be effective:

- **Resistance to the antimicrobial agent.** Some people are resistant to certain antimicrobials, which is why you don't want to rely on a single natural agent. Some comprehensive stool panels (e.g., Genova Diagnostics and Doctor's Data) will list the bacteria and mycology sensitivity to both prescription and natural antimicrobials. For example, a "high" inhibition indicates a greater ability of the antimicrobial agent to limit microbial growth, while "low" inhibition suggests that there is less ability to limit growth. Assuming you don't have access to such information, you can simply take two or three natural antimicrobial agents at the same time, and, in some cases, you might want to consider rotating different antimicrobials to prevent resistance from developing.

- **Biofilms.** As I mentioned earlier in this chapter, bacteria and yeast commonly form biofilms, and if you follow an antimicrobial protocol without taking a biofilm disruptor, then this can be a reason why the infection doesn't get completely eradicated.

- **Dosage wasn't high enough.** While you want to be cautious about taking massive doses of natural antimicrobials, sometimes, smaller doses aren't too effective. Taking smaller doses of multiple natural agents might be effective in some cases, although every situation is different, and, sometimes, taking a higher dose is indicated.

- **Duration wasn't long enough.** One of the downsides of taking natural antimicrobials is that it almost always takes significantly longer than prescription antibiotics to achieve eradication of the infection. It's common for someone to be on the natural antimicrobials for a few months before the infection has completely been eradicated.

- **Make sure you do the appropriate retest.** For example, if you initially test positive for H. pylori in the blood and then take natural antimicrobials (or prescription antibiotics), after treatment, you will want to do either a urea breath test or a stool panel to confirm that the bacteria has been eradicated because the antibodies can remain in the blood for months after treatment is completed. As a result, if H. pylori has been recently eradicated, you still might test positive in the blood, but negative in the stool or on the urea breath test.

Reminder: The Goal Is to Improve the Health of Your Immune System

Although this chapter focused on eradicating infections, the overall goal should be to improve your immune system health, which will greatly prevent the recurrence of infections. While finding and removing infections can be an important step in order to achieve optimal immune system health for some people with Hashimoto's, it is also important to eat well, correct nutrient deficiencies, improve your stress-management skills, get sufficient sleep each night, balance your blood sugar levels, and minimize your exposure to environmental toxins.

Chapter Highlights:

- While taking antimicrobials can be an important part of eradicating infections, taking other measures to improve the health of your immune system is equally important.
- Some sources consider H. pylori and Blastocystis hominis to be commensal organisms, although they are also linked to thyroid autoimmunity.
- Although most medical doctors will recommend prescription drugs to eradicate infections, natural agents are also an option in many cases.
- Natural agents that can help with bacterial infections include goldenseal, oregano oil, garlic, mastic gum, yerba mansa, cat's claw, and colloidal silver.
- Natural agents that can help with viral infections include garlic, cat's claw, caprylic acid, colloidal silver, monolaurin, licorice, quercetin, and lysine
- Natural agents that can help with fungal infections include oregano oil, garlic, caprylic acid, and uva ursi.
- Natural agents that can help with parasites include oregano oil, garlic, wormwood, black walnut, and clove
- Many different microorganisms have biofilms, and some of the more common ones include H. pylori, Borrelia burgdorferi, Yersinia enterocolitica, Escherichia coli, Klebsiella pneumoniae, Mycoplasma, and Candida albicans.
- Some natural agents that can disrupt biofilm include NAC, proteolytic enzymes, colloidal silver, and lactoferrin.

CHAPTER 32

HOW TO OVERCOME INSOMNIA AND GET QUALITY SLEEP

MANY PEOPLE WITH HASHIMOTO'S have challenges with getting quality sleep. Some people have difficulty falling asleep, while others have problems staying asleep. Of course, some people with Hashimoto's have both problems. Getting sufficient sleep regularly is important, and in this chapter, I'll discuss some of the most common factors that cause sleep problems and give some suggestions to help improve your sleep.

The Most Common Factors That Interfere With Sleep

I'd like to start by discussing some of the most common factors that can interfere with sleep. Some of these factors will cause problems falling asleep, while other factors will increase the likelihood of waking up in the middle of the night. Some of these factors can cause both problems.

1. Elevated Nighttime Cortisol Levels. Having high cortisol levels can cause insomnia.[301] The best way to determine if someone has high cortisol levels is through testing. This is one of the downfalls of serum testing for cortisol, as this involves a one-sample test. With a saliva test, you can measure the cortisol levels throughout the day in order to get a complete picture of what's going on with the adrenals.

Certain urinary tests (e.g., the DUTCH test) can also measure cortisol levels throughout the day. With these types of tests, you even have the option of collecting a sample if you wake up in the middle of the night. High early morning cortisol levels can also interfere with sleep, and is something to consider testing for if you are able to fall asleep without a problem, but constantly wake up in the middle of the night and can't fall back asleep.

Cortisol responds to stress and inflammation; thus, whenever someone has elevated cortisol levels, it is important to address the underlying cause of these problems. Stress is one of the biggest factors, and studies show a correlation between stress and insomnia.[302,303]

Since getting sufficient sleep is extremely important, when someone has elevated cortisol levels at night, I will usually recommend for them to take something to help decrease cortisol. I discussed supplements and herbs that can help with high cortisol levels in Chapter 27, although I will reinforce this information later in this chapter. Imbalances in cortisol are usually caused by chronic stress; thus, while taking supplements temporarily is fine, it is also important to improve your stress-management skills, which I also discussed in Chapter 27.

2. Reactive Hypoglycemia. Problems with the blood sugar levels can potentially lead to insomnia. This seems to be more common with reactive hypoglycemia. Reactive hypoglycemia is an exaggerated fall in the blood glucose levels, and is due to excessive insulin secretion in response to a meal. Dr. Alan Gaby has dedicated a chapter to reactive hypoglycemia in his excellent textbook *Nutritional Medicine*, and he discusses how, if the blood glucose levels fall too rapidly, the body compensates by releasing adrenaline and other compounds, which raise the blood glucose levels.

This, in turn, results in "fight or flight" symptoms such as anxiety, panic attacks, hunger, palpitations, tachycardia, tremors, sweating, and even abdominal pain. In his book, Dr. Gaby also discusses the symptoms presented when the blood glucose levels fall slowly over a period of hours, as this can lead to symptoms such as headaches, fatigue, blurred vision, mental confusion, impaired memory, and even seizures. These symptoms usually are worse before meals and frequently are relieved by eating.

Evidence indicates that hypothyroidism can be a factor in hypoglycemia.[304] It is also possible that having hypoglycemia can inhibit the pituitary-thyroid (HPT) axis.[305] Thus, a vicious cycle can form in which hypothyroidism can lead to hypoglycemia, and hypoglycemia can inhibit the HPT axis, which can further exacerbate the hypothyroid condition.

Other potential causes of hypoglycemia include alcohol consumption,[306,307] adrenal insufficiency,[308,309] and, according to Dr. Gaby, food allergies or sensitivities.

When someone has reactive hypoglycemia, many times just changing their diet can help with this and help the person sleep better. If someone has this condition, they should start with a diet consisting of whole foods, cut out the refined foods and sugars, as well as the alcohol, and try not to go long periods without eating in order to help keep the blood sugar levels stable. Addressing weak adrenals and food allergies/sensitivities might also help with this condition.

3. Decreased Melatonin. Melatonin, a hormone produced by the pineal gland, plays an essential role in your sleep-wake cycle. Melatonin levels usually begin to rise later in the day, and should be at the highest levels throughout the night, before decreasing early in the morning.

Someone with decreased amounts of melatonin at night can have difficulty falling asleep. When this is the case, taking a melatonin supplement can be beneficial. Studies show that melatonin can help with age-related insomnia,[310] as melatonin production normally decreases as we age.

Although age can be a factor, it usually isn't the primary factor, and, ultimately, the cause of the decreased production of melatonin should be addressed. Melatonin production is greatest when it's dark, which is why you should sleep in a room that is completely dark, and not have the television on (or other electronics) while trying to fall asleep. Evidence indicates that electromagnetic fields (EMFs) can interfere with the production of melatonin.[311]

Studies show that exposure to artificial light before bedtime suppresses melatonin and thus can interfere with sleep.[312,313] Artificial lighting emits a blue wavelength, which is why such lighting is described as "blue lights." Blue light has a very short wavelength; thus, it produces a high amount of energy. Besides being indoors most of the time and not getting sufficient sunlight, many people spend too much of their waking hours in front of a computer, on their cell phone, etc. In other words, most people are exposed to too much blue light.

If the precursors of melatonin are deficient, then this will lead to low melatonin levels. Serotonin is a precursor to melatonin. Thus, if someone has an imbalance of this neurotransmitter, they are likely to have low melatonin. But why would someone have a serotonin imbalance?

Several nutrients are required for the production of serotonin. This includes the amino acid tryptophan, but the production of serotonin also requires nutrients such as iron, magnesium, and the B vitamins (especially vitamin B6, B12, and folate). If someone is deficient in one or more of these nutrients, then this can cause an imbalance of serotonin, which, in turn, can lead to low melatonin.

4. Progesterone deficiency. Progesterone exerts a sleep induction or hypnotic effect, and studies show that decreases in progesterone levels can cause disturbed sleep.[314,315] Other studies show that balancing the hormones estradiol and progesterone can help with sleep.[316] Many healthcare professionals will recommend bioidentical progesterone for those who have a deficiency. However, this doesn't address the underlying cause of the low progesterone levels, and a big factor that can lead to a decrease in progesterone is compromised adrenals, which is usually a result of dysregulation of the hypothalamic-pituitary-adrenal (HPA) axis. I discussed how to address adrenal and sex hormone imbalances in Chapter 27.

5. Mineral Deficiencies. Certain mineral deficiencies can also cause insomnia. While many people are aware that a magnesium deficiency can cause problems with sleep, I came across a study showing that taking zinc might also help with insomnia.[317] It's important to mention that all of the participants took a supplement consisting of zinc, magnesium, and melatonin; thus, it's possible that the magnesium and/or melatonin played a greater role in helping with the insomnia. Additional evidence suggests a relationship of dietary zinc and blood zinc status with sleep quality and quantity.[318]

Iron is one of the precursors of serotonin production, and evidence shows that iron can indirectly help with sleep due to its role in regulating neurotransmitters that are essential to the intrinsic sleep processes.[318,319] Many women with Hashimoto's have an iron deficiency (as well as some men with Hashimoto's). Taking a magnesium supplement and/or a low dose of zinc usually won't cause any harmful effects. However, unless if an iron deficiency has been confirmed, be cautious about taking iron supplements, as high levels of iron can cause oxidative stress, which I discussed in Chapter 13.

6. Caffeine. To no surprise, the consumption of caffeine can also cause insomnia in some people. Those who consume caffeine later in the day are even more likely to have problems with sleep. One study showed that several genes have been identified as potentially influencing caffeine-induced insomnia.[320] Caffeine is metabolized by the cytochrome P450 1A2 (CYP1A2) enzyme. Many people have a genetic polymorphism for this enzyme, and those with certain genetic polymorphisms of the CYP1A2 enzyme are "rapid" caffeine metabolizers, whereas those with other genetic polymorphisms of the CYP1A2 enzyme are "slow" caffeine metabolizers.[321]

Being a fast or slow metabolizer of caffeine is a big reason why one person who drinks a single cup of coffee per day might have problems sleeping due to the caffeine, while someone else who drinks multiple cups of coffee per day sleeps fine. Just like anything else, caffeine has a different effect on different people, and genetics can play a role. But insomniacs who consume caffeine regularly, whether it's in the form of coffee, soda, dark chocolate, or something else, might want to try avoiding these sources for at least a few weeks and see if they notice an improvement in their sleep.

7. Aspartame. Evidence shows that consuming aspartame can result in insomnia.[322] This should make you wonder how other artificial ingredients and chemicals might have a similar effect on your health, and thus may result in sleeping difficulties. Thus, you should not only avoid aspartame, but other artificial ingredients as well.

8. Alcohol Consumption. Drinking too much alcohol can also interfere with sleep. At all dosages, alcohol causes a reduction in sleep onset latency, a more consolidated first half sleep and an increase in sleep disruption in the second half of sleep.[323] While some people seem to sleep better when drinking alcohol, numerous experts suggest that chronic consumption is likely to lead to greater late night sleep disturbances.[324] Thus, in most cases, the quality of sleep is greatly reduced with regular alcohol consumption.

9. Neurotransmitter Imbalance. When imbalances in serotonin affect the production of melatonin, taking tryptophan, a precursor to serotonin, can help some people in this area.[325] 5-HTP is the immediate precursor of serotonin, and, therefore, also might benefit some people with insomnia. Increasing serotonin levels by taking 5-HTP can frequently help with sleep because serotonin is a precursor of melatonin. Low serotonin levels will usually lead to low melatonin levels. While someone can take a melatonin supplement, this isn't doing anything for the serotonin imbalance.

Gamma-aminobutyric acid (GABA) is another neurotransmitter that plays a role in sleep. GABA is the main inhibitory neurotransmitter of the central nervous system, and it is well established that activation of GABA receptors favors sleep.[325] Studies demonstrate a reduction of GABA in the brain in primary insomnia.[326,327] Many people take the herb valerian root to help them sleep, as this herb binds to the GABA receptors.[328,329] A few other herbs also appear to affect the GABA receptors, including kava, Scutellaria baicalensis, licorice root, and lemon balm.[330]

10. Certain infections. Although sleep deprivation can increase your susceptibility to viral, bacterial, and parasitic infections,[331] having certain infections can result in sleep disruption.[331,332] For example, certain parasites can cause a fragmented sleep by disrupting the circadian rhythm.[333] Also, evidence shows that the common cold can have detrimental effects on sleep.[334] Another study showed that the H1N1 influenza virus could cause narcolepsy-like sleep disruption.[335] Thus, addressing infections can play a big role in getting a better night's sleep each night.

Overcoming Sleep Issues Through Diet and Lifestyle Factors

In addition to addressing those factors I've discussed so far, what else can you do to help get quality sleep? Although I'll be discussing supplements that can help with sleep later in this chapter, you want to focus on modifying certain lifestyle factors, and only take nutritional supplements and herbs for sleep if absolutely necessary. I realize that some people will need to initially take supplements to assist with falling and/or staying asleep, and I will bring up a few supplements when discussing the lifestyle factors.

Balance your blood sugar levels. I've already discussed reactive hypoglycemia, but besides eating well throughout the day, I'll add that sometimes mild carbohydrate loading (i.e., 200 to 250 calories of carbohydrates) one hour to 90 minutes prior to going to bed will help someone to fall asleep, and especially can be helpful in preventing some people from waking up in the middle of the night.

Control the inflammation. I've already discussed reducing inflammation in this book, including some supplements that can help to reduce pro-inflammatory cytokines (e.g., vitamin D, turmeric, and fish oils). Eating an anti-inflammatory diet is essential, and doing things to improve your stress-management skills can also help to reduce inflammation.

Take a break from your supplements. If you started taking any nutritional supplements or herbs right before you began experiencing sleep difficulties, then consider stopping them for a while. It doesn't matter which supplements you're taking, as people respond differently to various supplements. Sometimes, it might not be the nutrients or herbs in the supplement that are responsible for the sleep problem, but someone might be sensitive to the fillers or other ingredients in the supplements, thus causing problems with sleep (along with other symptoms). So consider taking a break from your supplements for one week and see if this helps you to sleep better. If you are working with a healthcare professional, then before discontinuing any supplements I would run this by him or her.

Make sure your room is completely dark when sleeping…and avoid artificial light one to two hours before going to sleep. As I mentioned earlier in this chapter, melatonin production is optimal when it's completely dark. Also, for those who are having problems falling asleep, being exposed to artificial light from your house one to two hours prior to going to bed can have a negative impact. I mentioned earlier how studies show that being exposed to artificial light before bedtime can suppress melatonin.

Thus, you want to try to decrease your exposure to artificial light, especially at night. If you must use your computer or other devices, consider installing a program such as f.lux, as this will help to reduce the amount of blue light these electronic devices emit. Another option is to wear blue blocker glasses at night while at home, as a few studies show that they prevent the artificial lighting from suppressing melatonin production.[336,337]

It's also beneficial to get some sun exposure during the day. Besides trying to get sun exposure upon waking up, take a 20-minute walk in the early afternoon to get some sun. Doing this along with reducing your exposure to artificial light will have a positive impact on your circadian rhythm.

Improve your stress-management skills. Many studies show that stress can interfere with sleep. I dedicated an entire chapter (Chapter 27) showing you how to improve the health of your adrenals, and, while diet and supplementation can be important, perhaps the best way of doing this is to take measures to improve your stress-management skills daily.

Reduce caffeine, alcohol, and/or nicotine. I discussed caffeine earlier. As for alcohol, some people might sleep better when drinking a glass of wine at night; however, for many others, drinking alcohol at night can cause sleep disturbances. Nicotine also can interfere with sleep, as the research shows that cigarette smoking and nicotine dependence are associated with poor sleep quality.[338]

Reduce your exposure to EMFs in the bedroom. As I mentioned earlier in this chapter, evidence shows that electromagnetic fields (EMFs) can interfere with the production of melatonin. If you have tried doing everything to improve your sleep yet still have problems falling and/or staying asleep, then you should seriously consider reducing the EMFs in your bedroom. If you have electronic devices in your room, then either get them out of the bedroom or, if this isn't feasible, unplug all devices right before going to sleep. Simply turning them off isn't sufficient. If you must use a cell phone or alarm clock to wake you up in the morning, make sure it's at least six feet away. Better yet, put the cell phone/alarm clock in an adjacent room.

Sticking with the topic of EMFs, besides reducing your exposure to these in your bedroom, you want to stop using all electronics two hours before going to sleep. For some people, watching television helps them to fall asleep. However, for many people, watching television or surfing the Internet right before going to bed can interfere with falling asleep. Even if watching television helps you to fall asleep, having the television on all night can have a negative effect on sleep quality. Once again, the EMFs from these electronics might affect the production of melatonin.

Make sure your mattress is comfortable. Many people don't put much thought into purchasing a bed and mattress, but when you consider how much time you spend in your bed, then it's wise to invest as much time into getting a bed and mattress as you would when purchasing a new car. Many people will spend weeks and, sometimes, even months test driving cars before making a decision, but won't spend enough time when it comes to purchasing a bed or mattress.

Since you spend so much time in your bed, it not only makes sense to get a good quality mattress that is comfortable, but you might also want to consider investing in an organic mattress, as it won't have all of the chemicals that a conventional mattress will have. Not only can the off-gassing of chemicals from your mattress be a factor in sleep, but they can have a negative effect on your overall health. In Chapter 8, I discussed how flame retardants from furniture alone can cause hormone disruption, cancer, and neurological toxicity. For the same reason you want to consider getting natural bedding (e.g., blankets, pillows).

Use aromatherapy. A few studies show that using aromatherapy can have a positive effect on sleep quality.[339,340,341] Although a few different essential oils can help with sleep, lavender oil is probably the one most commonly used to help some people get better quality sleep. Chamomile is widely regarded as a mild tranquillizer and sleep-inducer[342] and should also be considered.

Purchase an air purification system. In some cases, the air quality can interfere with your sleep. Evidence shows that air pollution can lead to sleep-disordered breathing, which can affect up to 17% of adults.[343] Thus, investing in a quality air purification system can be beneficial and might help you to sleep better. Even if it doesn't improve your sleep, it will benefit your health in other ways. I list some of my favorite air purification systems on the resources page of my website, which is **www.naturalendo-crinesolutions.com/resources**.

Take a hot bath 2 hours before going to bed. A few small studies have shown that taking a hot bath 1.5 to 2 hours before going to bed can help to improve sleep.[344,345] A big reason for this seems to be the change in body temperature, although taking a hot bath can also be very relaxing and a way to manage stress. You might also want to consider adding some Epsom salt, along with a few drops of lavender oil.

Adjust the temperature of your home. If the temperature in your bedroom is either too hot or too cold, this can affect sleep quality. Try adjusting the temperature of your bedroom one degree at a time and see if this helps to improve sleep. Keeping it on the cooler side (i.e., below 70 degrees Fahrenheit) is usually recommended.

Eradicate any infections. While certain infections will make you drowsy and cause you to sleep more, earlier I also mentioned how some infections can cause sleep disruption. Thus, if you have any infections, then these might need to be addressed in order for you to get quality sleep each night.

Clear your mind before going to bed. The primary reason why many people have problems with sleep is because they have too many thoughts going through their mind. Frequently these thoughts are stressful in nature, as one might go to sleep worrying about financial issues, health problems, and other stressful factors. When this is the case, improving your stress-management skills will play a big role in this.

Nutritional Supplements and Herbs That Can Help With Falling Asleep

Melatonin. As mentioned already, this is a hormone that is secreted by the pineal gland. Its primary function is to help regulate the body's circadian rhythm.

Suggested Dosage: ½ to 1 mg 90 minutes before going to bed

Can Taking Melatonin Worsen Hashimoto's?

Some people are concerned that taking melatonin can exacerbate autoimmunity, and should thus be avoided by those people with Hashimoto's. The main reason for this concern is due to a clinical trial in 2007 involving patients with rheumatoid arthritis,[346] which showed that taking 10 mg of melatonin daily increased the concentration of some inflammatory indicators, such as erythrocyte sedimentation rate (ESR). However, the same study showed that melatonin didn't cause an increase in proinflammatory cytokines. Another thing to keep in mind is that 10 mg is a fairly high dosage of melatonin.

In addition, in 1997 a patient developed autoimmune hepatitis after taking melatonin for the treatment of insomnia.[347] Of course, there was no way to prove for certain that the melatonin supplement triggered the autoimmune condition. A recent review article showed that with most autoimmune conditions, melatonin actually was beneficial.[348] The author concluded by suggesting that the internal production of melatonin can be important in preventing the development of autoimmune disease, and that taking melatonin supplements might be beneficial in the treatment of autoimmune conditions. Although I don't frequently give melatonin to my patients, I have had some of my patients with Hashimoto's supplement with it, and I don't recall a situation where it worsened someone's condition.

Magnesium. This mineral is a cofactor in hundreds of enzymatic reactions, and it plays important roles in ATP metabolism, DNA and RNA synthesis, muscle contraction, blood pressure regulation, and insulin metabolism. Many people with sleep issues can benefit from taking magnesium. Some of the better forms of magnesium include magnesium citrate, glycinate, and malate, although magnesium taurate might be a better option in people with sleeping difficulties who also have insulin resistance, as, besides having a calming effect, one study shows that the combination of magnesium and taurine may improve insulin sensitivity.[349] However, it's important to mention that other forms of magnesium can also help with insulin sensitivity.[350]

Suggested Dosage: 200 to 400 mg of magnesium citrate, taurate, malate, or glycinate 30 minutes before bed

5-Hydroxytryptophan (5-HTP). Serotonin is probably the most well-known neurotransmitter, and this converts into melatonin. The amino acid tryptophan is a precursor of serotonin. Tryptophan is converted into 5-hydroxytryptophan, also known as 5-HTP, which, in turn, is converted into serotonin. Thus, to increase serotonin levels, you can take tryptophan or 5-HTP.

Suggested Dosage: 50 to 200mg 30 to 60 minutes before going to bed

GABA (gamma-aminobutyric acid). I mentioned earlier that this is the main inhibitory neurotransmitter of the nervous system, and low levels of GABA can lead to anxiety, depression, and insomnia. It's important to understand that GABA can't cross the blood brain barrier. Thus, taking GABA orally normally wouldn't increase the levels of this neurotransmitter in the CNS. However, eating foods rich in glutamic acid such as walnuts, almonds, rice, spinach, and beans can increase the GABA levels. If you choose to take it in supplement form then you want to take it with a phenyl group attached (also known as "Phenibut"), as this will allow it to pass through the blood brain barrier.

Suggested Dosage: 200 to 500 mg before going to bed

Valerian root. Valerian root is an herb that is commonly used for inducing sleep and improving sleep quality. Earlier I mentioned that valerian root binds to the GABA receptors.

Suggested Dosage: 250 to 500 mg 30 minutes before going to bed

L-theanine. This is a natural constituent in tea, and the research shows that it can reduce both psychological and physiological stress.[351] Animal studies show that L-theanine increases brain serotonin, dopamine, and GABA levels.[352] A few studies show that it can have beneficial effects in those with sleep disturbances.[353,354]

Suggested Dosage: Take 100 to 200 mg one hour before going to bed. Some people can also benefit from taking L-theanine throughout the day.

S-Adenosyl-l-methionine (SAMe). SAMe will support 200 enzyme reactions, and if taking this helps you to fall asleep then this means that you have problems with methylation.

Suggested Dosage: 250mg 20 to 30 minutes before going to bed

Nutritional Supplements and Herbs to Take if You Wake Up in the Middle of the Night

Phosphatidylserine. This is essential for nerve cell membranes, and also supports cognition, including the formation of short-term memory, the consolidation of long-term memory, the ability to create new memories, and the ability to retrieve memories.[355] Supplementation with phosphatidylserine has been shown to lower cortisol levels by normalizing stress-induced dysregulation of the hypothalamus-pituitary-adrenal axis.[356]

Suggested Dosage: 100 to 500g taken before each high cortisol episode

Ashwagandha. This is also known as Withania somnifera, and it is an adaptogenic herb. It supports both the HPA and hypothalamic-pituitary-thyroid (HPT) axes. Thus, it can help people who have HPA axis dysregulation because of chronic stress, and by supporting the HPT axis it can also benefit thyroid function. As I mentioned in Chapter 27, ashwagandha is part of the nightshade (Solanaceae) family, and nightshades are excluded from an autoimmune Paleo diet. Ashwagandha can help with sleep issues by lowering cortisol levels, although one study showed that this herb might help with insomnia by increasing levels of the neurotransmitter GABA.[357]

Suggested Dosage: 250 to 500mg taken before each high cortisol episode

Relora. This involves a combination of the herbs Magnolia and Phellodendron amurense, and can help to reduce stress and anxiety. One study showed that 4 weeks of supplementation with Relora significantly lowered salivary cortisol when compared to a placebo.[358]

Suggested Dosage: 250 to 500mg taken before each high cortisol episode

Note: These natural agents I discussed can also help in some cases when people have problems falling asleep. Phosphatidylserine, ashwagandha, and relora can help with high cortisol levels, and if someone has elevated cortisol levels late at night (i.e., between 10 p.m. and midnight), then this can cause problems falling asleep, and taking these agents before bed can help.

Nutritional Supplements and Herbs for Blood Sugar Support

Many people who have blood sugar imbalances will fall asleep okay, but it's common for them to wake up in the middle of the night and have a difficult time going back to sleep. I find that taking supplements for hypoglycemia isn't too effective, as the best way to address this is through diet and lifestyle factors. Of course, one can make the argument that diet and lifestyle is the best way to address all other imbalances as well, but, with many conditions, taking nutritional supplements and herbs can help aid in the recovery process.

Sometimes high blood sugar levels can also be a factor when someone has sleep issues, and in addition to making dietary changes, here are a few nutritional supplements and herbs that can be beneficial:

Chromium. Chromium is a mineral that can help in the regulation of insulin and, therefore, improve blood glucose control.[359]

Suggested Dosage: 250 to 1,000 mcg/day

Food Sources: Broccoli, green beans, tomatoes, romaine lettuce

Gymnema sylvestre. This is an herb that has potent anti-diabetic properties by causing insulin secretion from the beta cells of the pancreas.[360]

Suggested Dosage: 250 to 450 mg/day

Berberine. Berberine is the main active ingredient of traditional Chinese medicines Coptis Root and Cortex Phellodendri, and research shows that it can regulate blood glucose levels and reduce blood lipid levels.[361]

Suggested Dosage: 250 to 500 mg 3x/day

Alpha lipoic acid. This is an antioxidant that can help to decrease insulin resistance and improve glucose metabolism.[362]
   Suggested Dosage: 200 to 600 mg/day

Bitter melon. Also known as Momordica charantia, this is a plant that has antidiabetic effects.
   Suggested Dosage: 250 to 1,000 mg/day

Cinnamon. This spice has many different benefits, but one of the primary benefits is helping to regulate blood glucose levels. Cinnamon also can modulate the immune system by increasing regulatory T cells and potentially suppressing Th17 cells.[363]

Sleep Case Study

Mark was able to fall asleep relatively easy, but he would always wake up in the middle of night between 2 and 3am. In addition to cleaning up his diet he took numerous nutritional supplements and herbs, including melatonin, valerian root, and 5-HTP. Even though he cleaned up his diet I asked for him to put together a food diary, and he also ordered an adrenal saliva test. His cortisol levels were elevated in the morning and evening, and while he was eating a good diet overall, he was eating a lot of fruit, and seemed to overindulge in AIP-friendly snacks such as sweet potato chips (with coconut oil). I asked for him to reduce his daily fruit intake to no more than two small servings of low glycemic fruits, and to cut down on the AIP-friendly snacks. I also had him take an herbal formulation to help with the elevated cortisol levels, and he started practicing meditation on a daily basis. Two weeks later he reported back that he was still waking up in the middle of the night, but instead of waking up between 2 and 3am he would wake up an hour or two later. I told him that this was a good sign and recommended that he continue with the diet, cortisol-lowering supplements, and mind-body medicine, and one month later he was consistently sleeping throughout the night without any interruption.

Chapter Highlights:

- Having high cortisol levels can cause problems falling and/or staying asleep, and this can be determined through testing.
- Reactive hypoglycemia is an exaggerated fall in the blood glucose levels, which can also lead to sleeping difficulties.
- Melatonin is a hormone that is made by the pineal gland, and it plays a very important role in your sleep-wake cycle.
- Progesterone exerts a sleep induction or hypnotic effect, and studies show that decreases in progesterone levels can cause disturbed sleep.
- Certain mineral deficiencies can also cause insomnia, including magnesium, zinc, and iron.
- The consumption of caffeine can also cause insomnia in some people.
- Drinking too much alcohol can also interfere with sleep.
- Imbalances in the neurotransmitters serotonin and GABA can lead to insomnia.
- Although supplements can help many people who have problems falling and/or staying asleep, you first want to focus on modifying certain lifestyle factors.
- Some of the supplements that can help with falling asleep include melatonin, magnesium, 5-HTP, GABA, valerian root, L-theanine, and SAMe.
- The following supplements can help with those who have problems falling and/or staying asleep due to high cortisol levels: phosphatidylserine, ashwagandha, and relora.

CHAPTER 33

OVERCOMING CHALLENGING TRIGGERS: LYME DISEASE, TOXIC MOLD, AND SIBO

THIS CHAPTER IS GOING to focus on overcoming some of the most challenging triggers of Hashimoto's thyroiditis, specifically Lyme disease, toxic mold, and small intestinal bacterial overgrowth (SIBO). Not all of these are direct triggers of Hashimoto's. Borrelia burgdorferi (Lyme disease) can be a potential direct trigger through a molecular mimicry mechanism; however, both mycotoxins and SIBO can lead to Hashimoto's through indirect mechanisms, such as causing an increase in intestinal permeability (a leaky gut).

I'll start by discussing both conventional and alternative treatments of Lyme disease. I'm not a Lyme disease specialist; thus, if you have an acute or chronic case of Lyme disease, it's probably best to work with someone who focuses on this. I'll then discuss the different treatment options for toxic mold, followed by conventional and natural treatment options for SIBO.

Conventional Treatment Options for Acute Lyme Disease

When Lyme disease is initially diagnosed, antibiotics are recommended by most medical doctors. The benefit of taking antibiotics is that if the infection is caught early, two to four weeks of antibiotics might help to completely eradicate it. The downside is that antibiotics have a negative effect on the good bacteria of the gut. Candida overgrowth is also a common consequence of taking antibiotics. This is why when someone takes antibiotics for Lyme disease, many medical doctors will also prescribe anti-fungals such as nystatin or fluconazole to help prevent the development of a Candida overgrowth.

In some cases of acute Lyme disease, taking a single antibiotic might not be sufficient to eradicate the infection because Borrelia burgdorferi can have several forms, including the cell wall form and the cystic form. In addition, there can also be biofilm (discussed in Chapter 31), protecting the organism from eradication through the antibiotics. Thus, different types of antibiotics might be required, and biofilm disruptors should be considered. If the infection hasn't spread, then taking doxycycline for two to four weeks might help to eradicate it, but if the infection has spread and/or the infection is in a cystic form, then taking this antibiotic alone probably won't be sufficient.

Conventional Treatment Options for Chronic Lyme Disease

Just as is the case with acute Lyme disease, most medical doctors will also recommend antibiotics for chronic Lyme disease. However, antibiotics are much less effective for chronic cases of Lyme disease. This is especially true when associated co-infections are also present. This doesn't mean that antibiotics can't help with some cases of chronic Lyme disease, but giving antibiotics alone usually won't be effective in those with this condition.

Recently, I was working with a patient who has Hashimoto's and chronic Lyme disease. She had been working with one of the leading Lyme disease experts for a couple of years, and, even though this doctor takes a functional medicine approach, she continued to receive antibiotics. The antibiotics were helping with her neurological symptoms, which was why she continued to take them. However, they obviously didn't address the cause of the problem, and, of course, taking antibiotics long term has a damaging effect on the gut microbiota, and can increase gut permeability.

Can a Natural Treatment Approach Help With Lyme Disease and Co-Infections?

Although antibiotics are without question overused and abused, if someone has a confirmed or suspected acute case of Lyme disease, antibiotics very well might be the best treatment option. However, the later stages of Lyme disease are much more difficult to treat; thus, while I can recommend natural antimicrobials for an acute case of Lyme disease, along with supplements for immune system support, if I knew for sure that it was an acute case of Lyme disease, I probably would advise taking a course of antibiotics. If I wasn't certain of this, I'm not sure if I would prescribe the antibiotics. Of course, if I did recommend antibiotics I would also recommend taking a probiotic supplement (at least two hours away from the antibiotic), eating more fermented foods, etc.

What if someone has a chronic case of Lyme disease, along with accompanying co-infections? Since antibiotics are not as effective in chronic Lyme disease, it makes sense to at least try following a natural treatment approach. A few natural treatment protocols have helped many people with Lyme disease and related co-infections. I'm not going to discuss these protocols here, as there is plenty of information online that lists the components, and you can also visit **www.naturalendocrinesolutions. com/resources** for more information. However, I will list three of the more well-known alternative protocols for Lyme disease:

1. The Zhang Protocol
2. The Cowden Protocol
3. The Buhner Protocol

These protocols are quite extensive, and while you can do a search online and find out the products recommended by each practitioner, if you have chronic Lyme disease you should work with a Lyme disease specialist. As for which of these protocols are more effective, it does seem to vary from person to person. Some people have received great results after following the Cowden protocol, while others claimed to have followed it strictly and didn't receive good results. The same is true with the other protocols I mentioned.

While certain antimicrobial herbs can be beneficial, I have also worked with some Lyme disease patients who did poorly on some of the herbal formulations aimed at treating Lyme disease. Not surprisingly, since everyone is different, there isn't a specific protocol for Lyme disease that is suitable for everyone.

Besides the three common protocols I listed, other natural approaches can be equally effective. For example, Byron White has some formulations that can help with many cases of Lyme disease and its coinfections. The same is true with the company Bio-Botanical Research. However, if you have a suspected or confirmed case of Lyme disease, work with a healthcare professional who has a lot of experience seeing Lyme disease patients, especially if you have chronic Lyme disease.

How long do you need to follow the protocol that you choose? This depends on the person, as no two people will respond exactly alike. As an example, Dr. Lee Cowden recommends to stay on the Cowden protocol until the person feels well for two consecutive months. Not surprisingly, having one or more coinfections will usually result in a longer duration of treatment.

Treatment Options for Mold Toxicity/CIRS

What are some of the different treatment options if someone has chronic inflammatory response syndrome (CIRS) associated with a mold toxicity? With this condition, it is important that you take measures in a certain sequence as follows in the order of importance:

1. Eliminate the source of the mold. Getting rid of the source of the mold is the most important step that needs to be taken if you've been diagnosed with mold toxicity/CIRS. If you skip this step, then you won't get rid of the mold toxicity. Of course, before eliminating the source of the mold, you need to confirm that there is a mold problem either at home, at work, or at school. Once this has been confirmed, then the next step is usually either 1) mold remediation, or 2) relocating.

If remediation isn't an option, or if it doesn't help with the mold toxicity, then the next step is to avoid the source. Unfortunately, this might involve moving to a different home, quitting your job, or attending a different school. I realize this is an extreme measure to take, but if remediation doesn't provide a solution to the mold toxicity problem, then the best option is to do whatever is necessary to completely avoid the source.

2. Eliminate the mycotoxins from your body. This can be accomplished through either prescription drugs or natural agents.

Cholestyramine. This is an FDA-approved medication used to lower elevated levels of cholesterol. Dr. Ritchie Shoemaker accidentally discovered how cholestyramine binds to mycotoxins in the small intestine (along with cholesterol and bile salts). The recommended dosage is 9 grams, taken four times per day on an empty stomach. Some forms of cholestyramine include aspartame, so you might want to consider getting a compounded form. Constipation is a common side effect; thus, you want to make sure to stay well hydrated and to consume plenty of fiber.

Here are some natural treatment options for binding mycotoxins:

Bentonite clay, zeolite, and activated charcoal. These natural agents can bind to aflatoxins,[364] which we're commonly exposed to through the food. However, according to Dr. Shoemaker, these natural agents aren't effective when binding to other mycotoxins. Thus, while you can always start by taking these natural binding agents, if you don't notice a significant improvement in your symptoms, then you should consider taking cholestyramine.

One of the products I have used with success for binding to mycotoxins is GI Detox, which is manufactured by the company Bio-Botanical Research. This product consists of 75% pyrophyllite clay and 25% activated charcoal. This can help to bind to not only mycotoxins but also other types of toxins, including bacterial endotoxins (e.g., lipopolysaccharides), heavy metals, and by-products of yeast and bacteria.

Glutathione. The CYP450 enzymes convert mycotoxins into reactive intermediates, and glutathione S-transferase catalyzes the conjugation of these intermediates with reduced glutathione, which leads to the excretion of the mycotoxin. Thus, having healthy glutathione levels is essential to eliminate mycotoxins from your body. You can take a precursor to glutathione such as N-acetylcysteine, or an acetylated or liposomal form of glutathione.

Air purifier. A good quality HEPA air purification system won't eliminate mycotoxins from your body, although it might be able to help reduce airborne mycotoxins. However, if someone is dealing with CIRS, then getting an air purification system alone probably won't be sufficient.

Ozone machine. Some studies show that ozone can degrade certain mycotoxins.[365,366] Just as is the case with an air purification system, it won't eliminate mycotoxins from your body, but instead will help to reduce airborne mycotoxins.

3. Address MARCoNS. These are strains of staphyloccoci bacteria, and they colonize the nasopharynx. MARCoNS can create biotoxins, which can further increase the inflammation associated with CIRS. If this is an issue, it needs to be addressed in order to overcome CIRS. Eradication of MAR-CoNS is typically done using a compounded nasal spray.

4. Reduce Inflammation and Correct Hormone Imbalances. The final steps involve addressing the inflammatory process and hormone imbalances associated with CIRS. While removing the source of the mold exposure and using binders to eliminate mycotoxins can help, this doesn't always suppress the inflammatory response, and it won't address the hormone imbalances I discussed earlier.

Just as with Lyme disease, it is a good idea to work with a competent healthcare professional who has a lot of experience working with patients who have CIRS/toxic mold. Dr. Richie Shoemaker is an expert on mold toxicity, and if you visit his website **www.survivingmold.com**, you can perform a search for a physician who has completed the Shoemaker Certification Protocol. Before contacting this physician, you can first choose to do some of the testing I mentioned in Chapter 11, as this can help to confirm if you have a mold toxicity problem. If this is the case, you can then contact a physician who has completed Dr. Shoemaker's certification for CIRS/toxic mold.

Treatment Options for Small Intestinal Bacterial Overgrowth

The third and final challenging case I'd like to discuss is small intestinal bacterial overgrowth (SIBO). There are a few challenges with treating SIBO. First, SIBO involves different bacteria, and not all bacteria respond to the same type of treatment. Second, when taking a natural treatment approach, most practitioners don't use high enough doses of antimicrobials, which is something I was guilty of in the past. Third, most cases of SIBO are caused by an autoimmune process involving the migrating motor complex (MMC), which I discussed in Chapter 21. When this is the case, after the overgrowth has been addressed, the person will need to take a prokinetic for a long time in order to prevent a relapse from occurring.

Three Ways to Eradicate SIBO

Three main methods are used to eradicate SIBO: taking prescription antibiotics, natural antimicrobials, and the elemental diet. Let's look at the pros and cons of each of these treatment methods.

Eradication Option #1: Prescription antibiotics. Rifaximin is the antibiotic most commonly recommended for SIBO. Xifaxan is a brand name of Rifaximin that is commonly prescribed. While I'm not a big fan of antibiotics, Rifaximin is different than most other antibiotics. First, it is a nonabsorbable antibiotic whose activity is localized to the small intestine due to its minimal systemic absorption. Thus, unlike most other antibiotics, Rifaximin doesn't go through the bloodstream, but only acts in the small intestine and won't harm the bacteria of the large intestine.

Evidence shows that Rifaximin might actually increase good bacteria (e.g., bifidobacteria) in the large intestine.[367] In addition, bacterial resistance isn't too common when using Rifaximin. However, some people with SIBO will respond to Rifaximin, and they will need to consider either the elemental diet or herbal antimicrobials. Also, if someone has high methane levels, Rifaximin alone usually won't successfully eradicate SIBO, which is why most medical doctors will recommend an additional antibiotic, such as metronidazole or neomycin.

One study showed that taking partially hydrolyzed guar gum makes Rifaximin more effective.[368] The study involved 77 patients with SIBO, and it showed that the eradication rate was 62.1% in those who took Rifaximin alone, and 85% effective in those who took Rifaximin combined with partially hydrolyzed guar gum.

Eradication Option #2: Herbal antimicrobials. I personally prefer to use herbal antimicrobials when dealing with SIBO. Here are some of the natural agents that can help to eradicate SIBO:

- Berberine
- Oregano oil
- Neem
- Thyme
- Uva Ursi
- Grapefruit seed extract
- Allicin

You'll notice that allicin is one of the antimicrobials listed, and, since garlic is a high FODMAP food, this might be confusing to some people with SIBO who were told to avoid garlic. However, most people with SIBO can tolerate an allicin supplement. If someone has high methane levels and chooses a natural antimicrobial approach, then taking allicin is indicated, along with at least one additional herbal antimicrobial.

Are the herbs as effective as Rifaximin? One study showed that herbal therapy is equivalent to Rifaximin for treating SIBO.[369] However, just as is the case with Rifaximin, not everyone with SIBO will respond to the herbal antimicrobials. Also, in most cases, the herbal antimicrobials will take longer to work.

If you read the study I just referred to, you'll see that a combination of herbal products were used. While these can be effective, the downside is that if someone has a severe case of SIBO, then the treatment duration will usually be at least a few months, and the bacteria can eventually become resistant to the herbs. Thus, if someone has very high methane and/or hydrogen levels on a breath test, they might want to consider using one or two of the individual herbs I listed earlier, rather than a combination formula. This way, they can rotate the herbs if necessary.

Sample Natural Treatment Protocol for SIBO

Although I'm listing a sample natural treatment protocol for SIBO, keep in mind that not everyone with this condition will respond to the same treatment. The sample given involves someone who has elevated methane levels, which is why I included allicin. It's also important to mention that while higher doses of berberine can be effective for SIBO, side effects are common with this high of a dosage, including nausea and stomach cramps. Thus, it probably is a good idea to start by taking a smaller dose.

It's also important to understand that berberine decreases the activity of the following cytochrome P450 enzymes: CYP2D6, CYP2C9, and CYP3A4.[370] These cytochrome P450 enzymes are involved in the metabolism of many different medications; thus, you need to exercise caution when taking berberine with certain medications. Fortunately, there are no interactions between berberine and thyroid hormone replacement.

Berberine: 500 to 1,000 mg 3x/day
Oregano oil: 150 to 300 mg 3x/day
Allicin: 450 to 900 mg 2x/day

Eradication Option #3: Elemental diet. The elemental diet can be the most effective diet for alleviating the symptoms of SIBO because it can lower gas levels to a much greater extent when compared to using prescription drugs and natural antimicrobials. However, it is a very challenging diet to follow. It's considered to be an antimicrobial approach because the goal is to starve the bacteria while simultaneously supplying the person with sufficient nutrients in an easily absorbed form.

The elemental diet essentially consists of protein, fat, carbohydrates, amino acids, vitamins, minerals, and either glucose or maltodextrin. You can get a premade formula from a company such as Integrative Thera-peutics, or if you visit the resources page at **www.siboinfo.com**, you can get a recipe to make your own. The elemental diet can help to lower both methane and hydrogen levels, and you want to follow it for usually two or three weeks, and then do another breath test immediately upon completion of it.

How Long Do You Need to Treat SIBO?

How long SIBO needs to be treated with prescription antibiotics or natu-ral antimicrobials depends on the individual. Although the severity of symptoms doesn't always correlate with the severity of the gas levels, the duration of treatment frequently does. Thus, those with very high hydrogen or methane levels will usually need to receive treatment for a longer period compared to those with lower gas levels.

One course of treatment with prescription antibiotics is two weeks, while one course of treatment with the natural antimicrobials is four weeks. Frequently, more than one course of treatment is necessary with either prescription antibiotics or natural antimicrobials. As for how to determine how many courses of treatment you need, doing another breath test is a very good idea, although if your symptoms have com-pletely resolved, then you can usually assume that the SIBO has been eradicated.

However, it's important to keep in mind that not everyone will achieve 100% resolution of their symptoms, which is especially true if their con-dition is due to an autoimmune process involving the MMC. The good news is that even when this is the case, most people can get significant relief from their symptoms, and, sometimes, complete resolution. The bad news is that if SIBO is caused by an autoimmune process, then the person will need to take a prokinetic for a prolonged period to prevent a relapse from occurring.

What to Do When Rifaximin or the Natural Antimicrobials Don't Work

What should be done if someone with SIBO takes either Rifaximin or the natural agents and their condition doesn't improve? It's important to do another SIBO breath test after completing a round of treatment. On the retest, if the gas levels have decreased but are still high, then it makes sense to do another round of the Rifaximin or natural antimicrobials, regardless if the person's symptoms have improved or not. However, if the gas levels haven't improved, then it probably is wise to try a different treatment approach.

While taking prescription antibiotics and herbal antimicrobials are the most common treatment options, the elemental diet is also considered to be an antimicrobial approach. When doing a SIBO breath retest, if the gas levels have normalized and the person still has a lot of symptoms, then this is usually an indication that something else is going on besides SIBO, and additional testing might be indicated.

Using Atrantil to Lower Methane

I've had some success helping patients reduce methane levels using a natural product called Atrantil. Reducing the high methane can help to improve symptoms such as gas, bloating, stomach pain, and constipation. Atrantil has three active botanicals, which include peppermint leaf, Quebracho extract, and Conker Tree extract.

The Role of Prokinetics in Preventing a Relapse

Prokinetics help to stimulate the MMC, and, since most cases of SIBO are caused by a dysfunctional MMC, taking prokinetics can be important to prevent a relapse from occurring after receiving treatment for SIBO. The MMC works in a fasting state; thus, while many people in general eat regularly throughout the day, those with SIBO probably shouldn't snack in between meals, and should go at least 12 hours overnight without eating.

Here are some of the prokinetics that can be used:

- Iberogast
- Ginger
- 5-HTP
- Low-dose naltrexone (LDN)
- Low-dose erythromycin
- Low-dose Prucalopride

As for what prokinetic you should specifically take, Iberogast is an herbal formulation I have recommended to patients, and it has been used by many other healthcare professionals as well. Ginger can be a good prokinetic, and 5-HTP can be helpful. Keep in mind that some people with Gastroesophageal reflux disease (GERD) don't do well when taking ginger, and thus might want to be cautious about using it as a prokinetic.

Many reading this are familiar with low-dose naltrexone, which can also act as a prokinetic. Erythromycin is commonly used as an antibiotic, but, in very low doses, it can also help to stimulate the MMC and, therefore, be an effective prokinetic.[371]

How long should someone take a prokinetic after SIBO has been eradicated? It depends on the person, as most people will need to take a prokinetic for at least 3 to 6 months. If someone has autoimmunity to vinculin, they might have to take prokinetics permanently. In Chapter 21, I mentioned how if someone has the CDT-b toxins, these harm the Interstitial cells of Cajal, and in a case of mistaken identity, the immune system attacks vinculin. Until we figure out how to stop this autoimmune process, then the person will most likely have to continuously take prokinetics.

SIBO and Visceral Manipulation
Some cases of SIBO are caused by structural problems, such as adhesions to the abdomen due to trauma, a surgical procedure, or endometriosis. Thus, some cases respond well to visceral manipulation or other types of body work. While most people with SIBO will respond to the other treatment methods, if this isn't the case, then visceral manipulation should be considered.

Natural Treatment Options for Small Intestinal Fungal Overgrowth (SIFO)
How is SIFO treated? Since SIFO involves the presence of yeast, it makes sense that antifungal treatment would be necessary. While antibiotics such as Rifaximin won't eradicate SIFO, some of the natural antimicrobials used for treating SIBO also have antifungal properties, such as oregano oil. Thus, there is a chance that taking the natural antimicrobials that can help with SIBO can also help to eradicate SIFO. However, there is also the chance that this isn't the case, and prescription antifungals such as nystatin or fluconazole might be needed.

Maintaining a State of Remission After Eradication of SIBO

I mentioned the importance of prokinetics in preventing a relapse from occurring. This is especially true for those who have damage to the MMC due to an autoimmune process. However, you will want to do two other things after eradicating SIBO. First, although most people don't have to be as restrictive with the diet after eradicating SIBO, you still want to be cautious about eating a lot of highly fermentable foods. In addition, meal spacing can also help benefit the MMC, and, according to Dr. Allison Siebecker, you should eat approximately every four hours throughout the day and go at least twelve hours at night without eating.

Once again, this is especially true for those who have damage to the MMC due to an autoimmune process. If the MMC is permanently damaged then there is a very good chance that SIBO will return if you don't take a prokinetic and space your meals. Although not all cases of SIBO are caused by an autoimmune process involving the MMC, this seems to be the most common cause.

Chapter Highlights:

- While antibiotics might be indicated in acute Lyme disease, they usually aren't as effective in cases of chronic Lyme disease.
- With chronic Lyme disease it makes sense to initially try following a natural treatment approach.
- Three of the more well-known alternative protocols for Lyme disease include 1) the Zhang protocol, 2) The Cowden protocol, 3) the Buhner protocol.
- Eliminating the source of the mold is the most important thing that needs to be done in someone who has already been diagnosed with mold toxicity/CIRS.
- Some of the different methods of eliminating mycotoxins from your body include 1) using cholestyramine, 2) using bentonite clay, zeolite, and activated charcoal, and 3) increasing glutathione levels.
- Three ways of eradicating SIBO include 1) taking prescription antibiotics, 2) herbal antimicrobials, 3) and the elemental diet.
- Not everyone with SIBO will respond to the same treatment.
- Some of the natural antimicrobials that can be effective with SIBO include berberine, oregano oil, neem, and allicin.
- Prokinetics help to stimulate the migrating motor complex and can be important to prevent a relapse after receiving treatment for SIBO.

. SECTION FIVE

QUESTIONS YOU MIGHT HAVE
ABOUT HASHIMOTO'S

H OPEFULLY MOST OF YOUR questions have been answered within the first four sections of this book. However, you may have some remaining questions. Thus, I thought it would be best to include a separate section that covers some of the common questions people with Hashimoto's have. I determined what questions to include in this section by sending out a survey to my email list. For example, one of the most common questions I was asked related to problems with losing weight. Thus there is a question that relates to this in this section, along with a comprehensive response.

I also included a few questions relating to topics that I thought were important to discuss. Some of the answers to the questions have a more detailed response than others. Part of this relates to the complexity of the question, although I also tend to spend more time on the questions that were frequently asked by those people I surveyed.

Here are the questions:

Will following the advice in this book help me to lose weight?
If losing weight is one of your goals, then following the advice in this book will most likely help you to lose weight. Let's briefly look at some of the main factors that can help someone to lose unwanted pounds:

1. Increase your thyroid hormone levels. The decrease in thyroid hormone levels is one of the main reasons why people with Hashimoto's have a difficult time losing weight. Although I'm about to discuss other factors, if you have low or depressed thyroid hormone levels then of course you should take measures to increase these.

2. Eat a clean diet. Ideally, you want to eat a diet consisting mostly of whole foods, and you especially want to minimize the consumption of refined carbohydrates and sugars. If you are eating a healthy diet, then I wouldn't worry about eating too many calories, and I definitely wouldn't cut out the fats. Some people will increase their protein consumption and reduce their fat intake, but eating healthy fats such as avocados and coconut oil shouldn't cause you to gain a lot of weight. Regardless of whether a patient of mine is trying to gain or lose weight, I encourage them to eat plenty of healthy fats, and to get most of their carbohydrates from vegetables.

3. Improve your stress-management skills. Evidence indicates that chronic stress and high cortisol levels can play a role in obesity.[1,2] While you won't be able to eliminate all of the stressors in your life, block out at least ten minutes each day to focus on stress management.

4. Reduce inflammation. There is some overlap between diet and inflammation. However, while eating an anti-inflammatory diet can greatly help, many times doing this isn't sufficient because other factors can cause inflammation, including stress, infections, and environmental toxins.

Having healthy vitamin D levels is important to reduce inflammation, and if you haven't been recently tested for vitamin D, then I would highly recommend doing so. If you are deficient, then regular sun exposure during safe hours and supplementation is recommended.

Speaking of supplementation, while you want to do as much as you can through diet, taking certain nutritional supplements can help to reduce inflammation, which I discussed in section one. Two of the most common supplements that can help accomplish this are fish oils and curcumin. But taking supplements will have a minimal impact if you aren't eating a healthy diet, improving your stress-management skills, and getting sufficient sleep.

5. Decrease insulin resistance/increase insulin sensitivity. Eating a lot of refined carbohydrates and sugars can be a factor in insulin resistance. Certain nutrients can help to increase insulin sensitivity, including chromium, magnesium, alpha lipoic acid, vanadium, and bitter melon. Berberine is also something to consider for those who have hyperglycemia and insulin resistance. While Metformin is commonly recommended for those with insulin resistance and type 2 diabetes, the research shows that berberine can also be a potent hypoglycemic agent. I also mentioned how regular exercise can help to increase insulin sensitivity and that inflammation is a factor; thus, you need to address this problem as well.

6. Balance the sex hormones. Imbalances of the sex hormones estrogen and progesterone can cause someone with Hashimoto's to gain weight. This is especially true when someone has estrogen dominance. Thus, make sure you refer to Chapter 27 on balancing sex hormones, including how to improve estrogen metabolism.

7. Get sufficient sleep each night. Everyone knows the importance of getting sufficient sleep, but many don't consider lack of sleep to be a potential cause of weight gain. In the literature, there is a correlation between short duration of sleep, poor sleep quality, and obesity.[3,4] This isn't to suggest that everyone who doesn't get adequate sleep will have problems losing weight, but if this is the case with you, then you want to do everything you can do to get sufficient sleep each night, which I discussed in section four.

8. Minimize your exposure to obesogens. Obesogens are endocrine disrupting chemicals that interfere with the body's adipose (fat) tissue biology and interact with the hormone receptors, which, in turn, disrupts the endocrine signaling pathways. Thus, it can be a factor in gaining weight.[5] Bisphenol A (BPA) and phthalates can contribute to weight gain, and other obesogens, including persistent organic pollutants (POPs), pesticides, polychlorinated biphenyls (PCBs), and polybrominated diphenyl ethers (PBDEs) have been shown to accumulate in adipose tissue after exposure.[5]

Therefore, you want to do everything you can to minimize your exposure to these chemicals. For example, avoid drinking water out of plastic bottles, as the xenoestrogens can be a factor. Similarly, if you are using body creams and lotions with some of the chemicals I listed earlier, then it's best to switch to a natural alternative.

9. Support the detoxification pathways. While minimizing your exposure to environmental toxins is important, you also want to take measures to detoxify these chemicals from your body. Eating a healthy diet with plenty of vegetables is essential, especially the cruciferous vegetables (e.g., broccoli, kale, cabbage, cauliflower). Taking supplements such as N-acetylcysteine (NAC) or a liposomal/acetylated form of glutathione can also help to support detoxification. Another thing to consider is infrared sauna therapy, which will help you to excrete toxins through sweat. I discussed detoxification in detail in section four.

10. Be active. I realize that some people with Hashimoto's don't have the energy to exercise, but, if at all possible, you want to avoid sitting for prolonged periods of time. I understand that, in some cases, this is difficult to accomplish, but even if you work a desk job Monday through Friday, you still want to try to take frequent breaks, go for a walk during lunch, etc. Getting a treadmill desk was one of the best investments I have made in order to stay active while working, although a standing desk is another option if you have the flexibility of working from home.

Do you ever recommend low-dose naltrexone to your patients?
For those reading this who aren't familiar with low-dose naltrexone (LDN), I'll give a brief explanation. Naltrexone is an FDA-approved medication, approved to help heroin and opium addicts by blocking opioid receptors. In 1985, Dr. Bernard Bihari experimented with lower doses of naltrexone and realized that it can modulate the immune system. Soon thereafter, it was found that LDN can benefit many people with autoimmune conditions, certain types of cancers, and some other chronic health conditions. While at times I recommend LDN to my patients, it's not something I jump into for the following reasons:

1. LDN doesn't do anything to address the cause of the problem. Although LDN can modulate the immune system, it doesn't do anything to address the underlying cause of Hashimoto's. However, some people choose to take LDN while simultaneously trying to detect and remove their triggers.

2. LDN isn't always effective. Although I can't say that I've had a lot of patients who have taken LDN, I've worked with enough people to see that LDN sometimes is effective, but, at other times, it doesn't seem to help at all.

3. LDN can have a negative effect on sleep. Initially, it is common for LDN to interfere with sleep. However, this seems to be more common in those people who start with a higher dosage (i.e., 4.5 mg); thus, if this occurs, you would want to lower the dosage. Better yet, start with a lower dosage of LDN and then gradually increase it if necessary.

When Do I Recommend Low-Dose Naltrexone?

In most cases, I will recommend a natural treatment approach first, and if the person isn't responding after a few months, then I'd consider LDN as an option. In addition, before someone takes LDN, it's important to address certain imbalances in order to increase its effectiveness. For example, low or depressed vitamin D levels should be corrected before someone starts taking LDN. In addition, according to some healthcare professionals, having a Candida overgrowth also can make LDN less effective.

Do you have any advice on overcoming fatigue?

Although finding and removing the autoimmune triggers while correcting other imbalances is very likely to help you to overcome fatigue, I'll specifically list a few things here that can help with fatigue. I'm not going to discuss each one in detail, as I've covered most of these areas in this book.

1. Balance your thyroid hormone levels. In most cases, low thyroid hormone levels related to hypothyroidism are associated with fatigue; thus, you obviously want to correct the hormone imbalance. Many people take thyroid hormone replacement to help with this, and, since thyroid hormone is so important, this usually is a good idea. However, while doing this, the goal should be to address the cause of the problem, which is what this book is about.

2. Improve the health of your adrenals/HPA axis. Refer to Chapter 27.

3. Get more sleep. Refer to Chapter 32.

4. Eradicate infections. Having an infection can cause fatigue, and I also discuss how to overcome infections in Chapter 31.

5. Correct nutrient deficiencies. Refer to Chapter 30.

6. Address blood sugar imbalances. Refer to Chapter 17 and Chapter 32.

7. Improve the health of your mitochondria. I briefly discussed the role of mitochondria in Chapter 13, and how the production of adenosine tri-phosphate (ATP) takes place in the mitochondria. ATP is important for energy production, and as a result, a decreased production of ATP can cause fatigue. Nutrient deficiencies play a big role in mitochondrial dys-function, although there can be other factors, including environmental toxins and infections.

How will I know when I'm in remission?

Here are three signs that you have achieved a state of remission:

1. Complete resolution of symptoms. One of the main goals is for your symp-toms to resolve. Of course, the primary way to eliminate your symp-toms is by finding and removing the autoimmune triggers, which you have learned about by reading this book. In some scenarios, someone might not achieve complete resolution of their symptoms. For example, if someone with Hashimoto's has small intestinal bacterial overgrowth (SIBO) due to damage to the migrating motor complex, which, in turn, is caused by an autoimmune process, they will not have complete resolu-tion of their symptoms. This doesn't mean that tremendous improvement isn't possible, but a person in this situation might still have some mild symptoms after treating their SIBO, and in order to prevent SIBO from coming back, they probably would need to take prokinetics after treat-ment, which I discussed in Chapter 33.

2. Normalization of your thyroid panel and other blood tests. When I say "thyroid panel," I'm not only referring to the TSH and thyroid hormones, but the thyroid antibodies as well. Other markers that were out of range initially should normalize as well, including vitamin D, an iron panel, etc.

3. Normalization of other tests. This includes adrenal saliva testing, the sex hormones, if someone tests positive for infections then these should be eradicated, etc.

I've followed a strict AIP diet for a few months and have worked with a few different healthcare professionals, yet my thyroid antibodies are still high. Why is this?

There are a few reasons why someone can follow a natural treatment protocol for Hashimoto's and still have elevated thyroid antibodies. Here are a few of the more common reasons:

1. Not enough time has passed since starting the natural treatment protocol. Achieving a state of remission takes time, and you need to have realistic expectations. The truth is that everyone is different, and, while some people achieve remission within 6 to 12 months, other people take longer. However, while it's great to see the thyroid antibodies decrease and eventually normalize, the primary thing you want to notice is overall progress. In other words, if you're feeling better, your thyroid panel is improving, other imbalances are also improving (e.g., adrenals), and if the thyroid antibodies are lower than when you first started the natural treatment protocol, then these are all excellent signs that you are headed in the right direction.

2. The patient didn't follow the recommendations. Sometimes, the patient intentionally doesn't follow the recommendations due to numerous reasons; other times, they might have misunderstood the recommendations. Although I always give my recommendations in writing, every now and then, a patient will still be confused. While most will usually ask me for some clarification, some don't.

3. The autoimmune trigger hasn't been detected and/or removed. If the patient was strictly following the recommendations for a sufficient amount of time, yet their thyroid antibodies remain high and aren't decreasing, this usually indicates that the autoimmune trigger hasn't been detected, or perhaps it has been detected but it hasn't been removed. Also, it's possible to have multiple triggers. Thus, one or more potential triggers may have been detected, but another one might not have been, and more testing might be necessary.

Another thing to keep in mind is that no test is perfect. For example, someone might have had a comprehensive stool panel that was negative and think that they don't have any parasites or other pathogenic infections. However, false negatives are possible with these and other tests.

4. The gut isn't fully healed. Besides removing the autoimmune trigger, it is necessary to heal the gut in order to get into remission and lower the antibodies. If the gut hasn't been healed, this usually means that the leaky gut trigger hasn't been detected and removed. If you are wondering how to know if your gut has been healed, another question addresses this in this section.

Is it possible to get off of thyroid hormone replacement?

Some people need to be on thyroid hormone permanently. It depends on the person, as, if there is extensive damage to the thyroid gland, then the person might need to remain on thyroid hormone for life. However, in some cases, it is possible to get off of thyroid hormone replacement.

This brings up the following question: Is it possible for the thyroid gland to regenerate? Many think that the thyroid gland doesn't have the ability to regenerate. This isn't completely true, although, without question, different areas of the body will heal at a much faster rate, and the cells of thyroid gland regenerate at a slower rate when compared to other areas. For example, the liver has a remarkable regenerative capacity after a partial hepatectomy.[6] After a partial thyroidectomy, the thyroid gland exhibits hypertrophy and hyperplasia,[7] but it doesn't return to its original weight as the liver does.

However, hyperplasia is an increase in cell production; thus, this suggests that regeneration of the thyroid gland is possible, although it's not a quick process when compared to other parts of the body. It also depends on how much damage takes place to the thyroid gland, as I'm not suggesting that someone who has received a partial thyroidectomy can expect complete regeneration to occur.

Can cold laser therapy regenerate my thyroid gland?

Therapies exist that can help speed up the healing process, or cause tissue regeneration to occur when it normally wouldn't happen on its own. An example of this is cold laser therapy.

A few small studies showed that using cold laser therapy can help improve vascularization and perhaps regeneration of the thyroid cells in some people with hypothyroidism. One of these studies involved 43 patients with autoimmune thyroiditis who were on thyroid hormone replacement (levothyroxine). Results showed that low-level laser therapy (LLLT) can improve thyroid parenchyma vascularization.[8] The same study showed a significant difference in the average levothyroxine dose required between those who received the treatment, and those who received a placebo treatment.[8]

The group treated by LLLT also had lower thyroid peroxidase antibodies, although there wasn't a change in the thyroglobulin antibodies. Another study involving fifteen patients with Hashimoto's showed that LLLT promotes the improvement of thyroid function, as patients experienced a decreased need for levothyroxine, a reduction in the TPO antibodies, and an increase in parenchymal echogenicity.[9]

Additional studies need to be conducted to show further proof of the benefits of LLLT on thyroid health, but these results are very encouraging. One important thing to keep in mind is that even if LLLT can help to regenerate the tissue of the thyroid gland, it still won't do anything to remove the underlying cause. For example, if someone has Hashimoto's due to an infection, which, in turn, caused a leaky gut, both the infection and the leaky gut need to be addressed.

Why am I presenting with thyroid symptoms even though I have a normal thyroid panel?

This is a very common question, and an entire book has been written on this by Dr. Datis Kharrazin entitled *Why Do I Still Have Thyroid Symptoms…When My Lab Tests Are Normal?* This is an excellent book that I highly recommend, but if you recall from Chapter 24, the "lab" reference ranges are different from the "optimal" reference ranges. It's very common for people with Hashimoto's to have a TSH and thyroid hormones that fall within the lab reference range, but are outside of the optimal range.

For example, let's take a look at someone with the following thyroid panel:

TSH: 3.5 uIU/ml
Free T4: 0.9 ng/dL
Free T3: 2.5 pg/ml

According to most laboratories, these values would be within the "normal" lab reference range. However, they are outside of the optimal range, as the TSH is higher than we'd like to see, and both thyroid hormone levels are lower than we'd like to see, especially the free T3 levels. Unfortunately, what frequently happens is that someone will have a thyroid panel that looks similar to this, so the medical doctor will tell the patient that the levels are normal, and many patients won't question their doctor.

If the same doctor were to test the thyroid antibodies, they most likely would see them elevated, and would realize that the person has the antibodies for Hashimoto's. The problem is that many medical doctors don't test the thyroid antibodies unless the TSH or thyroid hormone levels are out of range according to the lab they use.

I'm not suggesting that all medical doctors make this mistake, but many do. Sometimes, the person with a subclinical thyroid problem will go many years before they either seek another opinion or see the same doctor, but, at this time, one or more of the markers will fall outside of the lab reference range.

To summarize, many people feel lousy when their blood tests look normal because one or more markers are outside of the optimal range. Thus, you can't rely on the lab reference ranges, which is why it's important to either understand how to read these blood tests, or hire a functional medicine doctor who knows how to do this.

How can I tell if my leaky gut has been healed?

I frequently get asked this question, and there are a few different ways to know if your gut has been healed:

1. Not having frequent digestive symptoms. Although the lack of digestive symptoms alone doesn't rule out gut problems, if someone is having frequent digestive symptoms (e.g., gas, bloating, abdominal pain) then they can be confident that they don't have a healthy gut.

2. Having at least one daily bowel movement. Someone with a healthy gut should move their bowels daily. At minimum, you want to have at least one daily bowel movement, although two or three is even better.

3. Having well-formed stools. In addition to having at least one healthy bowel movement, your stools should be well formed. For example, you don't want to see any undigested food, and your stools shouldn't be too hard or soft.

4. Test negative for a leaky gut. Although I used to frequently recommend leaky gut testing to my patients, these days, I don't commonly recommend such testing. However, this is yet another way to confirm that you have a healthy gut, as if you don't have digestive symptoms, have daily bowel movements and well-formed stools, and on top of this test negative for a leaky gut, then there is a pretty good chance that you have a healthy gut. I discussed leaky gut testing in Chapter 25.

5. Have a negative stool panel. Instead of or in addition to doing a leaky gut test, you can do a comprehensive stool panel. Some people do a stool panel initially, but either way, if there were any positive findings, then you might choose to do a follow-up stool panel at some point. This is especially true if you tested positive for pathogens such as parasites, pathogenic bacteria, and/or a Candida overgrowth. Most comprehensive stool panels test for other factors, such as markers of gut inflammation. I discussed stool testing in section three.

Do you have any advice on overcoming brain fog?

Brain fog is very common in people with Hashimoto's. Some of the symptoms associated with this condition include slow thinking, difficulty focusing, confusion, lack of concentration, forgetfulness, or a haziness in thought processes. Just as is the case with fatigue, following the advice given in this book should help with most cases of brain fog. However, I'll also list a few specific things you can do here:

1. Normalize the thyroid hormones. Having low thyroid hormone levels can lead to many different symptoms, and brain fog is one of them.

2. Correct neurotransmitter imbalances. In many cases, having imbalances in serotonin, GABA, or acetylcholine can cause brain fog. High levels of certain neurotransmitters such as epinephrine and norepinephrine can also lead to brain fog symptoms. To correct neurotransmitter imbalances, many doctors will recommend taking the neurotransmitter precursors if they suspect a certain deficiency. For example, if they suspect an imbalance of serotonin then they commonly will recommend tryptophan or 5-HTP.

I have taken this approach in the past, but what's important to keep in mind is that certain nutrients are required for the enzyme reactions that produce these neurotransmitters. For example, many people have low iron levels, yet iron is necessary for the conversion of tryptophan to

5-HTP. In addition, since most of the neurotransmitters are produced in the gut, it is important to have a healthy gut.

3. Decrease cortisol levels and improve your stress-management skills. I discussed how to improve the health of the adrenals in Chapter 27.

4. Reduce your toxic load. In Chapter 8, I discussed how heavy metals, such as aluminum, mercury, and cadmium, can cause an increase in permeability of the blood brain barrier.[10,11,12,13] Other harmful chemicals can also disrupt the integrity of the blood brain barrier, such as PCBs.[14,15] There is even evidence that exposure to electromagnetic fields can disrupt the permeability of the blood brain barrier.[16]

5. Correct blood sugar imbalances. This also has been covered in this book.

6. Repair the blood brain barrier and eliminate brain inflammation. There can be numerous causes of brain inflammation. Obviously, a head trauma can lead to neuroinflammation, but other factors include blood sugar imbalances, a gluten sensitivity, environmental toxins, and a leaky blood brain barrier. In this book, I have discussed a leaky gut many times, which is when the integrity of the intestinal barrier system is compromised. Similarly, one can have a leaky blood brain barrier, which can cause the symptoms associated with brain fog.

How does someone develop a leaky blood brain barrier? Well, some of the same factors that can cause a leaky gut can also cause a "leaky brain." This includes stress,[17,18] a gluten sensitivity,[19] excess alcohol consumption,[20,21] and certain infections.[22] Certain environmental chemicals can also disrupt the blood brain barrier. Thus, these factors need to be addressed, and I have discussed most of them in this book.

How can you determine if you have a leaky blood brain barrier? The company Cyrex Labs has a blood brain barrier permeability test, which tests for antibodies found when someone has a compromised blood brain barrier. Another method is through something called the GABA challenge, which I learned through the work of Dr. Datis Kharrazian.

This involves swallowing a 1,000 mg GABA supplement during the day, and if you feel either a calming effect or more anxious then this is an indication that you have a compromised blood brain barrier. The reason for this is because most GABA supplements normally don't cross the blood brain barrier. Thus, if someone takes GABA and has an intact blood brain barrier they shouldn't feel any different.

How do you detect and address a T4 to T3 conversion problem?

The thyroid hormone thyroxine (T4) converts into triiodothyronine (T3). The enzyme 5'-deiodinase is responsible for this conversion process. Three forms of this enzyme include deodinase type I, deodinase type II, and deodinase type III. The type I and type II deiodinases are primarily responsible for the conversion of T4 to T3, whereas the type III deiodinase is mainly involved in the inactivation of T4 and T3.[23,24] Most of this conversion takes place in the liver, although some of the conversion also takes place in the gastrointestinal tract.

If someone has normal levels of T4 on a blood test, but low or depressed levels of T3, this is one indication of a conversion problem. Another indication is if reverse T3 is elevated or on the high end of the reference range. I mentioned earlier that most of the conversion takes place in the liver, although some of it takes place in the gut. These are the first two places to address when someone has a conversion problem.

Elevated cortisol levels can also affect the conversion of T4 to T3. Studies show that stress can inhibit both type I iodothyronine 5'-deiodinase activity,[25] as well as type II 5'-deiodinase activity.[26,27] In Chapter 27, I discussed how to improve the health of the adrenals, which will, in turn, help to normalize the cortisol levels.

A few other factors that can negatively affect the conversion of T4 to T3 include a selenium deficiency,[28,29] certain medications,[30] and even pro-inflammatory cytokines.[31] These are some of the factors that need to be addressed when someone has a conversion problem.

What should I do if I followed the AIP diet strictly for a few months and didn't experience an improvement in my symptoms?

Although some people with Hashimoto's feel a dramatic improvement in their symptoms upon following an AIP diet, this doesn't describe everyone. I've worked with many patients over the years who followed an AIP diet for a number of months without noticing any positive changes in their symptoms or blood tests. This can be frustrating if you visit some Hashimoto's forums or Facebook groups and come across some people who felt much better upon following an AIP diet. You might even have come across people who felt significantly better and/or experienced a reduction in their thyroid antibodies by only avoiding gluten.

Keep in mind that food isn't an autoimmune trigger in everyone. If you didn't notice any improvement in your symptoms or labs after following an AIP diet for at least 30 days, then it's probably safe to say that food isn't your primary trigger. However, keep in mind that one of the reasons for following an AIP diet is to avoid foods that can interfere with gut healing. Thus, even if you didn't feel better upon following an AIP diet, please don't feel like this was a waste of your time.

The truth is that the AIP diet is only one component of healing. While eating well and avoiding problematic foods are both important, there can be numerous other factors that triggered your condition, which is why I wrote this book. Sometimes, it can take some detective work to find your specific triggers. In section three, I discussed many of the different tests to help find the triggers of Hashimoto's. This can be complex, which is why many people can benefit from working with a natural healthcare professional to assist with this.

What can be done for hair loss?

Hair loss is one of the most frustrating symptoms many of my patients with Hashimoto's experience. It's common for the patient to be more concerned about the hair loss, even if they are experiencing other symptoms that many would consider to be more extreme. The good news is that most cases of hair loss are reversible, although it can take a good amount of time for the hair loss to stop and grow back.

Here are the most common causes of hair loss in people with Hashimoto's:

1. Low thyroid hormone levels. Keep in mind that it commonly takes a number of months after the thyroid hormones have normalized for the hair loss to stop.

2. Nutrient deficiencies. About 30% of women before the age of 50 have hair loss due to some type of nutritional deficiency, with depleted iron stores being the most common cause.[32] A suboptimal intake of the amino acid lysine can also be a factor.[32] I discussed correcting nutrient deficiencies in detail in Chapter 30.

3. Sex hormone imbalances. One study showed that a low estrogen to androgen ratio (ratio of estradiol to free testosterone) might be responsible for triggering hair loss in women.[33] Problems with the estrogen and progesterone receptors can also be a factor in some people.[34] High levels of androgens in postmenopause can result in hair loss.[35,36] High levels of prolactin can also cause hair loss.[37]

4. Stress. Evidence shows that neurohormones, neurotransmitters, and pro-inflammatory cytokines released during the stress response may also significantly influence the hair cycle.[38,39,40] In addition, acute emotional stress may cause alopecia areata by activating corticotropin-releasing hormone receptors around the hair follicles, leading to intense local inflammation.[41]

5. Alopecia Areata. This is an autoimmune condition that involves damage of the hair follicles. It usually begins with one or two patches of hair loss on the scalp, although hair loss can also occur in the eyebrows, arms, and legs.[42] Some people will experience hair loss of the entire scalp, which is known as alopecia totalis.[43] If it involves the whole body, this is known as alopecia universalis.[43] For some people, the hair will eventually grow back, although this isn't the case with everyone.

In most people with Hashimoto's, hair loss is caused by one of the first four factors. Thus, it is essential to balance the thyroid and sex hormones, correct any nutrient deficiencies, and to improve your stress-management skills.

What treatment approach do you recommend for someone who has the antibodies for both Hashimoto's and Graves' disease?

Some people with Hashimoto's also have the antibodies for Graves' disease. These are called TSH receptor antibodies, with the most common type being thyroid stimulating immunoglobulins.

Over the years, I have worked with many patients who had both the antibodies to Graves' disease and Hashimoto's. While, sometimes, they will fluctuate back and forth between hypothyroidism and hyperthyroidism, a common pattern is for someone to initially become hyperthyroid due to the immune system stimulating the TSH receptors, thus causing the excessive release of thyroid hormone.

In addition to having Graves' disease antibodies, if someone also has thyroid peroxidase and/or thyroglobulin antibodies, then, over time, the immune system will damage the thyroid gland. If the autoimmune component isn't addressed, then this is likely to lead to hypothyroidism over time.

When addressing the autoimmune component of Graves' disease and Hashimoto's, the approach will be similar. With both conditions, you want to detect and remove the trigger, heal the gut, and balance other compromised areas of the body. However, if you have the antibodies for both of these conditions, keep the following two things in mind:

1. When it comes to symptom management, the treatment approach will depend on whether the person presents with hyperthyroidism or hypothyroidism. For example, if someone has the antibodies for both Graves' disease and Hashimoto's, but their recent symptoms are exclusively hypothyroid, and their blood tests show an elevated TSH and thyroid hormone levels that are low or depressed, then, in this situation, it makes sense for the person to take thyroid hormone replacement. However, if their symptoms are predominantly hyperthyroid and their blood tests present with a depressed TSH and elevated thyroid hormone levels, then giving thyroid hormone replacement would be a big mistake, and you would want to take measures to lower the thyroid hormone levels while addressing the cause of the problem.

2. Different autoimmune conditions will have different triggers. Just to clarify, most of the triggers I listed in this book will apply to other autoimmune conditions, and not just Hashimoto's. However, certain triggers are more likely to be found in Graves' disease than Hashimoto's thyroiditis, and the reverse is true. For example, Blastocystis Hominis seems to be a more common trigger in those with Hashimoto's, although I've also seen this parasite in some people with Graves' disease. Similarly, H. pylori seems to be a more common trigger in people with Graves' disease, although it can also be a factor in those with Hashimoto's.

Can I get into remission without taking any supplements?

Although I do give supplement recommendations in section four, I also try to give plenty of food options. Without question, you want to try to do as much as you can through diet. Eating whole healthy foods is essential to restore your health back to normal. However, I find that taking supplements are an important component of the recovery process. When I was diagnosed with Graves' disease, I took numerous nutritional supplements and herbs. While I followed a strict diet at the time, I'm confident that I wouldn't have received the same results without taking the supplements and herbs.

However, taking more supplements isn't necessarily better. I've consulted with patients for the first time who were taking dozens of supplements with very little improvement in their condition. What I do initially is have my patients focus more on the diet, and I give a few general supplement recommendations. Then, once I receive the results of any recommended tests, I make more specific supplement recommendations. Getting back to the original question, although you might be able to get into remission without taking any supplements, I find that supplements are an important component of the natural treatment protocol, although I don't think that most people need to take dozens of nutritional supplements and herbs to get into remission.

Can breast implants trigger Hashimoto's?

Over the years, I have worked with some patients with breast implants, as well as those who had their breast implants removed. However, it's hard to make the connection between these and autoimmunity. As I mentioned when I discussed the autoimmunity timeline in Chapter 1, the development of thyroid autoantibodies can occur years before the onset of symptoms. In many cases, a person with Hashimoto's won't get diagnosed until 5 to 10 years after the formation of these antibodies. Thus, if someone received silicone breast implants 5 to 10 years prior to being diagnosed and has no other obvious triggers, then while we still wouldn't know with certainty if the breast implants were the primary trigger, in this scenario, it would seem likely.

What does the research show? A couple of case reports involved Hashimoto's and silicone breast implants.[44] One patient was a 45-year-old woman who had silicone breast implants in 1976, and in 1991, she developed Hashimoto's. The implants were painful, and, in 1996, they were removed. The second patient was a 55-year-old woman who had silicone breast implants in 1994, and, in 1995, she developed Hashimoto's. In 1996, the implants were painful and the patient developed positive antinuclear antibodies. As I mentioned earlier, there is no way to know for certain that the silicone breast implants were the cause of Hashimoto's, but, since these case reports were in the literature, I figured I'd mention them.

I also came across a journal article that brought up a possible link between breast implants and an increased risk for autoimmune disease, although it focused on connective tissue diseases such as scleroderma, along with syndromes such as fibromyalgia and chronic fatigue syndrome.[45] I also found a study in which the authors investigated the immunological mechanisms underlying peri-silicone implant capsule formation, which is the most common complication in patients receiving silicone mammary implants.[46] The results of the study indicated that silicone implants activated Th1 and Th17 cells, which are associated with autoimmune conditions such as Hashimoto's.

What recommendations do you have for someone who can't afford to buy organic food?

Although eating organic food is ideal, this doesn't mean that doing so is essential to get into remission. The most important thing you can do is to eat mostly whole foods, including plenty of vegetables, while trying to avoid the refined foods and sugars, along with fast food. Sure, eating mostly organic is best for your health over the long term, and, of course, your future health needs to be considered. However, I realize that many people can't ignore their current financial situation.

At the very least, try to purchase organic meat, fruit, and vegetables. If you initially follow an AIP diet and then reintroduce eggs in the future, try to make sure these are organic as well. What if you still can't afford to purchase these foods as organic or don't have access to organic food where you live? In the latter situation, perhaps you can order organic food online, as some companies will ship organic fruits and vegetables to you, and other companies will ship 100% grass fed beef, organic free range chicken, etc.

If you absolutely can't afford to purchase all fruits, vegetables, meat, and eggs organic, then you can still eat whole foods, and I'll also remind you about the Dirty Dozen and Clean Fifteen lists provided by the Environmental Working group. As I mentioned earlier in this book, these lists aren't perfect, as they don't take into account the fact that some pesticides are more toxic than others; thus, it's not just the concentration of pesticides that's a concern.

However, I still think these lists are valuable, and until a better option comes along, I would recommend not to purchase any non-organic fruits or vegetables that are on the Dirty Dozen list. However, if you can't afford organic fruits and vegetables, then feel free to eat fruits and vegetables that are on the Clean Fifteen list. I also should add that the 2017 Clean Fifteen list includes a few foods that are excluded from an AIP diet (sweet corn and eggplant); thus, if following this diet, you, of course, would want to avoid these. Papaya is also on this list, and non-organic corn and papaya can be produced from genetically modified seeds. Thus, also avoid non-organic foods that are on the list of genetically modified foods I included in section two.

Can essential oils help with Hashimoto's?

Essential oils can benefit many people with Hashimoto's. Two of the more beneficial essential oils are myrrh and frankincense, as both of these have been shown to benefit the health of the immune system. A few studies demonstrated how myrrh and frankincense can benefit immune system health and reduce inflammation.[47,48,49]

While I didn't find any studies showing that either of these essential oils can directly affect thyroid health, some people have found that rubbing a few drops of myrrh oil around the thyroid gland can be beneficial in reducing goiters. Some people have claimed to have used essential oils as a substitute for thyroid hormone replacement, although I can't say that this is common.

Other essential oils can be beneficial as well. For example, lavender has a calming effect and therefore can help some people who have sleep issues. Research also shows that lavender has some antimicrobial properties,[50] which is the case with many other essential oils, including tea tree oil and geranium.

Keep in mind that you usually only need one or two drops of these essential oils to get a therapeutic effect. In most cases, you'll want to dilute these essential oils with a carrier oil, such as coconut oil, olive oil, or avocado oil, which reduces the chances of skin irritation occurring when applying the essential oils topically.

How strict do I need to be when following the AIP Diet?

This question is worded in many different ways, as some will ask if they can occasionally "stray" from the AIP diet, while others will ask if they can have a "cheat day" every now and then. The truth is that everyone is different, and some people can get away with straying from the diet, while others can't. This is why I recommend trying to be strict with the diet.

Whether or not someone's progress will be affected when straying from the diet also depends on which "forbidden" foods they eat. For example, if someone has a "cheat day" once a week where they eat pizza and ice cream then chances are this will be more problematic when compared with someone who eats eggs and nuts. However, this depends on the person, as some people have problems with eggs, nuts, and seeds, which is why they are excluded from an AIP diet.

Remember, you're not expected to follow the AIP diet for a prolonged period, which is why I discuss the reintroduction of foods in section three. I would try to be strict with the AIP diet for at least the first 30 days, which, ideally, means no "cheat days" or straying from the diet. Because of this, you want to try your best to choose a start date where you're confident that you'll be successful with sticking to the diet. For example, if you plan on going on vacation within the next 30 days, then it probably is best to start the AIP diet when you get back.

Just don't postpone following the AIP diet for too long, as, while certain times of the year are more challenging than others, the truth is that, throughout the year, there are many occasions when you can try to justify straying from the diet.

Do you recommend for people with Hashimoto's to take thyroid hormone replacement?

Many of my patients are already taking synthetic or natural thyroid hormone prior to speaking with me for the first time. Many people with Hashimoto's do need to take thyroid hormone replacement. If someone has depressed thyroid hormone levels, then it usually is wise for the person to take thyroid hormone replacement while trying to address the cause of the problem. That's the key, as most doctors who prescribe thyroid hormone to their Hashimoto's patients don't do anything to improve the health of the immune system or correct other imbalances.

Some people become surprised when I discuss how some people need to take thyroid hormone replacement. Since I encourage people with Hashimoto's to take a natural treatment approach, they wonder why I don't recommend an alternative to thyroid hormone medication. First, even though I sometimes use the word *medication,* probably the more appropriate term is thyroid hormone *replacement.* After all, someone is taking thyroid hormone as a replacement for the hormone that is produced naturally by their own body. Thus, it's not exactly the same as taking other types of medication such as antibiotics, statins, acid blockers, etc.

I'll also add that if someone has a thyroid hormone deficiency, then there is no nutritional supplement or herb you can take in place of thyroid hormone. Some herbs can help to stimulate the production of thyroid hormone by affecting the hypothalamic-pituitary-thyroid (HPT) axis (i.e., ashwagandha), but these aren't always effective, and they usually aren't a long-term solution to the problem. If someone is deficient in a nutrient important for the formation of thyroid hormone such as iodine or tyrosine, then this can help with the production of thyroid hormone. However, while many people with Hashimoto's have nutrient deficiencies, most cases of low thyroid hormone levels aren't directly caused by these deficiencies.

How about thyroid glandulars? Some thyroid glandulars include small amounts of thyroid hormone, along with some nutrients and/or herbs (e.g., zinc, selenium, ashwagandha), and many people can take these instead of synthetic or natural thyroid hormone and do fine. However, glandulars without thyroid hormone might provide some support to the thyroid gland, but if someone has low or depressed thyroid hormone levels, then this probably won't be sufficient.

Although many people do fine on levothyroxine, which is synthetic T4, if I had to take thyroid hormone replacement, I'm pretty certain that I would at least try to take desiccated thyroid hormone, such as Nature-Throid or WP Thyroid, with Armour being another option. These include both T4 and T3, in addition to T1, T2, and calcitonin. From a symptomatic perspective, many people do better on desiccated thyroid hormone. If someone does need to be on synthetic thyroid hormone, then Tirosint is something to consider, as this is a hypoallergenic form of synthetic T4. Another option is compounded T4 and T3 through a compounding pharmacist, although this usually is more expensive.

Is there a relationship between histamine intolerance and Hashimoto's?

Research shows that histamine can play a role in the pathogenesis of autoimmune conditions.[51,52] Histamine apparently affects the Th1/Th2 cytokine balance.[53] In section one, I discussed how Hashimoto's is typically a Th1 dominant condition, and histamine enhances the secretion of Th2 cytokines and inhibits the production of Th1 cytokines. Based on this information, it is possible that increased histamine levels might shift the balance towards Th2 dominant conditions such as Graves' disease.

This doesn't mean that people with Hashimoto's can't have conditions such as histamine intolerance and mast cell activation syndrome. Some of the potential causes of histamine intolerance include intestinal dysbiosis, impaired methylation, and certain medications that can inhibit the enzyme diamine oxidase (DAO), which is primarily responsible for the metabolism of ingested histamine, although another enzyme called histamine N-methyl transferase (HNMT) also breaks down histamine. While many people with a histamine intolerance will eat low histamine foods, you want to try to address the cause of the problem. For example, if intestinal dysbiosis is the problem, then this needs to be corrected. If impaired methylation is a factor, then this should be addressed.

Do I need to work with a natural healthcare professional to get into remission?

I think it's wise for most people with Hashimoto's who are looking to restore their health to work with a competent natural healthcare professional because autoimmunity can be complex, and it's challenging to get into remission on your own. Of course, some things you can do on your own, including making dietary and lifestyle changes. However, finding the autoimmune triggers does take some detective work, and, while some of the information provided in this book can no doubt help you with this, it's beneficial to work with someone who has a lot of experience working with Hashimoto's patients.

There is no shortage of natural healthcare professionals, including holistic medical doctors, chiropractors, naturopaths, etc. While the healthcare professional you work with doesn't need to exclusively deal with Hashimoto's patients, in my opinion, it's a good idea to work with someone who works with these patients every week, if not every day.

A functional medicine practitioner will address the underlying cause of the condition. While most medical doctors no doubt want to help their patients, unfortunately, most don't do anything to address the cause of the problem for those who have Hashimoto's, as well as other chronic health conditions. Many medical doctors who practice functional medicine still recommend prescription medication to some of their patients, but a good practitioner will only do so when absolutely necessary.

What type of natural healthcare practitioner should you work with? This depends on your specific situation. For example, if you are taking thyroid hormone replacement, then you might prefer working with a medical doctor who practices functional medicine so that they not only can help you address the cause of your problem but also prescribe thyroid hormone. Such a doctor will usually be more open to writing a prescription for desiccated thyroid (i.e., Armour, Nature-Throid, WP-Thyroid).

Regardless of the type of practitioner you choose to work with, in order to make sure they have a good amount of experience with Hashimoto's patients, do a little bit of research. Visit their website and see if they have patient testimonials from people with Hashimoto's, or perhaps the healthcare professional you're thinking about seeing has written a number of articles or recorded some videos on helping people with Hashimoto's. Call their office and ask the front desk person who answers the phone the following question: "What are the top three conditions your practice deals with?" If one of the top three conditions don't relate to thyroid conditions or Hashimoto's, then you might want to cross this office of your list.

I received my IFMCP certification from the Institute for Functional Medicine, and they do have an online directory where you can search for a functional medicine practitioner in your area. Their website is **https://www.ifm.org**. I should add that not everyone listed on their website is certified, although everyone has at least attended the Applying Functional Medicine in Clinical Practice conference.

Do you have any advice for pregnant women who have Hashimoto's?

In section two, I dedicated a chapter on postpartum thyroiditis (Chapter 16); thus, women who are pregnant should read this chapter if you haven't done so already. Overall, most of the same "rules" apply, as you want eat a healthy diet consisting of whole foods, improve your stress-management skills, minimize your exposure to environmental toxins, etc.

Some pregnant women are concerned that the AIP diet will be too restrictive, and might not provide enough nutrients to both her and the baby. Besides meat being very nutrient dense, if you eat a wide variety of vegetables each day, then getting enough nutrients shouldn't be a problem. Most women will also take a prenatal vitamin.

Speaking of which, some pregnant women with Hashimoto's become concerned about taking a prenatal with iodine. While iodine can be problematic in some people with Hashimoto's, this mineral is critically important to the developing fetus. Iodine deficiency isn't something to take lightly, and studies demonstrate the importance of iodine sufficiency during pregnancy.

Thus, I'm in favor of pregnant women with Hashimoto's taking a prenatal vitamin with iodine. In most cases, we're talking about a small dose of iodine, which usually isn't going to cause problems. In addition, taking iodine in the presence of other nutrients in the prenatal vitamin will usually minimize any negative effects of the iodine, although it might be a good idea to take extra selenium, making sure you don't exceed a total of 250 mcg/day. While some people seem to have problems tolerating even small doses of iodine, remember that we're discussing risks vs. benefits here, and in those women with Hashimoto's, the risk of completing avoiding iodine during pregnancy is, in most cases, greater than the risk of having a small amount of iodine in the form of a prenatal vitamin.

For those with Hashimoto's who aren't currently pregnant but plan on conceiving in the near future, while I've had patients with elevated autoantibodies have successful pregnancies, I would take at least a few months to improve your health. While it would be great to get into remission before getting pregnant, at the very least, make sure to correct your nutrient deficiencies and take measures to reduce your toxic load prior to conceiving.

The reason for this should be obvious, as you will have an even greater requirement for nutrients during pregnancy; thus, you definitely want to work on this prior to getting pregnant. Also, you won't be able to detoxify while pregnant or breastfeeding since any chemicals in your body will be passed onto the baby. Thus, it makes sense to do what you can to eliminate toxins prior to conception. I discussed how to reduce your total toxic load in Chapter 29.

How can I maintain a state of wellness after getting into remission?

Once you have achieved a state of remission, how can you maintain your health? I admit that maintaining a state of wellness can be a challenge, especially initially. Even after being in remission for many years, there still is always a chance of a relapse. However, doing the following will greatly increase the chances of maintaining a state of wellness:

1. Continue to eat well most of the time. What do I mean by "most of the time"? For example, is it okay for people who are in remission to eat well during the week but then have a cheat day or two on the weekend? This depends on the person, as some people are able to indulge more than others, while others need to be more strict with their diet in order to maintain a state of wellness.

2. Always work on stress management. Stress is a big factor with most people. In fact, chronic stress that is not properly managed can lead to a relapse. This is why continuing to improve your stress-management skills is essential. Please refer to Chapter 27 for more information on this.

3. Minimize your exposure to triggers. I discuss this in detail in section four.

4. Get sufficient sleep. I discussed this in Chapter 32, but I'll emphasize it here again. Once you achieve a state of remission, in order to maintain a state of wellness, you also want to get sufficient sleep consistently. This doesn't mean that staying up late once in a while will cause you to relapse, but you should aim to get at least six or seven hours sleep each night, and many people do better getting seven or eight hours of sleep each night. Keep in mind that "catching up" on sleep doesn't work. For example, if you only get four hours sleep Monday through Friday, and then sleep 10 to 12 hours on Saturday and Sunday, the extra sleep on the weekend isn't going to compensate for the sleep deprivation during the week.

BIBLIOGRAPHY

**Special thanks to my wonderful wife Cindy for helping to put this bibliography together

SECTION ONE

[1] https://www.aarda.org/news-information/statistics/

[2] Katja Zaletel and Simona Gaberšcek, Hashimoto's Thyroiditis: From Genes to the Disease; Curr Genomics. 2011 Dec; 12(8): 576–588

[3] Tandon N, Zhang L, Weetman AP, HLA associations with Hashimoto's thyroiditis; Clin Endocrinol (Oxf). 1991 May;34(5):383-6

[4] Beth L. Cobb, MBA,a ChristopherJ. Lessard, BS,a,b John B. Harley, MD, PhD,a,c,d and Kathy L. Moser, PhD, Genes and Sjögren's Syndrome; Rheum Dis Clin North Am. 2008 Nov; 34(4): 847–vii.

[5] Konca Degertekin C, Aktas Yilmaz B, Balos Toruner F, Kalkanci A, Turhan Iyidir O, Fidan I, Yesilyurt E, Cakır N, Kustimur S, Arslan M; Circulating Th17 cytokine levels are altered in Hashimoto's thyroiditis; Cytokine. 2016 Apr;80:13-7.

[6] Li D1, Cai W, Gu R, Zhang Y, Zhang H, Tang K, Xu P, Katirai F, Shi W, Wang L, Huang T, Huang B, Th17 cell plays a role in the pathogenesis of Hashimoto's thyroiditis in patients; Clin Immunol. 2013 Dec;149(3):411-20.

[7] Figueroa-Vega N, Alfonso-Pérez M, Benedicto I, Sánchez-Madrid F, González-Amaro R, Marazuela M, Increased circulating pro-inflammatory cytokines and Th17 lymphocytes in Hashimoto's thyroiditis; J Clin Endocrinol Metab. 2010 Feb;95(2):953-62.

[8] Lauren Anderson, William D. Middleton, Sharlene A. Teefey, Carl C. Reading, Hashimoto Thyroiditis: Part 1, Sonographic Analysis of the Nodular Form of Hashimoto Thyroiditis; AJR Am J Roentgenol. 2010 Jul;195(1):208-15.

[9] Friedman M, Shimaoka K, Rao U, Tsukada Y, Gavigan M, Tamura K, Diagnosis of chronic lymphocytic thyroiditis (nodular presentation) by needle aspiration; Acta Cytol. 1981 Sep-Oct;25(5):513-22

[10] Galland, Leo; Textbook of Functional Medicine; Chapter 8: Patient-centered Care: Antecedents, Triggers, and Mediators; Page 81

[11] Chen Y, Zhang J, Ge X, Du J, Deb DK, Li YC, Vitamin D receptor inhibits nuclear factor ?B activation by interacting with I?B kinase ß protein; J Biol Chem. 2013 Jul 5;288(27):19450-8.

[12] Cohen-Lahav M, Shany S, Tobvin D, Chaimovitz C, Douvdevani A, Vitamin D decreases NFkappaB activity by increasing IkappaBalpha levels; Nephrol Dial Transplant. 2006 Apr;21(4):889-97. Epub 2006 Feb 2.

[13] Kim JH1, Gupta SC, Park B, Yadav VR, Aggarwal BB, Turmeric (Curcuma longa) inhibits inflammatory nuclear factor (NF)-?B and NF-?B-regulated gene products and induces death receptors leading to suppressed proliferation, induced chemosensitization, and suppressed osteoclastogenesis; Mol Nutr Food Res. 2012 Mar;56(3):454-65.

[14] Bengmark S, Curcumin, an atoxic antioxidant and natural NFkappaB, cyclooxygenase-2, lipooxygenase, and inducible nitric oxide synthase inhibitor: a shield against acute and chronic diseases; JPEN J Parenter Enteral Nutr. 2006 Jan-Feb;30(1):45-51.

[15] Shakibaei M, John T, Schulze-Tanzil G, Lehmann I, Mobasheri A, Suppression of NF-kappaB activation by curcumin leads to inhibition of expression of cyclo-oxygenase-2 and matrix metalloproteinase-9 in human articular chondrocytes: Implications for the treatment of osteoarthritis; Biochem Pharmacol. 2007 May 1;73(9):1434-45. Epub 2007 Jan 7.

[16] Shoba G1, Joy D, Joseph T, Majeed M, Rajendran R, Srinivas PS, Influence of piperine on the pharmacokinetics of curcumin in animals and human volunteers; Planta Med. 1998 May;64(4):353-6.

[17] Ralf Jäger,corresponding author1 Ryan P Lowery, Allison V Calvanese, Jordan M Joy, Martin Purpura, and Jacob M Wilson, Comparative absorption of curcumin formulations; Published online 2014 Jan 24.

[18] Cuomo J, Appendino G, Dern AS, Schneider E, McKinnon TP, Brown MJ, Togni S, Dixon BM; Comparative absorption of a standardized curcuminoid mixture and its lecithin formulation; J Nat Prod. 2011 Apr 25;74(4):664-9.

[19] Di Lorenzo C, Dell'Agli M, Sangiovanni E, Dos Santos A, Uberti F, Moro E, Bosisio E, Restani P, Correlation between catechin content and NF-?B inhibition by infusions of green and black tea; Plant Foods Hum Nutr. 2013 Jun;68(2):149-54.

[20] Park HJ, Lee JY, Chung MY, Park YK, Bower AM, Koo SI, Giardina C, Bruno RS, Green tea extract suppresses NF?B activation and inflammatory responses in diet-induced obese rats with nonalcoholic steatohepatitis; J Nutr. 2012 Jan;142(1):57-63. doi: 10.3945/jn.111.148544. Epub 2011 Dec 7.

[21] http://www.mayoclinic.org/healthy-living/nutrition-and-healthy-eating/in-depth/caffeine/art-20049372

[22] Henning SM, Fajardo-Lira C, Lee HW, Youssefian AA, Go VL, Heber D, Catechin content of 18 teas and a green tea extract supplement correlates with the antioxidant capacity; Nutr Cancer. 2003;45(2):226-35.

[23] Hsu SP, Wu MS, Yang CC, Huang KC, Liou SY, Hsu SM, Chien CT, Chronic green tea extract supplementation reduces hemodialysis-enhanced production

of hydrogen peroxide and hypochlorous acid, atherosclerotic factors, and proinflammatory cytokines; Am J Clin Nutr. 2007 Nov;86(5):1539-47.

[24] Dario A. A. Vignali, Lauren W. Collison, and Creg J. Workman, How regulatory T cells work; Nat Rev Immunol. 2008 Jul; 8(7): 523–532.

[25] Cebula A1, Seweryn M, Rempala GA, Pabla SS, McIndoe RA, Denning TL, Bry L, Kraj P, Kisielow P, Ignatowicz L, Thymus-derived regulatory T cells contribute to tolerance to commensal microbiota; Nature. 2013 May 9;497(7448):258-62.

[26] Waite JC1, Skokos D, Th17 response and inflammatory autoimmune diseases; Int J Inflam. 2012;2012:819467. Epub 2011 Nov 15.

[27] Bedoya SK, Lam B, Lau K, Larkin J 3rd, Th17 cells in immunity and autoimmunity; Clin Dev Immunol. 2013;2013:986789. doi: 10.1155/2013/986789. Epub 2013 Dec 26.

[28] Han L, Yang J, Wang X, Li D, Lv L, Li B; Th17 cells in autoimmune diseases; Front Med. 2015 Mar;9(1):10-9.

[29] Li D1, Cai W, Gu R, Zhang Y, Zhang H, Tang K, Xu P, Katirai F, Shi W, Wang L, Huang T, Huang B; Th17 cell plays a role in the pathogenesis of Hashimoto's thyroiditis in patients; Clin Immunol. 2013 Dec;149(3):411-20.

[30] Liu Y, Tang X, Tian J, Zhu C, Peng H, Rui K, Wang Y, Mao C, Ma J, Lu L, Xu H, Wang S; Th17/Treg cells imbalance and GITRL profile in patients with Hashimoto's thyroiditis; Int J Mol Sci. 2014 Nov 25;15(12):21674-86.

[31] Dayanne da Silva Borges Betiati, Paula Fernanda de Oliveira, Carolina de Quadros Camargo, Everson Araújo Nunes, and Erasmo Benício Santos de Moraes Trindade; Effects of omega-3 fatty acids on regulatory T cells in hematologic neoplasms; Rev Bras Hematol Hemoter. 2013; 35(2): 119-125.

[32] Issazadeh-Navikas S, Teimer R, Bockermann R., Influence of dietary components on regulatory T cells; Mol Med. 2012 Feb 10;18:95-110.

[33] Zhao HM1, Huang XY, Zuo ZQ, Pan QH, Ao MY, Zhou F, Liu HN, Liu ZY, Liu DY, Probiotics increase T regulatory cells and reduce severity of experimental colitis in mice; World J Gastroenterol. 2013 Feb 7;19(5):742-9.

[34] Smits HH, Engering A, van der Kleij D, de Jong EC, Schipper K, van Capel TM, Zaat BA, Yazdanbakhsh M, Wierenga EA, van Kooyk Y, Kapsenberg ML, Selective probiotic bacteria induce IL-10-producing regulatory T cells in vitro by modulating dendritic cell function through dendritic cell-specific intercellular adhesion molecule 3-grabbing nonintegrin; J Allergy Clin Immunol. 2005 Jun;115(6):1260-7.

[35] Kim CH, Regulation of FoxP3 regulatory T cells and Th17 cells by retinoids; Clin Dev Immunol. 2008;2008:416910.

[36] Kozela E, Juknat A, Kaushansky N, Rimmerman N, Ben-Nun A, Vogel Z, Cannabinoids decrease the th17 inflammatory autoimmune phenotype; J Neuroimmune Pharmacol. 2013 Dec;8(5):1265-76.

[37] Galland, Leo; Textbook of Functional Medicine; Chapter 8: Patient-centered Care: Antecedents, Triggers, and Mediators; Page 82

[38] Sung Hee Lee, Intestinal Permeability Regulation by Tight Junction: Implication on Inflammatory Bowel Diseases; Intest Res. 2015 Jan; 13(1): 11–18.

[39] Jeroen Visser,a Jan Rozing,a Anna Sapone,b Karen Lammers,b and Alessio Fasano, Tight Junctions, Intestinal Permeability, and Autoimmunity Celiac Disease and Type 1 Diabetes Paradigms; Ann N Y Acad Sci. 2009 May; 1165: 195–205.

[40] Justin Hollon,,* Elaine Leonard Puppa, Bruce Greenwald, Eric Goldberg, Anthony Guerrerio, and Alessio Fasano, Effect of Gliadin on Permeability of Intestinal Biopsy Explants from Celiac Disease Patients and Patients with Non-Celiac Gluten Sensitivity; Nutrients. 2015 Mar; 7(3): 1565–1576 Published online 2015 Feb 27.

[41] Mingming Zhang, Qian Zhou, Robert G. Dorfman, Xiaoli Huang, Tingting Fan, Hao Zhang, Jun Zhang,corresponding author and Chenggong Yu, Butyrate inhibits interleukin-17 and generates Tregs to ameliorate colorectal colitis in rats; BMC Gastroenterol. 2016; 16: 84. Published online 2016 Jul 30.

[42] Jeongho Park, Myunghoo Kim, Seung G. Kang, Amber Hopf Jannasch, Bruce Cooper, John Patterson, and Chang H. Kim, Short chain fatty acids induce both effector and regulatory T cells by suppression of histone deacetylases and regulation of the mTOR-S6K pathway; Mucosal Immunol. 2015 Jan; 8(1): 80–93.

[43] John R. Kelly, Paul J. Kennedy, John F. Cryan, Timothy G. Dinan, Gerard Clarke,* and Niall P. Hyland, Breaking down the barriers: the gut microbiome, intestinal permeability and stress-related psychiatric disorders; Front Cell Neurosci. 2015; 9: 392.

[44] Monica Vera-Lise Tulstrup, Ellen Gerd Christensen, Vera Carvalho, Caroline Linninge, Siv Ahrné, Ole Højberg, Tine Rask Licht, and Martin Iain Bahl, Antibiotic Treatment Affects Intestinal Permeability and Gut Microbial Composition in Wistar Rats Dependent on Antibiotic Class; PLoS One. 2015; 10(12): e0144854.

[45] G Sigthorsson, J Tibble, J Hayllar, I Menzies, A Macpherson, R Moots, D Scott, M Gumpel, and I Bjarnason, Intestinal permeability and inflammation in patients on NSAIDs; Gut. 1998 Oct; 43(4): 506–511.

[46] Wang Y, Tong J, Chang B, Wang B, Zhang D, Wang B, Effects of alcohol on intestinal epithelial barrier permeability and expression of tight junction-associated proteins; Mol Med Rep. 2014 Jun;9(6):2352-6.

[47] Stephan C Bischoff,corresponding author Giovanni Barbara, Wim Buurman, Theo Ockhuizen, Jörg-Dieter Schulzke, Matteo Serino, Herbert Tilg, Alastair Watson, and Jerry M Wells, Intestinal permeability—a new target for disease prevention and therapy; BMC Gastroenterol. 2014; 14: 189. Published online 2014 Nov 18.

[48] Hurley JC, Endotoxemia: methods of detection and clinical correlates; Clin Microbiol Rev. 1995 Apr;8(2):268-92.

[49] Rossol M, Heine H, Meusch U, Quandt D, Klein C, Sweet MJ, Hauschildt S, LPS-induced cytokine production in human monocytes and macrophages; Crit Rev Immunol. 2011;31(5):379-446.

[50] Guo S, Al-Sadi R, Said HM, Ma TY, Lipopolysaccharide causes an increase in intestinal tight junction permeability in vitro and in vivo by inducing enterocyte membrane expression and localization of TLR-4 and CD14; Am J Pathol. 2013 Feb;182(2):375-87.

[51] Guo S, Nighot M, Al-Sadi R, Alhmoud T, Nighot P, Ma TY, Lipopolysaccharide Regulation of Intestinal Tight Junction Permeability Is Mediated by TLR4 Signal Transduction Pathway Activation of FAK and MyD88; J Immunol. 2015 Nov 15;195(10):4999-5010.

[52] Alessio Fasano, Zonulin, regulation of tight junctions, and autoimmune diseases; Ann N Y Acad Sci. 2012 Jul; 1258(1): 25–33.

[53] Andrew B. Shreiner, John Y. Kao, and Vincent B. Young, The gut microbiome in health and in disease; Curr Opin Gastroenterol. 2015 Jan; 31(1): 69–75.

[54] Scott T. Weiss, M.D, Eat Dirt — The Hygiene Hypothesis and Allergic Diseases; N Engl J Med 2002; 347:930-931September 19, 2002DOI: 10.1056/NEJMe020092

[55] SF Bloomfield,* R Stanwell-Smith,† RWR Crevel,‡ and J Pickup, Too clean, or not too clean: the Hygiene Hypothesis and home hygiene; Clin Exp Allergy. 2006 Apr; 36(4): 402–425.

[56] Amy M. Romano, MSN, CNM, Research Summaries for Normal Birth; J Perinat Educ. 2005 Spring; 14(2): 52–55.

[57] Josef Neu, MDa,b,a,b and Jona Rushing, MD, Cesarean versus Vaginal Delivery: Long term infant outcomes and the Hygiene Hypothesis; Clin Perinatol. 2011 Jun; 38(2): 321–331.

[58] Vaccines & Immunizations; http://www.cdc.gov/vaccines/vac-gen/additives.htm

[59] Fang JL, Stingley RL, Beland FA, Harrouk W, Lumpkins DL, Howard P, Occurrence, efficacy, metabolism, and toxicity of triclosan; J Environ Sci Health C Environ Carcinog Ecotoxicol Rev. 2010 Jul;28(3):147-71.

[60] Dann AB1, Hontela A, Triclosan: environmental exposure, toxicity and mechanisms of action; J Appl Toxicol. 2011 May;31(4):285-311.

[61] Yazdankhah SP, Scheie AA, Høiby EA, Lunestad BT, Heir E, Fotland TØ, Naterstad K, Kruse H, Triclosan and antimicrobial resistance in bacteria: an overview; Microb Drug Resist. 2006 Summer;12(2):83-90.

[62] Suller MT, Russell AD, Triclosan and antibiotic resistance in Staphylococcus aureus; J Antimicrob Chemother. 2000 Jul;46(1):11-8.

[63] Wang CF, Tian Y, Reproductive endocrine-disrupting effects of triclosan: Population exposure, present evidence and potential mechanisms; Environ Pollut. 2015 Nov;206:195-201.

[64] Stoker TE, Gibson EK, Zorrilla LM, Triclosan exposure modulates estrogen-dependent responses in the female wistar rat; Toxicol Sci. 2010 Sep;117(1):45-53.

[65] Rodríguez PE, Sanchez MS, Maternal exposure to triclosan impairs thyroid homeostasis and female pubertal development in Wistar rat offspring; J Toxicol Environ Health A. 2010;73(24):1678-88.

[66] Cullinan MP, Palmer JE, Carle AD, West MJ, Seymour GJ, Long term use of triclosan toothpaste and thyroid function; Sci Total Environ. 2012 Feb 1;416:75-9.

[67] Trombelli L, Farina R, Efficacy of triclosan-based toothpastes in the prevention and treatment of plaque-induced periodontal and peri-implant diseases; Minerva Stomatol. 2013 Mar;62(3):71-88.

[68] Lee HR, Hwang KA, Nam KH, Kim HC, Choi KC, Progression of breast cancer cells was enhanced by endocrine-disrupting chemicals, triclosan and octylphenol, via an estrogen receptor-dependent signaling pathway in cellular and mouse xenograft models; Chem Res Toxicol. 2014 May 19;27(5):834-42.

[69] Kim SH, Hwang KA, Shim SM, Choi KC, Growth and migration of LNCaP prostate cancer cells are promoted by triclosan and benzophenone-1 via an androgen receptor signaling pathway; Environ Toxicol Pharmacol. 2015 Mar;39(2):568-76.

[70] Yueh MF, Taniguchi K, Chen S, Evans RM, Hammock BD, Karin M, Tukey RH, The commonly used antimicrobial additive triclosan is a liver tumor promoter; Proc Natl Acad Sci U S A. 2014 Dec 2;111(48):17200-5.

[71] Teplova VV, Belosludtsev KN, Kruglov AG, Mechanism of triclosan toxicity: Mitochondrial dysfunction including complex II inhibition, superoxide release and uncoupling of oxidative phosphorylation; Toxicol Lett. 2017 Jun 5;275:108-117.

[72] Polly Soo Xi Yap, Beow Chin Yiap, Hu Cai Ping, and Swee Hua Erin Lim, Essential Oils, A New Horizon in Combating Bacterial Antibiotic Resistance; Open Microbiol J. 2014; 8: 6–14.

[73] Gnatta JR, Pinto FM, Bruna CQ, Souza RQ, Graziano KU, Silva MJ, Comparison of hand hygiene antimicrobial efficacy: Melaleuca alternifolia essential oil versus triclosan; Rev Lat Am Enfermagem. 2013 Nov-Dec;21(6):1212-9.

[74] Päivi M. Salo, PhD and Darryl C. Zeldin, MD, Does exposure to cats and dogs decrease the risk of developing allergic sensitization and disease?; J Allergy Clin Immunol. 2009 Oct; 124(4): 751–752.

[75] Dharmage SC, Lodge CL, Matheson MC, Campbell B, Lowe AJ, Exposure to cats: update on risks for sensitization and allergic diseases; Curr Allergy Asthma Rep. 2012 Oct;12(5):413-23.

[76] Rick M. Maizels, PhDa,* and Henry J. McSorley, PhDb, Regulation of the host immune system by helminth parasites; J Allergy Clin Immunol. 2016 Sep; 138(3): 666–675.

[77] Hotez PJ, Brindley PJ, Bethony JM, King CH, Pearce EJ, Jacobson J, Helminth infections: the great neglected tropical diseases; J Clin Invest. 2008 Apr;118(4):1311-21.

[78] Maizels RM, McSorley HJ, Smyth DJ, Helminths in the hygiene hypothesis: sooner or later?; Clin Exp Immunol. 2014 Jul;177(1):38-46.

[79] McSorley HJ, Maizels RM, Helminth infections and host immune regulation; Clin Microbiol Rev. 2012 Oct;25(4):585-608.

[80] Lee SC, Tang MS, Lim YA, Choy SH, Kurtz ZD, Cox LM, Gundra UM, Cho I, Bonneau R, Blaser MJ, Chua KH, Loke P, Helminth colonization is associated with increased diversity of the gut microbiota; PLoS Negl Trop Dis. 2014 May 22;8(5):e2880.

[81] Weinstock JV1, Elliott DE, Translatability of helminth therapy in inflammatory bowel diseases; Int J Parasitol. 2013 Mar;43(3-4):245-51.

[82] McSorley HJ, Gaze S, Daveson J, Jones D, Anderson RP, Clouston A, Ruyssers NE, Speare R, McCarthy JS, Engwerda CR, Croese J, Loukas A; Suppression of

inflammatory immune responses in celiac disease by experimental hookworm infection; PLoS One. 2011;6(9):e24092.

[83] Fleming JO, Helminth therapy and multiple sclerosis; Int J Parasitol. 2013 Mar;43(3-4):259-74.

SECTION TWO

[1] George Janssen, Chantal Christis, Yvonne Kooy-Winkelaar, Luppo Edens, Drew Smith, Peter van Veelen, and Frits Koning; Ineffective Degradation of Immunogenic Gluten Epitopes by Currently Available Digestive Enzyme Supplements; PLoS One. 2015; 10(6): e0128065

[2] Hollon J, Puppa EL, Greenwald B, Goldberg E, Guerrerio A, Fasano A; Effect of gliadin on permeability of intestinal biopsy explants from celiac disease patients and patients with non-celiac gluten sensitivity; Nutrients. 2015 Feb 27;7(3):1565-76.

[3] Granzotto M, dal Bo S, Quaglia S, Tommasini A, Piscianz E, Valencic E, Ferrara F, Martelossi S, Ventura A, Not T; Regulatory T-cell function is impaired in celiac disease; Dig Dis Sci. 2009 Jul;54(7):1513-9.

[4] Shohreh Issazadeh-Navikas, Roman Teimer, and Robert Bockermann; Influence of Dietary Components on Regulatory T Cells; Mol Med. 2012; 18(1): 95–110.

[5] http://www.fda.gov/NewsEvents/Newsroom/PressAnnouncements/ucm265838.htm

[6] Di Cagno R, Barbato M, Di Camillo C, Rizzello CG, De Angelis M, Giuliani G, De Vincenzi M, Gobbetti M, Cucchiara S; Gluten-free sourdough wheat baked goods appear safe for young celiac patients: a pilot study; J Pediatr Gastroenterol Nutr. 2010 Dec;51(6):777-83.

[7] Di Cagno R, De Angelis M, Auricchio S, Greco L, Clarke C, De Vincenzi M, Giovannini C, D'Archivio M, Landolfo F, Parrilli G, Minervini F, Arendt E, Gobbetti M; Sourdough bread made from wheat and nontoxic flours and started with selected lactobacilli is tolerated in celiac sprue patients; Appl Environ Microbiol. 2004 Feb;70(2):1088-96

[8] Niklas Engström, Ann-Sofie Sandberg, and Nathalie Scheers; Sourdough Fermentation of Wheat Flour does not Prevent the Interaction of Transglutaminase 2 with alpha2-Gliadin or Gluten; Nutrients. 2015 Apr; 7(4): 2134–2144

[9] Valentino R, Savastano S, Tommaselli AP, Dorato M, Scarpitta MT, Gigante M, Micillo M, Paparo F, Petrone E, Lombardi G, Troncone R; Prevalence of coeliac disease in patients with thyroid autoimmunity; Horm Res. 1999;51(3):124-7

[10] Metso S, Hyytiä-Ilmonen H, Kaukinen K, Huhtala H, Jaatinen P, Salmi J, Taurio J, Collin P; Gluten-free diet and autoimmune thyroiditis in patients with celiac disease. A prospective controlled study; Scand J Gastroenterol. 2012 Jan;47(1):43-8.

[11] Valentino R, Savastano S, Maglio M, Paparo F, Ferrara F, Dorato M, Lombardi G, Troncone R; Markers of potential coeliac disease in patients with Hashimoto's thyroiditis; Eur J Endocrinol. 2002 Apr;146(4):479-83

[12] Collins D, Wilcox R, Nathan M, Zubarik R; Celiac disease and hypothyroidism; Am J Med. 2012 Mar;125(3):278-82.

[13] Ansaldi N, Palmas T, Corrias A, Barbato M, D'Altiglia MR, Campanozzi A, Baldassarre M, Rea F, Pluvio R, Bonamico M, Lazzari R, Corrao G; Autoimmune thyroid disease and celiac disease in children; J Pediatr Gastroenterol Nutr. 2003 Jul;37(1):63-6

[14] van der Pals M, Ivarsson A, Norström F, Högberg L, Svensson J, Carlsson A; Prevalence of thyroid autoimmunity in children with celiac disease compared to healthy 12-year olds; Autoimmune Dis. 2014;2014:417356.

[15] Di Sabatino A, Vanoli A, Giuffrida P, Luinetti O, Solcia E, Corazza GR; The function of tissue transglutaminase in celiac disease; Autoimmun Rev. 2012 Aug;11(10):746-53.

[16] Martin W James, Brian B Scott; Endomysial antibody in the diagnosis and management of coeliac disease; Postgraduate Medical Journal Volume 76, Issue 898

[17] Kaukinen K, Partanen J, Mäki M, Collin P; HLA-DQ typing in the diagnosis of celiac disease; Am J Gastroenterol. 2002 Mar;97(3):695-9

[18] Tursi A, Giorgetti G, Brandimarte G, Rubino E, Lombardi D, Gasbarrini G; Prevalence and clinical presentation of subclinical/silent celiac disease in adults: an analysis on a 12-year observation; Hepatogastroenterology. 2001 Mar-Apr;48(38):462-4

[19] Verkasalo MA, Raitakari OT, Viikari J, Marniemi J, Savilahti E; Undiagnosed silent coeliac disease: a risk for underachievement?; Scand J Gastroenterol. 2005 Dec;40(12):1407-12

[20] Carlo Catassi, Julio C. Bai, Bruno Bonaz, Gerd Bouma, Antonio Calabrò, Antonio Carroccio, Gemma Castillejo, Carolina Ciacci, Fernanda Cristofori, Jernej Dolinsek, Ruggiero Francavilla, Luca Elli, Peter Green, Wolfgang Holtmeier, Peter Koehler, Sibylle Koletzko, Christof Meinhold, David Sanders, Michael Schumann, Detlef Schuppan, Reiner Ullrich, Andreas Vécsei, Umberto Volta, Victor Zevallos, Anna Sapone, and Alessio Fasano; Non-Celiac Gluten Sensitivity: The New Frontier of Gluten Related Disorders; Nutrients. 2013 Oct; 5(10): 3839–3853

[21] https://www.ncbi.nlm.nih.gov/gene/7052

[22] http://www.ncbi.nlm.nih.gov/gene/7053

[23] Thomas H, Beck K, Adamczyk M, Aeschlimann P, Langley M, Oita RC, Thiebach L, Hils M, Aeschlimann D; Transglutaminase 6: a protein associated with central nervous system development and motor function; Amino Acids. 2013 Jan;44(1):161-77.

[24] Tate PL, Bibb R, Larcom LL; Milk stimulates growth of prostate cancer cells in culture; Nutr Cancer. 2011 Nov;63(8):1361-6. doi: 10.1080/01635581.2011.609306. Epub 2011 Nov 1

[25] Macdonald LE, Brett J, Kelton D, Majowicz SE, Snedeker K, Sargeant JM; A systematic review and meta-analysis of the effects of pasteurization on milk vitamins, and evidence for raw milk consumption and other health-related outcomes; J Food Prot. 2011 Nov;74(11):1814-32.

[26] Pape-Zambito DA, Roberts RF, Kensinger RS; Estrone and 17beta-estradiol concentrations in pasteurized-homogenized milk and commercial dairy products; J Dairy Sci. 2010 Jun;93(6):2533-40.

[27] Michalski MC; On the supposed influence of milk homogenization on the risk of CVD, diabetes and allergy; Br J Nutr. 2007 Apr;97(4):598-610

[28] https://www.cambridge.org/core/product/identifier/S0007114507657900/type/ JOURNAL_ARTICLE

[29] Melnik B; Dietary intervention in acne: Attenuation of increased mTORC1 signaling promoted by Western diet; Dermatoendocrinol. 2012 Jan 1;4(1):20-32.

[30] Melnik BC, Zouboulis CC; Potential role of FoxO and mTORC1 in the pathogenesis of Western diet-induced acne; Exp Dermatol. 2013 May;22(5):311-5.

[31] Melnik BC; Excessive Leucine-mTORC1-Signalling of Cow Milk-Based Infant Formula: The Missing Link to Understand Early Childhood Obesity; J Obes. 2012;2012:197653.

[32] Arnberg K, Mølgaard C, Michaelsen KF, Jensen SM, Trolle E, Larnkjær A; Skim milk, whey, and casein increase body weight and whey and casein increase the plasma C-peptide concentration in overweight adolescents; J Nutr. 2012 Dec;142(12):2083-90.

[33] Melnik BC; Leucine signaling in the pathogenesis of type 2 diabetes and obesity; World J Diabetes. 2012 Mar 15;3(3):38-53. doi: 10.4239/wjd.v3.i3.38.

[34] Pópulo H, Lopes JM, Soares P; The mTOR signalling pathway in human cancer; Int J Mol Sci. 2012;13(2):1886-918.

[35] Hsieh AC, Liu Y, Edlind MP, Ingolia NT, Janes MR, Sher A, Shi EY, Stumpf CR, Christensen C, Bonham MJ, Wang S, Ren P, Martin M, Jessen K, Feldman ME, Weissman JS, Shokat KM, Rommel C, Ruggero D; The translational landscape of mTOR signalling steers cancer initiation and metastasis; Nature. 2012 Feb 22;485(7396):55-61.

[36] Bodo C Melnik, Swen Malte John, Pedro Carrera-Bastos and Loren Cord; The impact of cow's milk-mediated mTORC1-signaling in the initiation and progression of prostate cancer; Nutrition & Metabolism20129:74

[37] Kaminski S, Cieslinska A, Kostyra E; Polymorphism of bovine beta-casein and its potential effect on human health; J Appl Genet. 2007;48(3):189-98

[38] Hsueh-Chung Kao, R.T. Conner, H.C. Sherman; THE AVAILABILITY OF CALCIUM FROM CHINESE CABBAGE; March 1, 1938 The Journal of Biological Chemistry 123, 221-228

[39] Juan P. Ortiz-Sánchez, Francisco Cabrera-Chávez, and Ana M. Calderón de la Barca1; Maize Prolamins Could Induce a Gluten-Like Cellular Immune Response in Some Celiac Disease Patients; Nutrients. 2013 Oct; 5(10): 4174–4183.

[40] Doerge DR, Sheehan DM; Goitrogenic and estrogenic activity of soy isoflavones; Environ Health Perspect. 2002 Jun;110 Suppl 3:349-53.

[41] Divi RL, Chang HC, Doerge DR; Anti-thyroid isoflavones from soybean: isolation, characterization, and mechanisms of action; Biochem Pharmacol. 1997 Nov 15;54(10):1087-96.

[42] Hampl R, Ostatnikova D, Celec P, Putz Z, Lapcík O, Matucha P; Short-term effect of soy consumption on thyroid hormone levels and correlation with phytoestrogen level in healthy subjects; Endocr Regul. 2008 Jun;42(2-3):53-61

[43] Sathyapalan T, Manuchehri AM, Thatcher NJ, Rigby AS, Chapman T, Kilpatrick ES, Atkin SL; The effect of soy phytoestrogen supplementation on thyroid status and cardiovascular risk markers in patients with subclinical hypothyroidism: a randomized, double-blind, crossover study; J Clin Endocrinol Metab. 2011 May;96(5):1442-9.

[44] Hurrell RF, Juillerat MA, Reddy MB, Lynch SR, Dassenko SA, Cook JD; Soy protein, phytate, and iron absorption in humans; Am J Clin Nutr. 1992 Sep;56(3):573-8.

[45] Heaney RP, Weaver CM, Fitzsimmons ML; Soybean phytate content: effect on calcium absorption; Am J Clin Nutr. 1991 Mar;53(3):745-7.

[46] Pam Tangvoranuntakul,* Pascal Gagneux,* Sandra Diaz,* Muriel Bardor,* Nissi Varki,* Ajit Varki,*† and Elaine Muchmore; Human uptake and incorporation of an immunogenic nonhuman dietary sialic acid; Proc Natl Acad Sci U S A. 2003 Oct 14; 100(21): 12045–12050.

[47] Samraj AN, Pearce OM, Läubli H, Crittenden AN, Bergfeld AK, Banda K, Gregg CJ, Bingman AE, Secrest P, Diaz SL, Varki NM, Varki A; A red meat-derived glycan promotes inflammation and cancer progression; Proc Natl Acad Sci U S A. 2015 Jan 13;112(2):542-7.

[48] Eleftheriou P, Kynigopoulos S, Giovou A, Mazmanidi A, Yovos J, Skepastianos P, Vagdatli E, Petrou C, Papara D, Efterpiou M; Prevalence of anti-Neu5Gc antibodies in patients with hypothyroidism; Biomed Res Int. 2014;2014:963230.

[49] Ponnampalam EN, Mann NJ, Sinclair AJ; Effect of feeding systems on omega-3 fatty acids, conjugated linoleic acid and trans fatty acids in Australian beef cuts: potential impact on human health; Asia Pac J Clin Nutr. 2006;15(1):21-9.

[50] Daley CA, Abbott A, Doyle PS, Nader GA, Larson S; A review of fatty acid profiles and antioxidant content in grass-fed and grain-fed beef; Nutr J. 2010 Mar 10;9:10.

[51] Bjorklund EA, Heins BJ, Dicostanzo A, Chester-Jones H; Fatty acid profiles, meat quality, and sensory attributes of organic versus conventional dairy beef steers; J Dairy Sci. 2014 Mar;97(3):1828-34.

[52] McAfee AJ, McSorley EM, Cuskelly GJ, Fearon AM, Moss BW, Beattie JA, Wallace JM, Bonham MP, Strain JJ; Red meat from animals offered a grass diet increases plasma and platelet n-3 PUFA in healthy consumers; Br J Nutr. 2011 Jan;105(1):80-9.

[53] Suez J, Korem T, Zeevi D, Zilberman-Schapira G, Thaiss CA, Maza O, Israeli D, Zmora N, Gilad S, Weinberger A, Kuperman Y, Harmelin A, Kolodkin-Gal I, Shapiro H, Halpern Z, Segal E, Elinav E; Artificial sweeteners induce glucose intolerance by altering the gut microbiota; Nature. 2014 Oct 9;514(7521):181-6.

[54] Jotham Suez, Tal Korem, Gili Zilberman-Schapira, Eran Segal, and Eran Elinav; Non-caloric artificial sweeteners and the microbiome: findings and challenges; Gut Microbes. 2015; 6(2): 149–155.

[55] Xiaoming Bian, Liang Chi, Bei Gao, Pengcheng Tu, Hongyu Ru, and Kun Lu; The artificial sweetener acesulfame potassium affects the gut microbiome and body weight gain in CD-1 mice; PLoS One. 2017; 12(6): e0178426.

56 Xiaoming Bian, Liang Chi, Bei Gao, Pengcheng Tu, Hongyu Ru, and Kun Lu; The artificial sweetener acesulfame potassium affects the gut microbiome and body weight gain in CD-1 mice; PLoS One. 2017; 12(6): e0178426.

57 Yingfeng Wei, Chong Lu, Jianing Chen, Guangying Cui, Lin Wang, Tianming Yu, Yue Yang, Wei Wu, Yulong Ding, Lanjuan Li, Toshimitsu Uede, Zhi Chen, and Hongyan Diao; High salt diet stimulates gut Th17 response and exacerbates TNBS-induced colitis in mice; Oncotarget. 2017 Jan 3; 8(1): 70–82.

58 Markus Kleinewietfeld Arndt Manzel, Jens Titze, Heda Kvakan, Nir Yosef, Ralf A. Linker, Dominik N. Muller, and David A. Hafler; Sodium Chloride Drives Autoimmune Disease by the Induction of Pathogenic Th17 Cells; Nature. 2013 Apr 25; 496(7446): 518–522.

59 Chen GQ, Chen YY, Wang XS, Wu SZ, Yang HM, Xu HQ, He JC, Wang XT, Chen JF, Zheng RY; Chronic caffeine treatment attenuates experimental autoimmune encephalomyelitis induced by guinea pig spinal cord homogenates in Wistar rats; Brain Res. 2010 Jan 14;1309:116-25.

60 Amy Yang, Abraham A. Palmer, and Harriet de Witcorresponding author; Genetics of caffeine consumption and responses to caffeine; Psychopharmacology (Berl). 2010 Aug; 211(3): 245–257.

61 Palatini P, Benetti E, Mos L, Garavelli G, Mazzer A, Cozzio S, Fania C, Casiglia E; Association of coffee consumption and CYP1A2 polymorphism with risk of impaired fasting glucose in hypertensive patients; Eur J Epidemiol. 2015 Mar;30(3):209-17.

62 Cornelis MC, El-Sohemy A, Kabagambe EK, Campos H; Coffee, CYP1A2 genotype, and risk of myocardial infarction; JAMA. 2006 Mar 8;295(10):1135-41.

63 Sicherer SH, Sampson HA; Food allergy: recent advances in pathophysiology and treatment; Annu Rev Med. 2009;60:261-77.

64 Bauer ME; Stress, glucocorticoids and ageing of the immune system; Stress. 2005 Mar;8(1):69-83.

65 Rehman Q, Lane NE; Effect of glucocorticoids on bone density; Med Pediatr Oncol. 2003 Sep;41(3):212-6.

66 Ferris HA, Kahn CR; New mechanisms of glucocorticoid-induced insulin resistance: make no bones about it; J Clin Invest. 2012 Nov;122(11):3854-7.

67 Masuzaki H, Yamamoto H, Kenyon CJ, Elmquist JK, Morton NM, Paterson JM, Shinyama H, Sharp MG, Fleming S, Mullins JJ, Seckl JR, Flier JS; Transgenic amplification of glucocorticoid action in adipose tissue causes high blood pressure in mice; J Clin Invest. 2003 Jul;112(1):83-90.

68 Heyma P, Larkins RG; Glucocorticoids decrease in conversion of thyroxine into 3, 5, 3'-tri-iodothyronine by isolated rat renal tubules; Clin Sci (Lond). 1982 Feb;62(2):215-20.

69 Golshiri P, Pourabdian S, Najimi A, Zadeh HM, Hasheminia J; Job stress and its relationship with the level of secretory IgA in saliva: a comparison between nurses working in emergency wards and hospital clerks; J Pak Med Assoc. 2012 Mar;62(3 Suppl 2):S26-30.

[70] Satoshi Tsujita, Kanehisa Morimoto; Secretory IgA in saliva can be a useful stress marker; Environ Health Prev Med. 1999 Apr; 4(1): 1–8.

[71] Firdaus S. Dhabhar; Enhancing versus Suppressive Effects of Stress on Immune Function: Implications for Immunoprotection and Immunopathology; Neuroimmunomodulation. 2009 Jun; 16(5): 300–317.

[72] Phillips AC, Carroll D, Evans P, Bosch JA, Clow A, Hucklebridge F, Der G; Stressful life events are associated with low secretion rates of immunoglobulin A in saliva in the middle aged and elderly; Brain Behav Immun. 2006 Mar;20(2):191-7. Epub 2005 Aug 1

[73] Radosavljevic VR, Jankovic SM, Marinkovic JM; Stressful life events in the pathogenesis of Graves' disease; Eur J Endocrinol. 1996 Jun;134(6):699-701

[74] Mizokami T, Wu Li A, El-Kaissi S, Wall JR; Stress and thyroid autoimmunity; Thyroid. 2004 Dec;14(12):1047-55

[75] Harris T, Creed F, Brugha TS; Stressful life events and Graves' disease; Br J Psychiatry. 1992 Oct;161:535-41

[76] Tsatsoulis A; The role of stress in the clinical expression of thyroid autoimmunity; Ann N Y Acad Sci. 2006 Nov;1088:382-95.

[77] Blaise Corthésy; Multi-Faceted Functions of Secretory IgA at Mucosal Surfaces; Front Immunol. 2013; 4: 185.

[78] Nicholas J. Mantis, PhD, Nicolas Rol, MSc, and Blaise Corthésy, PhD; Secretory IgA's Complex Roles in Immunity and Mucosal Homeostasis in the Gut; Mucosal Immunol. 2011 Nov; 4(6): 603–611.

[79] Mizokami T, Wu Li A, El-Kaissi S, Wall JR; Stress and thyroid autoimmunity; Thyroid. 2004 Dec;14(12):1047-55.

[80] Olff M, Güzelcan Y, de Vries GJ, Assies J, Gersons BP; HPA- and HPT-axis alterations in chronic posttraumatic stress disorder; Psychoneuroendocrinology. 2006 Nov;31(10):1220-30. Epub 2006 Nov 1.

[81] Helmreich DL, Parfitt DB, Lu XY, Akil H, Watson SJ; Relation between the hypothalamic-pituitary-thyroid (HPT) axis and the hypothalamic-pituitary-adrenal (HPA) axis during repeated stress; Neuroendocrinology. 2005;81(3):183-92. Epub 2005 Jul 11.

[82] Mastorakos G, Pavlatou MG, Mizamtsidi M; The hypothalamic-pituitary-adrenal and the hypothalamic- pituitary-gonadal axes interplay; Pediatr Endocrinol Rev. 2006 Jan;3 Suppl 1:172-81.

[83] Rivier C, Rivest S; Effect of stress on the activity of the hypothalamic-pituitary-gonadal axis: peripheral and central mechanisms; Biol Reprod. 1991 Oct;45(4):523-32.

[84] Jones TH, Kennedy RL; Cytokines and hypothalamic-pituitary function; Cytokine. 1993 Nov;5(6):531-8.

[85] Dunn AJ; Cytokine activation of the HPA axis; Ann N Y Acad Sci. 2000;917:608-17.

[86] Turnbull AV, Rivier C; Regulation of the HPA axis by cytokines; Brain Behav Immun. 1995 Dec;9(4):253-75.

[87] Heesen C, Gold SM, Huitinga I, Reul JM; Stress and hypothalamic-pituitary-adrenal axis function in experimental autoimmune encephalomyelitis and multiple sclerosis—a review; Psychoneuroendocrinology. 2007 Jul;32(6):604-18. Epub 2007 Jun 29.

[88] Foster SC, Daniels C, Bourdette DN, Bebo BF Jr; Dysregulation of the hypothalamic-pituitary-gonadal axis in experimental autoimmune encephalomyelitis and multiple sclerosis; J Neuroimmunol. 2003 Jul;140(1-2):78-87.

[89] Heisler LK, Pronchuk N, Nonogaki K, Zhou L, Raber J, Tung L, Yeo GS, O'Rahilly S, Colmers WF, Elmquist JK, Tecott LH; Serotonin activates the hypothalamic-pituitary-adrenal axis via serotonin 2C receptor stimulation; J Neurosci. 2007 Jun 27;27(26):6956-64.

[90] Sorenson AN, Sullivan EC2, Mendoza SP2, Capitanio JP2, Higley JD; Serotonin transporter genotype modulates HPA axis output during stress: effect of stress, dexamethasone test and ACTH challenge; Transl Dev Psychiatry. 2013 Sep 9;1:21130.

[91] Szymanska M, Budziszewska B, Jaworska-Feil L, Basta-Kaim A, Kubera M, Leskiewicz M, Regulska M, Lason W; The effect of antidepressant drugs on the HPA axis activity, glucocorticoid receptor level and FKBP51 concentration in prenatally stressed rats; Psychoneuroendocrinology. 2009 Jul;34(6):822-32.

[92] Sullivan RM, Dufresne MM; Mesocortical dopamine and HPA axis regulation: role of laterality and early environment; Brain Res. 2006 Mar 3;1076(1):49-59. Epub 2006 Feb 17.

[93] de Oliveira AR, Reimer AE, Reis FM, Brandão ML; Conditioned fear response is modulated by a combined action of the hypothalamic-pituitary-adrenal axis and dopamine activity in the basolateral amygdala; Eur Neuropsychopharmacol. 2013 May;23(5):379-89.

[94] Cullinan WE, Ziegler DR, Herman JP; Functional role of local GABAergic influences on the HPA axis; Brain Struct Funct. 2008 Sep;213(1-2):63-72.

[95] Keivan Gohari Moghaddam, Negin Rashidi, Hamidreza Aghaei Meybodi,1 Nader Rezaie, Mahdi Montazeri, Ramin Heshmat,1 and Zohreh Annabestani; The effect of inhaled corticosteroids on hypothalamic-pituitary-adrenal axis; Indian J Pharmacol. 2012 May-Jun; 44(3): 314–318.

[96] Casale TB, Nelson HS, Stricker WE, Raff H, Newman KB; Suppression of hypothalamic-pituitary-adrenal axis activity with inhaled flunisolide and fluticasone propionate in adult asthma patients; Ann Allergy Asthma Immunol. 2001 Nov;87(5):379-85.

[97] Bryan R. Haugen, MD; DRUGS THAT SUPPRESS TSH OR CAUSE CENTRAL HYPOTHYROIDISM; Best Pract Res Clin Endocrinol Metab. 2009 Dec; 23(6): 793–800.

[98] Kondo K, Harbuz MS, Levy A, Lightman SL; Inhibition of the hypothalamic-pituitary-thyroid axis in response to lipopolysaccharide is independent of changes in circulating corticosteroids; Neuroimmunomodulation. 1997 Jul-Aug;4(4):188-94.

[99] Roger D. Stanworth, BMEDSCI,1,2 Dheeraj Kapoor, MD,1 Kevin S. Channer, MD,3 and T. Hugh Jones, MD; Statin Therapy Is Associated With Lower Total but Not

Bioavailable or Free Testosterone in Men With Type 2 Diabetes; Diabetes Care. 2009 Apr; 32(4): 541–546.

[100] Anam K, Amare M, Naik S, Szabo KA, Davis TA; Severe tissue trauma triggers the autoimmune state systemic lupus erythematosus in the MRL/++ lupus-prone mouse; Lupus. 2009 Apr;18(4):318-31.

[101] O'Donovan A, Cohen BE, Seal KH, Bertenthal D, Margaretten M, Nishimi K, Neylan TC; Elevated risk for autoimmune disorders in iraq and afghanistan veterans with posttraumatic stress disorder; Biol Psychiatry. 2015 Feb 15;77(4):365-74.

[102] Boscarino JA; Posttraumatic stress disorder and physical illness: results from clinical and epidemiologic studies; Ann N Y Acad Sci. 2004 Dec;1032:141-53.

[103] Mladen Jergovic, Kreso Bendelja, Andelko Vidovic, Ana Savic, Valerija Vojvoda, Neda Aberle, Sabina Rabatic, Tanja Jovanovic, and Ante Sabioncello; Patients with posttraumatic stress disorder exhibit an altered phenotype of regulatory T cells; Allergy Asthma Clin Immunol. 2014; 10(1): 43.

[104] Dube SR, Fairweather D, Pearson WS, Felitti VJ, Anda RF, Croft JB; Cumulative childhood stress and autoimmune diseases in adults; Psychosom Med. 2009 Feb;71(2):243-50

[105] Moog NK, Heim CM2, Entringer S3, Kathmann N4, Wadhwa PD5, Buss C6; Childhood maltreatment is associated with increased risk of subclinical hypothyroidism in pregnancy; Psychoneuroendocrinology. 2017 Oct;84:190-196.

[106] Mesnage R, Bernay B, Séralini GE; Ethoxylated adjuvants of glyphosate-based herbicides are active principles of human cell toxicity; Toxicology. 2013 Nov 16;313(2-3):122-8.

[107] Song M, Kim YJ, Park YK, Ryu JC; Changes in thyroid peroxidase activity in response to various chemicals; J Environ Monit. 2012 Aug;14(8):2121-6.

[108] Yamasaki K, Ishii S, Kikuno T, Minobe Y; Endocrine-mediated effects of two benzene related compounds, 1-chloro-4-(chloromethyl)benzene and 1,3-diethyl benzene, based on subacute oral toxicity studies using rats; Food Chem Toxicol. 2012 Aug;50(8):2635-42.

[109] Knox SS, Jackson T, Frisbee SJ, Javins B, Ducatman AM; Perfluorocarbon exposure, gender and thyroid function in the C8 Health Project; J Toxicol Sci. 2011 Aug;36(4):403-10.

[110] Yamasaki K, Ishii S, Kikuno T, Minobe Y; Endocrine-mediated effects of two benzene related compounds, 1-chloro-4-(chloromethyl)benzene and 1,3-diethyl benzene, based on subacute oral toxicity studies using rats; Food Chem Toxicol. 2012 Aug;50(8):2635-42.

[111] Koeppe ES, Ferguson KK, Colacino JA, Meeker JD; Relationship between urinary triclosan and paraben concentrations and serum thyroid measures in NHANES 2007-2008; Sci Total Environ. 2013 Feb 15;445-446:299-305.

[112] Goldner WS, Sandler DP, Yu F, Hoppin JA, Kamel F, Levan TD; Pesticide use and thyroid disease among women in the Agricultural Health Study; Am J Epidemiol. 2010 Feb 15;171(4):455-64.

[113] Rathore M1, Bhatnagar P, Mathur D, Saxena GN; Burden of organochlorine pesticides in blood and its effect on thyroid hormones in women; Sci Total Environ. 2002 Aug 5;295(1-3):207-15.

[114] Khan DA, Ahad K, Ansari WM, Khan H; Pesticide exposure and endocrine dysfunction in the cotton crop agricultural workers of southern Punjab, Pakistan; Asia Pac J Public Health. 2013 Mar;25(2):181-91.

[115] Duntas LH; Environmental factors and thyroid autoimmunity; Ann Endocrinol (Paris). 2011 Apr;72(2):108-13.

[116] Burek CL, Talor MV; Environmental triggers of autoimmune thyroiditis; J Autoimmun. 2009 Nov-Dec;33(3-4):183-9.

[117] Burek CL, Talor MV; Environmental triggers of autoimmune thyroiditis; J Autoimmun. 2009 Nov-Dec;33(3-4):183-9.

[118] Mitro SD, Johnson T2, Zota AR3; Cumulative Chemical Exposures During Pregnancy and Early Development; Curr Environ Health Rep. 2015 Dec;2(4):367-78.

[119] Konieczna A, Rutkowska A, Rachon D; Health risk of exposure to Bisphenol A (BPA); Rocz Panstw Zakl Hig. 2015;66(1):5-11.

[120] 120 La-or Chailurkit, Wichai Aekplakorn, and Boonsong Ongphiphadhanakul; The Association of Serum Bisphenol A with Thyroid Autoimmunity; Int J Environ Res Public Health. 2016 Nov; 13(11): 1153.

[121] Datis Kharrazian; The Potential Roles of Bisphenol A (BPA) Pathogenesis in Autoimmunity; Autoimmune Dis. 2014; 2014: 743616.

[122] Datis Kharrazian, Aristo Vojdani; Correlation between antibodies to bisphenol A, its target enzyme protein disulfide isomerase and antibodies to neuron-specific antigens; J Appl Toxicol. 2017 Apr; 37(4): 479–484.

[123] Carpenter DO; Polychlorinated biphenyls (PCBs): routes of exposure and effects on human health; Rev Environ Health. 2006 Jan-Mar;21(1):1-23.

[124] Langer P, Tajtáková M, Kocan A, Petrík J, Koska J, Ksinantová L, Rádiková Z, Ukropec J, Imrich R, Hucková M, Chovancová J, Drobná B, Jursa S, Vlcek M, Bergman A, Athanasiadou M, Hovander L, Shishiba Y, Trnovec T, Sebökova E, Klimes I; Thyroid ultrasound volume, structure and function after long-term high exposure of large population to polychlorinated biphenyls, pesticides and dioxin; Chemosphere. 2007 Aug;69(1):118-27. Epub 2007 May 29.

[125] Schell LM, Gallo MV, Ravenscroft J, DeCaprio AP; Persistent organic pollutants and anti-thyroid peroxidase levels in Akwesasne Mohawk young adults; Environ Res. 2009 Jan;109(1):86-92.

[126] Iglesias ML, Schmidt A2, Ghuzlan AA1, Lacroix L1, Vathaire F1,3, Chevillard S4, Schlumberger M; Radiation exposure and thyroid cancer: a review; Arch Endocrinol Metab. 2017 Mar-Apr;61(2):180-187.

[127] Jereczek-Fossa BA, Alterio D, Jassem J, Gibelli B, Tradati N, Orecchia R; Radiotherapy-induced thyroid disorders; Cancer Treat Rev. 2004 Jun;30(4):369-84.

[128] Hancock SL, Cox RS, McDougall IR; Thyroid diseases after treatment of Hodgkin's disease; N Engl J Med. 1991 Aug 29;325(9):599-605.

[129] Frederick W. Miller,corresponding authora Lars Alfredsson,b Karen H. Costenbader,c Diane L. Kamen,d Lorene Nelson,e Jill M. Norris,f and Anneclaire J. De Roos; Epidemiology of Environmental Exposures and Human Autoimmune Diseases: Findings from a National Institute of Environmental Health Sciences Expert Panel Workshop; J Autoimmun. 2012 Dec; 39(4): 259–271. Published online 2012 Jun 25.

[130] Kasatkina EP, Shilin DE, Rosenbloom AL, Pykov MI, Ibragimova GV, Sokolovskaya VN, Matkovskaya AN, Volkova TN, Odoud EA, Bronshtein MI, Poverenny AM, Mursankova NM; Effects of low level radiation from the Chernobyl accident in a population with iodine deficiency; Eur J Pediatr. 1997 Dec;156(12):916-20.

[131] Tronko MD, Brenner AV, Olijnyk VA, Robbins J, Epstein OV, McConnell RJ, Bogdanova TI, Fink DJ, Likhtarev IA, Lubin JH, Markov VV, Bouville AC, Terekhova GM, Zablotska LB, Shpak VM, Brill AB, Tereshchenko VP, Masnyk IJ, Ron E, Hatch M, Howe GR; Autoimmune thyroiditis and exposure to iodine 131 in the Ukrainian cohort study of thyroid cancer and other thyroid diseases after the Chornobyl accident: results from the first screening cycle (1998-2000); J Clin Endocrinol Metab. 2006 Nov;91(11):4344-51. Epub 2006 Aug 15.

[132] Fukata S, Kuma K, Sugawara M; Relationship between cigarette smoking and hypothyroidism in patients with Hashimoto's thyroiditis; J Endocrinol Invest. 1996 Oct;19(9):607-12.

[133] Vestergaard P, Rejnmark L, Weeke J, Hoeck HC, Nielsen HK, Rungby J, Laurberg P, Mosekilde L; Smoking as a risk factor for Graves' disease, toxic nodular goiter, and autoimmune hypothyroidism; Thyroid. 2002 Jan;12(1):69-75.

[134] Hegediüs L, Brix TH, Vestergaard P; Relationship between cigarette smoking and Graves' ophthalmopathy; J Endocrinol Invest. 2004 Mar;27(3):265-71.

[135] Katsoyiannis A, Leva P, Kotzias D; VOC and carbonyl emissions from carpets: a comparative study using four types of environmental chambers; J Hazard Mater. 2008 Apr 1;152(2):669-76. Epub 2007 Jul 25.

[136] Tunga Salthammer, Sibel Mentese,‡ and Rainer Marutzky; Formaldehyde in the Indoor Environment; Chem Rev. 2010 Apr 14; 110(4): 2536–2572.

[137] Katsoyiannis A, Leva P, Kotzias D; VOC and carbonyl emissions from carpets: a comparative study using four types of environmental chambers; J Hazard Mater. 2008 Apr 1;152(2):669-76. Epub 2007 Jul 25.

[138] Bahn AK, Mills JL, Snyder PJ, Gann PH, Houten L, Bialik O, Hollmann L, Utiger RD; Hypothyroidism in workers exposed to polybrominated biphenyls; N Engl J Med. 1980 Jan 3;302(1):31-3.

[139] C. Lynne Burek and Monica V. Talor; Environmental Triggers of Autoimmune Thyroiditis; J Autoimmun. 2009 Nov–Dec; 33(3-4): 183–189.

[140] Turyk ME, Persky VW, Imm P, Knobeloch L, Chatterton R, Anderson HA; Hormone disruption by PBDEs in adult male sport fish consumers; Environ Health Perspect. 2008 Dec;116(12):1635-41.

[141] Chen YP, Zheng YJ, Liu Q, Ellison AM, Zhao Y, Ma QY; PBDEs (polybrominated diphenyl ethers) pose a risk to captive giant pandas; Environ Pollut. 2017 Jul;226:174-181.

[142] Smith-Spangler C1, Brandeau ML, Hunter GE, Bavinger JC, Pearson M, Eschbach PJ, Sundaram V, Liu H, Schirmer P, Stave C, Olkin I, Bravata DM; Are organic foods safer or healthier than conventional alternatives?: a systematic review; Ann Intern Med. 2012 Sep 4;157(5):348-66.

[143] Wissem Mnif, Aziza Ibn Hadj Hassine, Aicha Bouaziz, Aghleb Bartegi, Olivier Thomas, and Benoit Roig; Effect of Endocrine Disruptor Pesticides: A Review; Int J Environ Res Public Health. 2011 Jun; 8(6): 2265–2303.

[144] Buranatrevedh S, Roy D; Occupational exposure to endocrine-disrupting pesticides and the potential for developing hormonal cancers; J Environ Health. 2001 Oct;64(3):17-29.

[145] Ejaz S, Akram W, Lim CW, Lee JJ, Hussain I; Endocrine disrupting pesticides: a leading cause of cancer among rural people in Pakistan; Exp Oncol. 2004 Jun;26(2):98-105.

[146] A M Soto, K L Chung, and C Sonnenschein; The pesticides endosulfan, toxaphene, and dieldrin have estrogenic effects on human estrogen-sensitive cells; Environ Health Perspect. 1994 Apr; 102(4): 380–383.

[147] Tamura H, Yoshikawa H, Gaido KW, Ross SM, DeLisle RK, Welsh WJ, Richard AM; Interaction of organophosphate pesticides and related compounds with the androgen receptor; Environ Health Perspect. 2003 Apr;111(4):545-52.

[148] Ricardo Persaud, George Garas, Sanjeev Silva, Constantine Stamatoglou, Paul Chatrath, and Kalpesh Patel; An evidence-based review of botulinum toxin (Botox) applications in non-cosmetic head and neck conditions; JRSM Short Rep. 2013 Feb; 4(2): 10.

[149] Gregoric E, Gregoric JA, Guarneri F, Benvenga S; Injections of Clostridium botulinum neurotoxin A may cause thyroid complications in predisposed persons based on molecular mimicry with thyroid autoantigens; Endocrine. 2011 Feb;39(1):41-7.

[150] http://www.environmentalhealthnews.org/ehs/newscience/2012/01/2012-0320-mercury-linked-thyroid-antibody

[151] Hybenova M, Hrda P, Procházková J, Stejskal V, Sterzl; The role of environmental factors in autoimmune thyroiditis; Neuro Endocrinol Lett. 2010;31(3):283-9.

[152] Drasch G, Schupp I, Höfl H, Reinke R, Roider G; Mercury burden of human fetal and infant tissues; Eur J Pediatr. 1994 Aug;153(8):607-10.

[153] Eggleston DW, Nylander M; Correlation of dental amalgam with mercury in brain tissue; J Prosthet Dent. 1987 Dec;58(6):704-7.

[154] Masahiro Kawahara,* and Midori Kato-Negishi; Link between Aluminum and the Pathogenesis of Alzheimer's Disease: The Integration of the Aluminum and Amyloid Cascade Hypotheses; Int J Alzheimers Dis. 2011; 2011: 276393.

[155] Ferreira PC, Piai Kde A, Takayanagui AM, Segura-Muñoz SI; Aluminum as a risk factor for Alzheimer's disease; Rev Lat Am Enfermagem. 2008 Jan-Feb;16(1):151-7.

[156] Tomljenovic L, Shaw CA; Do aluminum vaccine adjuvants contribute to the rising prevalence of autism?; J Inorg Biochem. 2011 Nov;105(11):1489-99.

[157] Tomljenovic L, Shaw CA; Mechanisms of aluminum adjuvant toxicity and autoimmunity in pediatric populations; Lupus. 2012 Feb;21(2):223-30.

[158] Tomljenovic L, Shaw CA; Mechanisms of aluminum adjuvant toxicity and autoimmunity in pediatric populations; Lupus. 2012 Feb;21(2):223-30.

[159] Vahter ME; Interactions between arsenic-induced toxicity and nutrition in early life; J Nutr. 2007 Dec;137(12):2798-804.

[160] Hojsak I, Braegger C, Bronsky J, Campoy C, Colomb V, Decsi T, Domellöf M, Fewtrell M, Mis NF, Mihatsch W, Molgaard C, van Goudoever J; Arsenic in rice: a cause for concern; J Pediatr Gastroenterol Nutr. 2015 Jan;60(1):142-5.

[161] Ciarrocca M, Tomei F, Caciari T, Cetica C, Andrè JC, Fiaschetti M, Schifano MP, Scala B, Scimitto L, Tomei G, Sancini A; Exposure to arsenic in urban and rural areas and effects on thyroid hormones; Inhal Toxicol. 2012 Aug;24(9):589-98.

[162] Jennifer C. Davey, Athena P. Nomikos, Manida Wungjiranirun, Jenna R. Sherman, Liam Ingram, Cavus Batki, Jean P. Lariviere, and Joshua W. Hamilton; Arsenic as an Endocrine Disruptor: Arsenic Disrupts Retinoic Acid Receptor–and Thyroid Hormone Receptor–Mediated Gene Regulation and Thyroid Hormone–Mediated Amphibian Tail Metamorphosis; Environ Health Perspect. 2008 Feb; 116(2): 165–172.

[163] Järup L; Cadmium overload and toxicity; Nephrol Dial Transplant. 2002;17 Suppl 2:35-9.

[164] Aimin Chen,corresponding author Stephani S. Kim, Ethan Chung, and Kim N. Dietrich; Thyroid Hormones in Relation to Lead, Mercury, and Cadmium Exposure in the National Health and Nutrition Examination Survey, 2007–2008; Environ Health Perspect. 2013 Feb; 121(2): 181–186.

[165] Hammouda F, Messaoudi I, El Hani J, Baati T, Saïd K, Kerkeni A; Reversal of cadmium-induced thyroid dysfunction by selenium, zinc, or their combination in rat; Biol Trace Elem Res. 2008 Winter;126(1-3):194-203. doi: 10.1007/s12011-008-8194-8. Epub 2008 Aug 8.

[166] Bigazzi PE; Autoimmunity and heavy metals; Lupus. 1994 Dec;3(6):449-53.

[167] Liang QR, Liao RQ, Su SH, Huang SH, Pan RH, Huang JL; [Effects of lead on thyroid function of occupationally exposed workers]; Zhonghua Lao Dong Wei Sheng Zhi Ye Bing Za Zhi. 2003 Apr;21(2):111-3.

[168] Robins JM, Cullen MR, Connors BB, Kayne RD; Depressed thyroid indexes associated with occupational exposure to inorganic lead; Arch Intern Med. 1983 Feb;143(2):220-4.

[169] Mishra KP; Lead exposure and its impact on immune system: a review; Toxicol In Vitro. 2009 Sep;23(6):969-72.

[170] Koyu A, Cesur G, Ozguner F, Akdogan M, Mollaoglu H, Ozen S; Effects of 900 MHz electromagnetic field on TSH and thyroid hormones in rats; Toxicol Lett. 2005 Jul 4;157(3):257-62. Epub 2005 Apr 11.

[171] Seyed Mortavazi, Asadollah Habib, Amir Ganj-Karami, Razieh Samimi-Doost, Atefe Pour-Abedi, and Ali Babaie; Alterations in TSH and Thyroid Hormones following Mobile Phone Use; Oman Med J. 2009 Oct; 24(4): 274–278.

[172] Paolo Boscolo, Raffaele Iovene, and Gabriele Paiardini; Electromagnetic fields and autoimmune diseases; 2014 February; 3(2): 79–83. ISSN: 2240-2594

[173] Shin Ohtani, Akira Ushiyama, Machiko Maeda, Yuki Ogasawara, Jianqing Wang, Naoki Kunugita, and Kazuyuki Ishii; The effects of radio-frequency electromagnetic fields on T cell function during development; J Radiat Res. 2015 May; 56(3): 467–474.

[174] Rajaei F, Borhani N, Sabbagh-Ziarani F, Mashayekhi F; Effects of extremely low-frequency electromagnetic field on fertility and heights of epithelial cells in pre-implantation stage endometrium and fallopian tube in mice; Zhong Xi Yi Jie He Xue Bao. 2010 Jan;8(1):56-60.

[175] Carpenter DO; Electromagnetic fields and cancer: the cost of doing nothing; Rev Environ Health. 2010 Jan-Mar;25(1):75-80.

[176] Knight SC, Stagg AJ; Antigen-presenting cell types; Curr Opin Immunol. 1993 Jun;5(3):374-82.

[177] Gerard E Kaiko, Jay C Horvat, Kenneth W Beagley, and Philip M Hansbro; Immunological decision-making: how does the immune system decide to mount a helper T-cell response?; Immunology. 2008 Mar; 123(3): 326–338.

[178] Fischer M1, Ehlers M; Toll-like receptors in autoimmunity; Ann N Y Acad Sci. 2008 Nov;1143:21-34.

[179] Marshak-Rothstein A; Toll-like receptors in systemic autoimmune disease; Nat Rev Immunol. 2006 Nov;6(11):823-35.

[180] Chen JQ, Szodoray P, Zeher M; Toll-Like Receptor Pathways in Autoimmune Diseases; Clin Rev Allergy Immunol. 2016 Feb;50(1):1-17.

[181] Cusick MF, Libbey JE, Fujinami RS; Molecular mimicry as a mechanism of autoimmune disease; Clin Rev Allergy Immunol. 2012 Feb;42(1):102-11.

[182] Cornaby C, Gibbons L, Mayhew V, Sloan CS, Welling A, Poole BD; B cell epitope spreading: mechanisms and contribution to autoimmune diseases; Immunol Lett. 2015 Jan;163(1):56-68.

[183] Tuohy VK, Kinkel RP; Epitope spreading: a mechanism for progression of autoimmune disease; Arch Immunol Ther Exp (Warsz). 2000;48(5):347-51.

[184] A M Ercolini and S D Miller; The role of infections in autoimmune disease; Clin Exp Immunol. 2009 Jan; 155(1): 1–15.

[185] Mori K, Yoshida K; Viral infection in induction of Hashimoto's thyroiditis: a key player or just a bystander?; Curr Opin Endocrinol Diabetes Obes. 2010 Oct;17(5):418-24.

[186] Chey WD, Leontiadis GI, Howden CW, Moss SF; ACG Clinical Guideline: Treatment of Helicobacter pylori Infection; Am J Gastroenterol. 2017 Feb;112(2):212-239.

[187] Rimbara E, Fischbach LA, Graham DY; Optimal therapy for Helicobacter pylori infections; Nat Rev Gastroenterol Hepatol. 2011 Feb;8(2):79-88.

[188] De Francesco V, Giorgio F, Hassan C, Manes G, Vannella L, Panella C, Ierardi E, Zullo A; Worldwide H. pylori antibiotic resistance: a systematic review; J Gastrointestin Liver Dis. 2010 Dec;19(4):409-14.

[189] Vilaichone RK, Gumnarai P, Ratanachu-Ek T, Mahachai V; Nationwide survey of Helicobacter pylori antibiotic resistance in Thailand; Diagn Microbiol Infect Dis. 2013 Dec;77(4):346-9.

[190] http://www.cdc.gov/epstein-barr/about-ebv.html

[191] Toussirot E, Roudier J; Epstein-Barr virus in autoimmune diseases; Best Pract Res Clin Rheumatol. 2008 Oct;22(5):883-96.

[192] Janegova A, Janega P, Rychly B, Kuracinova K, Babal P; The role of Epstein-Barr virus infection in the development of autoimmune thyroid diseases; Endokrynol Pol. 2015;66(2):132-6.

[193] Vrbikova J, Janatkova I, Zamrazil V, Tomiska F, Fucikova T; Epstein-Barr virus serology in patients with autoimmune thyroiditis; Exp Clin Endocrinol Diabetes. 1996;104(1):89-92.

[194] http://www.cdc.gov/std/herpes/stdfact-herpes.htm

[195] Robyn S Klein, MD, PhD; Treatment of herpes simplex virus type 1 infection in immunocompetent patients; UpToDate

[196] Di Crescenzo V, D'Antonio A, Tonacchera M, Carlomagno C, Vitale M; Human herpes virus associated with Hashimoto's thyroiditis; Infez Med. 2013 Sep;21(3):224-8.

[197] http://www.cdc.gov/hepatitis/hcv/

[198] http://www.cdc.gov/hepatitis/C/

[199] http://www.who.int/mediacentre/factsheets/fs164/en/

[200] B. Wagner, H. Vierhapper, and H. Hofmann; Prevalence of hepatitis C virus infection in Hashimoto's thyroiditis; BMJ. 1996 Mar 9; 312(7031): 640–641.

[201] Zohreh Jadali; Autoimmune thyroid disorders in hepatitis C virus infection: Effect of interferon therapy; Indian J Endocrinol Metab. 2013 Jan-Feb; 17(1): 69–75.

[202] http://www.ncbi.nlm.nih.gov/pmc/articles/PMC2548497/pdf/bmj00575-0062e.pdf

[203] http://www.cdc.gov/parvovirusb19/about-parvovirus.html

[204] http://www.cdc.gov/parvovirusB19/fifth-disease.html

[205] Lehmann HW, Lutterbüse N, Plentz A, Akkurt I, Albers N, Hauffa BP, Hiort O, Schoenau E, Modrow S.; Association of parvovirus B19 infection and Hashimoto's thyroiditis in children.; Viral Immunol. 2008 Sep;21(3):379-83. doi: 10.1089/vim.2008.0001.

[206] David T Scadden, MDAndrew R Freedman, FRCPPaul Robertson, MRCP, FRCPath; http://www.uptodate.com/contents/human-t-lymphotropic-virus-type-i-virology-pathogenesis-and-epidemiology%20

[207] Akamine H, Takasu N, Komiya I, Ishikawa K, Shinjyo T, Nakachi K, Masuda M.; Association of HTLV-I with autoimmune thyroiditis in patients with adult T-cell leukaemia (ATL) and in HTLV-I carriers.; Clin Endocrinol (Oxf). 1996 Oct;45(4):461-6.

[208] Matsuda T, Tomita M, Uchihara JN, Okudaira T, Ohshiro K, Tomoyose T, Ikema T, Masuda M, Saito M, Osame M, Takasu N, Ohta T, Mori N.; Human T cell leukemia virus type I-infected patients with Hashimoto's thyroiditis and Graves' disease.; J Clin Endocrinol Metab. 2005 Oct;90(10):5704-10. Epub 2005 Aug 2.

[209] Chatzipanagiotou S, Legakis JN, Boufidou F, Petroyianni V, Nicolaou C.; Prevalence of Yersinia plasmid-encoded outer protein (Yop) class-specific antibodies in patients with Hashimoto's thyroiditis.; Clin Microbiol Infect. 2001 Mar;7(3):138-43.

[210] Aghili R1, Jafarzadeh F, Ghorbani R, Khamseh ME, Salami MA, Malek M.; The association of Helicobacter pylori infection with Hashimoto's thyroiditis.; Acta Med Iran. 2013 May 30;51(5):293-6.

[211] Yun Mi Choi, Tae Yong Kim, Eui Young Kim, Eun Kyung Jang, Min Ji Jeon, Won Gu Kim, Young Kee Shong, and Won Bae Kim; Association between thyroid autoimmunity and Helicobacter pylori infection; Korean J Intern Med. 2017 Mar; 32(2): 309–313.

[212] Delitala AP1, Pes GM, Errigo A, Maioli M, Delitala G, Dore MP.; Helicobacter pylori CagA antibodies and thyroid function in latent autoimmune diabetes in adults.; Eur Rev Med Pharmacol Sci. 2016 Oct;20(19):4041-4047.

[213] Francesco Franceschi, Tortora Annalisa, Di Rienzo Teresa, D'Angelo Giovanna, Gianluca Ianiro, Scaldaferri Franco, Gerardi Viviana, Tesori Valentina, Lopetuso Loris Riccardo, and Gasbarrini Antonio; Role of Helicobacter pylori infection on nutrition and metabolism; World J Gastroenterol. 2014 Sep 28; 20(36): 12809–12817.

[214] Benvenga S, Guarneri F, Vaccaro M, Santarpia L, Trimarchi F.; Homologies between proteins of Borrelia burgdorferi and thyroid autoantigens.; Thyroid. 2004 Nov;14(11):964-6.

[215] Beyhan YE, Yilmaz H, Cengiz ZT, Ekici A.; Clinical significance and prevalence of Blastocystis hominis in Van, Turkey.; Saudi Med J. 2015 Sep;36(9):1118-21.

[216] Mei Xing Lim,a,b Chin Wen Png,a,b Crispina Yan Bing Tay,a,b Joshua Ding Wei Teo,a Huipeng Jiao,a,b Norbert Lehming,a Kevin Shyong Wei Tan,corresponding authora and Yongliang Zhangcorresponding authora,b; Differential Regulation of Proinflammatory Cytokine Expression by Mitogen-Activated Protein Kinases in Macrophages in Response to Intestinal Parasite Infection; Infect Immun. 2014 Nov; 82(11): 4789–4801.

[217] Mei Xing Lim, Chin Wen Png,a,b Crispina Yan Bing Tay, Joshua Ding Wei Teo,a Huipeng Jiao, Norbert Lehming, Kevin Shyong Wei Tan, Yongliang Zhang; Differential Regulation of Proinflammatory Cytokine Expression by Mitogen-Activated Protein Kinases in Macrophages in Response to Intestinal Parasite Infection; Infect Immun. 2014 Nov; 82(11): 4789–4801.

[218] Puthia MK, Sio SW, Lu J, Tan KS.; Blastocystis ratti induces contact-independent apoptosis, F-actin rearrangement, and barrier function disruption in IEC-6 cells.; Infect Immun. 2006 Jul;74(7):4114-23.

[219] Rajic B, Arapovic J, Raguž K, Boškovic M, Babic SM, Maslac S.; Eradication of Blastocystis hominis prevents the development of symptomatic Hashimoto's thyroiditis: a case report.; J Infect Dev Ctries. 2015 Jul 30;9(7):788-91.

[220] Samudi Chandramathi, Kumar Suresh, Sinnadurai Sivanandam, and Umah Rani Kuppusamy; Stress Exacerbates Infectivity and Pathogenicity of Blastocystis hominis: In Vitro and In Vivo Evidences; PLoS One. 2014; 9(5): e94567.

[221] Gratacap RL, Rawls JF, Wheeler RT.; Mucosal candidiasis elicits NF-?B activation, proinflammatory gene expression and localized neutrophilia in zebrafish.; Dis Model Mech. 2013 Sep;6(5):1260-70.

[222] Zouali M, Drouhet E, Eyquem A.; Evaluation of auto-antibodies in chronic mucocutaneous candidiasis without endocrinopathy.; Mycopathologia. 1984 Feb 15;84(2-3):87-93.

[223] Mathur S, Melchers JT 3rd, Ades EW, Williamson HO, Fudenberg HH.; Anti-ovarian and anti-lymphocyte antibodies in patients with chronic vaginal candidiasis.; J Reprod Immunol. 1980 Dec;2(5):247-62.

[224] Vojdani A, Rahimian P, Kalhor H, Mordechai E.; Immunological cross reactivity between Candida albicans and human tissue.; J Clin Lab Immunol. 1996;48(1):1-15.

[225] Yan L, Yang C, Tang J.; Disruption of the intestinal mucosal barrier in Candida albicans infections.; Microbiol Res. 2013 Aug 25;168(7):389-95. doi: 10.1016/j. micres.2013.02.008. Epub 2013 Mar 30.

[226] A. Whyte; HAPTENISATION OF SERUM PROTEINS BY ACETALDEHYDE; St John's College, Cambridge CB2 1TP Published: 06 December 1986

[227] N Yamaguchi, R Sugita, A Miki, N Takemura, J Kawabata, J Watanabe, and K Sonoyama; Gastrointestinal Candida colonisation promotes sensitisation against food antigens by affecting the mucosal barrier in mice; Gut. 2006 Jul; 55(7): 954–960.

[228] https://www.cdc.gov/lyme/stats/humancases.html

[229] Kosik-Bogacka DI, Kuzna-Grygiel W, Jaborowska M.; Ticks and mosquitoes as vectors of Borrelia burgdorferi s. l. in the forested areas of Szczecin.; Folia Biol (Krakow). 2007;55(3-4):143-6.

[230] Berghoff W.; Chronic Lyme Disease and Co-infections: Differential Diagnosis.; Open Neurol J. 2012;6:158-78.

[231] Edlow JA.; Erythema migrans.; Med Clin North Am. 2002 Mar;86(2):239-60.

[232] Sigal LH.; Early disseminated Lyme disease: cardiac manifestations.; Am J Med. 1995 Apr 24;98(4A):25S-28S; discussion 28S-29S.

[233] Fallon BA, Nields JA.; Lyme disease: a neuropsychiatric illness.; Am J Psychiatry. 1994 Nov;151(11):1571-83.

[234] Pachner AR.; Neurologic manifestations of Lyme disease, the new "great imitator".; Rev Infect Dis. 1989 Sep-Oct;11 Suppl 6:S1482-6.

[235] Adriana Marques, MD; Chronic Lyme Disease: An appraisal; Infect Dis Clin North Am. 2008 Jun; 22(2): 341–360. doi: 10.1016/j.idc.2007.12.011

[236] https://www.cdc.gov/lyme/postlds/

[237] Joanna Scieszka, Józefa Dabek, and Pawel Cieslik; Post-Lyme disease syndrome; Reumatologia. 2015; 53(1): 46–48.

[238] Seriburi V, Ndukwe N, Chang Z, Cox ME, Wormser GP.; High frequency of false positive IgM immunoblots for Borrelia burgdorferi in clinical practice.; Clin Microbiol Infect. 2012 Dec;18(12):1236-40.

[239] Adriana R. Marques, MD; Laboratory Diagnosis of Lyme Disease - Advances and Challenges; Infect Dis Clin North Am. 2015 Jun; 29(2): 295–307.

[240] Carolyn M. Nielsen, Matthew J. White, Martin R. Goodier, and Eleanor M. Riley,; Functional Significance of CD57 Expression on Human NK Cells and Relevance to Disease; Front Immunol. 2013; 4: 422.

[241] Stricker RB, Savely VR, Motanya NC, Giclas PC.; Complement split products c3a and c4a in chronic lyme disease.; Scand J Immunol. 2009 Jan;69(1):64-9.

[242] Chenggang Jin,,* Diana R. Roen,1 Paul V. Lehmann, and Gottfried H. Kellermann; An Enhanced ELISPOT Assay for Sensitive Detection of Antigen-Specific T Cell Responses to Borrelia burgdorferi; Cells. 2013 Sep; 2(3): 607–620.

[243] Krause PJ, Daily J, Telford SR, Vannier E, Lantos P, Spielman A.; Shared features in the pathobiology of babesiosis and malaria.; Trends Parasitol. 2007 Dec;23(12):605-10. Epub 2007 Nov 7.

[244] Ganguly S, Mukhopadhayay SK.; Tick-borne ehrlichiosis infection in human beings.; J Vector Borne Dis. 2008 Dec;45(4):273-80.

[245] Ricardo G. Maggi, B. Robert Mozayeni, Elizabeth L. Pultorak, Barbara C. Hegarty, Julie M. Bradley, Maria Correa, and Edward B. Breitschwerdt; Bartonella spp. Bacteremia and Rheumatic Symptoms in Patients from Lyme Disease–endemic Region; Emerg Infect Dis. 2012 May; 18(5): 783–791.

[246] Walter Berghoff; Chronic Lyme Disease and Co-infections: Differential Diagnosis; Open Neurol J. 2012; 6: 158–178. Sanjeev K Sahni, PhD† and Elena Rydkina, PhD

[247] Sanjeev K Sahni, PhD and Elena Rydkina, PhD; Host-cell interactions with pathogenic Rickettsia species; Future Microbiol. 2009 Apr; 4: 323–339.

[248] Paddock CD, Denison AM, Lash RR, Liu L, Bollweg BC, Dahlgren FS, Kanamura CT, Angerami RN, Pereira dos Santos FC, Brasil Martines R, Karpathy SE.; Phylogeography of Rickettsia rickettsii genotypes associated with fatal Rocky Mountain spotted fever.; Am J Trop Med Hyg. 2014 Sep;91(3):589-97.

[249] Surender Kashyap and Malay Sarkar; Mycoplasma pneumonia: Clinical features and management; Lung India. 2010 Apr-Jun; 27(2): 75–85.

[250] Walter Berghoff; Chronic Lyme Disease and Co-infections: Differential Diagnosis; Open Neurol J. 2012; 6: 158–178.

[251] Benvenga S, Guarneri F, Vaccaro M, Santarpia L, Trimarchi F; Homologies between proteins of Borrelia burgdorferi and thyroid autoantigens.; Thyroid. 2004 Nov;14(11):964-6.

[252] Benvenga S, Santarpia L, Trimarchi F, Guarneri F; Human thyroid autoantigens and proteins of Yersinia and Borrelia share amino acid sequence homology that includes binding motifs to HLA-DR molecules and T-cell receptor.; Thyroid. 2006 Mar;16(3):225-36.

[253] Chiuri RM, Matronola MF, Di Giulio C, Comegna L, Chiarelli F, Blasetti A.; Bartonella henselae infection associated with autoimmune thyroiditis in a child.; Horm Res Paediatr. 2013;79:185-8.

[254] Sack J, Zilberstein D, Barile MF, Lukes YG, Baker JR Jr, Wartofsky L, Burman KD.; Binding of thyrotropin to selected Mycoplasma species: detection of serum

antibodies against a specific Mycoplasma membrane antigen in patients with autoimmune thyroid disease.; J Endocrinol Invest. 1989 Feb;12(2):77-86.

[255] Keith Berndtson, MD; CHRONIC INFLAMMATORY RESPONSE SYNDROME Overview, Diagnosis, and Treatment; http://www.survivingmold.com/docs/Berndtson_essay_2_CIRS.pdf

[256] Cooper GS, Stroehla BC.; The epidemiology of autoimmune diseases.; Autoimmun Rev. 2003 May;2(3):119-25.

[257] Anatoly V. Rubtsov, Kira Rubtsova, John W. Kappler, and Philippa Marr; Genetic and hormonal factors in female-biased autoimmunity; Autoimmun Rev. 2010 May; 9(7): 494–498.

[258] DeLisa Fairweather and Noel R. Rose; Women and Autoimmune Diseases; Emerg Infect Dis. 2004 Nov; 10(11): 2005–2011. doi: 10.3201/eid1011.040367

[259] Whitacre CC.; Sex differences in autoimmune disease.; Nat Immunol. 2001 Sep;2(9):777-80.

[260] Xiong YH, Yuan Z, He L.; Effects of estrogen on CD4(+) CD25(+) regulatory T cell in peripheral blood during pregnancy.; Asian Pac J Trop Med. 2013 Sep;6(9):748-52.

[261] Jee H. Lee, John P. Lydon, and Chang H. Kim; Progesterone suppresses the mTOR pathway and promotes generation of induced regulatory T cells with increased stability; Eur J Immunol. 2012 Oct; 42(10): 2683–2696.

[262] Hughes GC.; Progesterone and autoimmune disease.; Autoimmun Rev. 2012 May;11(6-7):A502-14. doi: 10.1016/j.autrev.2011.12.003. Epub 2011 Dec 13.

[263] Xu L, Dong B, Wang H, Zeng Z, Liu W, Chen N, Chen J, Yang J, Li D, Duan Y.; Progesterone suppresses Th17 cell responses, and enhances the development of regulatory T cells, through thymic stromal lymphopoietin-dependent mechanisms in experimental gonococcal genital tract infection.; Microbes Infect. 2013 Nov;15(12):796-805.

[264] Lee JH, Ulrich B, Cho J, Park J, Kim CH.; Progesterone promotes differentiation of human cord blood fetal T cells into T regulatory cells but suppresses their differentiation into Th17 cells.; J Immunol. 2011 Aug 15;187(4):1778-87.

[265] Lateef A, Petri M.; Hormone replacement and contraceptive therapy in autoimmune diseases.; J Autoimmun. 2012 May;38(2-3):J170-6. doi: 10.1016/j.jaut.2011.11.002. Epub 2012 Jan 18.

[266] El-Etr M, Ghoumari A, Sitruk-Ware R, Schumacher M; Hormonal influences in multiple sclerosis: new therapeutic benefits for steroids; Maturitas. 2011 Jan;68(1):47-51.

[267] Beaber EF, Buist DS, Barlow WE, Malone KE, Reed SD, Li CI.; Recent oral contraceptive use by formulation and breast cancer risk among women 20 to 49 years of age.; Cancer Res. 2014 Aug 1;74(15):4078-89.

[268] Kumle M, Weiderpass E, Braaten T, Persson I, Adami HO, Lund E.; Use of oral contraceptives and breast cancer risk: The Norwegian-Swedish Women's Lifestyle and Health Cohort Study.; Cancer Epidemiol Biomarkers Prev. 2002 Nov;11(11):1375-81.

[269] Havrilesky LJ, Moorman PG, Lowery WJ, Gierisch JM, Coeytaux RR, Urrutia RP, Dinan M, McBroom AJ, Hasselblad V, Sanders GD, Myers ER.; Oral contraceptive pills as primary prevention for ovarian cancer: a systematic review and meta-analysis.; Obstet Gynecol. 2013 Jul;122(1):139-47.

[270] Palmery M, Saraceno A, Vaiarelli A, Carlomagno G.; Oral contraceptives and changes in nutritional requirements.; Eur Rev Med Pharmacol Sci. 2013 Jul;17(13):1804-13.

[271] Konieczna A, Rutkowska A1, Rachon D1.; Health risk of exposure to Bisphenol A (BPA).; Rocz Panstw Zakl Hig. 2015;66(1):5-11.

[272] Bittner GD, Yang CZ, Stoner MA.; Estrogenic chemicals often leach from BPA-free plastic products that are replacements for BPA-containing polycarbonate products.; Environ Health. 2014 May 28;13(1):41.

[273] Kim EJ1, Lee D, Chung BC, Pyo H, Lee J.; Association between urinary levels of bisphenol-A and estrogen metabolism in Korean adults.; Sci Total Environ. 2014 Feb 1;470-471:1401-7.

[274] Rochester JR, Bolden AL.; Bisphenol S and F: A Systematic Review and Comparison of the Hormonal Activity of Bisphenol A Substitutes.; Environ Health Perspect. 2015 Jul;123(7):643-50.

[275] Qiu W, Zhao Y, Yang M, Farajzadeh M, Pan C, Wayne NL.; Actions of Bisphenol A and Bisphenol S on the Reproductive Neuroendocrine System During Early Development in Zebrafish.; Endocrinology. 2016 Feb;157(2):636-47.

[276] Annette M. Hormann, Frederick S. vom Saal, Susan C. Nagel, Richard W. Stahlhut, Carol L. Moyer, Mark R. Ellersieck, Wade V. Welshons, Pierre-Louis Toutain, and Julia A. Taylor,; Holding Thermal Receipt Paper and Eating Food after Using Hand Sanitizer Results in High Serum Bioactive and Urine Total Levels of Bisphenol A (BPA); PLoS One. 2014; 9(10): e110509.

[277] Hsieh TH, Tsai CF, Hsu CY, Kuo PL, Lee JN, Chai CY, Wang SC, Tsai EM.; Phthalates induce proliferation and invasiveness of estrogen receptor-negative breast cancer through the AhR/HDAC6/c-Myc signaling pathway.; FASEB J. 2012 Feb;26(2):778-87.

[278] Lee HR, Hwang KA1, Choi KC1.; The estrogen receptor signaling pathway activated by phthalates is linked with transforming growth factor-ß in the progression of LNCaP prostate cancer models.; Int J Oncol. 2014 Aug;45(2):595-602.

[279] Zhang Y, Gaikwad NW, Olson K, Zahid M, Cavalieri EL, Rogan EG.; Cytochrome P450 isoforms catalyze formation of catechol estrogen quinones that react with DNA.; Metabolism. 2007 Jul;56(7):887-94.

[280] Cao K, Stack DE, Ramanathan R, Gross ML, Rogan EG, Cavalieri EL.; Synthesis and structure elucidation of estrogen quinones conjugated with cysteine, N-acetylcysteine, and glutathione.; Chem Res Toxicol. 1998 Aug;11(8):909-16.

[281] Naifeng Zhang; Epigenetic modulation of DNA methylation by nutrition and its mechanisms in animals; Animal Nutrition Volume 1, Issue 3, September 2015, Pages 144-151

[282] Koller LD, Exon JH.; The two faces of selenium-deficiency and toxicity—are similar in animals and man.; Can J Vet Res. 1986 Jul;50(3):297-306.

[283] Koller LD, Exon JH.; The two faces of selenium-deficiency and toxicity—are similar in animals and man.; Can J Vet Res. 1986 Jul;50(3):297-306.

[284] M. Rederstorff, A. Krol, and A. Lescure; Understanding the importance of selenium and selenoproteins in muscle function; Cell Mol Life Sci. 2006 Jan; 63(1): 52–59.

[285] Ms. Jennifer K. MacFarquhar, RN, MPH, Dr. Danielle L. Broussard, PhD, MPH, Dr. Paul Melstrom, PhD, Mr. Richard Hutchinson, Ms. Amy Wolkin, MPH, Ms. Colleen Martin, MPH, Dr. Raymond F. Burk, MD, Dr. John R. Dunn, DVM, PhD, Dr. Alice L. Green, MS, DVM, Dr. Roberta Hammond, PhD, Dr. William Schaffner, MD, and Dr. Timothy F. Jones, MD; Acute Selenium Toxicity Associated With a Dietary Supplement; Arch Intern Med. 2010 Feb 8; 170(3): 256–261.

[286] DePalo D, Kinlaw WB, Zhao C, Engelberg-Kulka H, St Germain DL.; Effect of selenium deficiency on type I 5'-deiodinase.; J Biol Chem. 1994 Jun 10;269(23):16223-8.

[287] G J Beckett, S E Beddows, P C Morrice, F Nicol, and J R Arthur; Inhibition of hepatic deiodination of thyroxine is caused by selenium deficiency in rats.; Biochem J. 1987 Dec 1; 248(2): 443–447.

[288] Gärtner R, Gasnier BC, Dietrich JW, Krebs B, Angstwurm MW.; Selenium supplementation in patients with autoimmune thyroiditis decreases thyroid peroxidase antibodies concentrations.; J Clin Endocrinol Metab. 2002 Apr;87(4):1687-91.

[289] Roberto Negro; Selenium and thyroid autoimmunity; Biologics. 2008 Jun; 2(2): 265–273.

[290] Rostami R, Aghasi MR, Mohammadi A, Nourooz-Zadeh J.; Enhanced oxidative stress in Hashimoto's thyroiditis: inter-relationships to biomarkers of thyroid function.; Clin Biochem. 2013 Mar;46(4-5):308-12.

[291] https://ods.od.nih.gov/factsheets/Selenium-HealthProfessional/

[292] Thomson CD, Chisholm A, McLachlan SK, Campbell JM.; Brazil nuts: an effective way to improve selenium status.; Am J Clin Nutr. 2008 Feb;87(2):379-84.

[293] Elisângela Colpo, Carlos Dalton de Avila Vilanova, Luiz Gustavo Brenner Reetz, Marta Maria Medeiros Frescura Duarte, Iria Luiza Gomes Farias, Edson Irineu Muller, Aline Lima Hermes Muller, Erico Marlon Moraes Flores, Roger Wagner, and João Batista Teixeira da Rocha; A Single Consumption of High Amounts of the Brazil Nuts Improves Lipid Profile of Healthy Volunteers; J Nutr Metab. 2013; 2013: 653185.

[294] Karina Pino-Lagos, Micah J. Benson, and Randolph J. Noelle; Retinoic Acid in the Immune System; Ann N Y Acad Sci. 2008 Nov; 1143: 10.1196/annals.1443.017.

[295] Sheng Xiao, Hulin Jin, Thomas Korn, Sue M. Liu, Mohamed Oukka, Bing Lim, and Vijay K. Kuchroo; Retinoic acid increases Foxp3+ regulatory T cells and inhibits development of Th17 cells by enhancing TGF-ß-driven Smad3 signaling and inhibiting IL-6 and IL-23 receptor expression; J Immunol. 2008 Aug 15; 181(4): 2277–2284.

[296] A Catharine Ross; Vitamin A and retinoic acid in T cell–related immunity1,2,3,4; Am J Clin Nutr. 2012 Nov; 96(5): 1166S–1172S.

[297] Nazanin Roohani, Richard Hurrell,1 Roya Kelishadi,2 and Rainer Schulin; Zinc and its importance for human health: An integrative review; J Res Med Sci. 2013 Feb; 18(2): 144–157.

[298] Prasad AS.; Clinical manifestations of zinc deficiency.; Annu Rev Nutr. 1985;5:341-63.

[299] Stoye D, Schubert C, Goihl A, Guttek K, Reinhold A, Brocke S, Grüngreiff K, Reinhold D.; Zinc aspartate suppresses T cell activation in vitro and relapsing experimental autoimmune encephalomyelitis in SJL/J mice.; Biometals. 2012 Jun;25(3):529-39.

[300] Kitabayashi C, Fukada T, Kanamoto M, Ohashi W, Hojyo S, Atsumi T, Ueda N, Azuma I, Hirota H, Murakami M, Hirano T.; Zinc suppresses Th17 development via inhibition of STAT3 activation.; Int Immunol. 2010 May;22(5):375-86.

[301] Mariam Mathew George, Kavitha Subramanian Vignesh, George S Deepe Jr; Zinc Induces Dendritic Cell Tolerogenic Phenotype and Skews Regulatory T Cell – Th17 Balance; J Immunol, 197 (5), 1864-1876 2016 Sep 1

[302] Randa Reda, Amal A. Abbas, Mai Mohammed, Shahira F. El Fedawy, Hala Ghareeb, Rania H. El Kabarity, Rania A. Abo-Shady, and Doaa Zakaria; The Interplay between Zinc, Vitamin D and, IL-17 in Patients with Chronic Hepatitis C Liver Disease; J Immunol Res. 2015; 2015: 846348.

[303] Rosenkranz E, Metz CH, Maywald M, Hilgers RD, Weßels I, Senff T, Haase H, Jäger M, Ott M, Aspinall R, Plümäkers B, Rink L.; Zinc supplementation induces regulatory T cells by inhibition of Sirt-1 deacetylase in mixed lymphocyte cultures.; Mol Nutr Food Res. 2016 Mar;60(3):661-71.

[304] Prasad AS, Beck FW, Bao B, Fitzgerald JT, Snell DC, Steinberg JD, Cardozo LJ.; Zinc supplementation decreases incidence of infections in the elderly: effect of zinc on generation of cytokines and oxidative stress.; Am J Clin Nutr. 2007 Mar;85(3):837-44.

[305] Shankar AH, Prasad AS.; Zinc and immune function: the biological basis of altered resistance to infection.; Am J Clin Nutr. 1998 Aug;68(2 Suppl):447S-463S.

[306] Fischer Walker C, Black RE.; Zinc and the risk for infectious disease.; Annu Rev Nutr. 2004;24:255-75.

[307] Zackular JP, Moore JL, Jordan AT, Juttukonda LJ, Noto MJ, Nicholson MR, Crews JD, Semler MW, Zhang Y, Ware LB1, Washington MK, Chazin WJ, Caprioli RM, Skaar EP.; Dietary zinc alters the microbiota and decreases resistance to Clostridium difficile infection.; Nat Med. 2016 Nov;22(11):1330-1334.

[308] Sonja Skrovanek, Katherine DiGuilio, Robert Bailey, William Huntington, Ryan Urbas, Barani Mayilvaganan, Giancarlo Mercogliano, and James M Mullin; Zinc and gastrointestinal disease; World J Gastrointest Pathophysiol. 2014 Nov 15; 5(4): 496–513.

[309] Mahmood A1, FitzGerald AJ, Marchbank T, Ntatsaki E, Murray D, Ghosh S, Playford RJ.; Zinc carnosine, a health food supplement that stabilises small bowel integrity and stimulates gut repair processes.; Gut. 2007 Feb;56(2):168-75. Epub 2006 Jun 15.

[310] Wegmüller R, Tay F, Zeder C, Brnic M, Hurrell RF.; Zinc absorption by young adults from supplemental zinc citrate is comparable with that from zinc gluconate and higher than from zinc oxide.; J Nutr. 2014 Feb;144(2):132-6.

[311] Schlegel P, Windisch W.; Bioavailability of zinc glycinate in comparison with zinc sulphate in the presence of dietary phytate in an animal model with Zn labelled rats.; J Anim Physiol Anim Nutr (Berl). 2006 Jun;90(5-6):216-22.

[312] DiSilvestro RA, Koch E, Rakes L.; Moderately High Dose Zinc Gluconate or Zinc Glycinate: Effects on Plasma Zinc and Erythrocyte Superoxide Dismutase Activities in Young Adult Women.; Biol Trace Elem Res. 2015 Nov;168(1):11-4.

[313] https://www.nhlbi.nih.gov/health/health-topics/topics/ida/signs

[314] Anthony Samsel and Stephanie Seneff; Glyphosate, pathways to modern diseases II: Celiac sprue and gluten intolerance; Interdiscip Toxicol. 2013 Dec; 6(4): 159–184.

[315] Uzel C, Conrad ME.; Absorption of heme iron.;Semin Hematol. 1998 Jan;35(1):27-34.

[316] Pizarro F, Olivares M, Hertrampf E, Mazariegos DI, Arredondo M.; Heme-iron absorption is saturable by heme-iron dose in women.; J Nutr. 2003 Jul;133(7):2214-7.

[317] Tamagno G, De Carlo E, Murialdo G, Scandellari C.; A possible link between genetic hemochromatosis and autoimmune thyroiditis.; Minerva Med. 2007 Dec;98(6):769-72.

[318] Edwards CQ, Kelly TM, Ellwein G, Kushner JP.; Thyroid disease in hemochromatosis. Increased incidence in homozygous men.; Arch Intern Med. 1983 Oct;143(10):1890-3.

[319] Puntarulo S.; Iron, oxidative stress and human health.; Mol Aspects Med. 2005 Aug-Oct;26(4-5):299-312.

[320] Zimmermann MB, Köhrle J.; The impact of iron and selenium deficiencies on iodine and thyroid metabolism: biochemistry and relevance to public health.; Thyroid. 2002 Oct;12(10):867-78.

[321] Hess SY, Zimmermann MB, Arnold M, Langhans W, Hurrell RF.; Iron deficiency anemia reduces thyroid peroxidase activity in rats.; J Nutr. 2002 Jul;132(7):1951-5.

[322] Schaible UE, Kaufmann SH.; Iron and microbial infection.; Nat Rev Microbiol. 2004 Dec;2(12):946-53.

[323] Bobby J. Cherayil; The role of iron in the immune response to bacterial infection; Immunol Res. 2011 May; 50(1): 1–9. doi: 10.1007/s12026-010-8199-1

[324] Bizzaro G, Shoenfeld Y.; Vitamin D and autoimmune thyroid diseases: facts and unresolved questions.; Immunol Res. 2015 Feb;61(1-2):46-52.

[325] Kivity S, Agmon-Levin N, Zisappl M, Shapira Y, Nagy EV, Dankó K, Szekanecz Z, Langevitz P, Shoenfeld Y.; Vitamin D and autoimmune thyroid diseases.; Cell Mol Immunol. 2011 May;8(3):243-7.

[326] Muscogiuri G, Tirabassi G, Bizzaro G, Orio F, Paschou SA, Vryonidou A, Balercia G, Shoenfeld Y, Colao A.; Vitamin D and thyroid disease: to D or not to D?; Eur J Clin Nutr. 2015 Mar;69(3):291-6.

[327] Mazokopakis EE, Papadomanolaki MG, Tsekouras KC, Evangelopoulos AD, Kotsiris DA, Tzortzinis AA.; Is vitamin D related to pathogenesis and treatment of Hashimoto's thyroiditis?; Hell J Nucl Med. 2015 Sep-Dec;18(3):222-7.

[328] Assa A, Vong L, Pinnell LJ, Avitzur N, Johnson-Henry KC, Sherman PM.; Vitamin D deficiency promotes epithelial barrier dysfunction and intestinal inflammation.; J Infect Dis. 2014 Oct 15;210(8):1296-305.

[329] Raftery T, Martineau AR, Greiller CL, Ghosh S, McNamara D, Bennett K, Meddings J, O'Sullivan M.; Effects of vitamin D supplementation on intestinal permeability, cathelicidin and disease markers in Crohn's disease: Results from a randomised double-blind placebo-controlled study.; United European Gastroenterol J. 2015 Jun;3(3):294-302.

[330] Hector F DeLuca; Overview of general physiologic features and functions of vitamin D; The American Journal of Clinical Nutrition, Volume 80, Issue 6, 1 December 2004, Pages 1689S–1696S, https://doi.org/10.1093/ajcn/80.6.1689S

[331] Kevin B. Comerford; Frequent Canned Food Use is Positively Associated with Nutrient-Dense Food Group Consumption and Higher Nutrient Intakes in US Children and Adults; Nutrients. 2015 Jul; 7(7): 5586–5600.

[332] Lisa A Houghton, Reinhold Vieth; The case against ergocalciferol (vitamin D2) as a vitamin supplement; The American Journal of Clinical Nutrition, Volume 84, Issue 4, 1 October 2006, Pages 694–697, https://doi.org/10.1093/ajcn/84.4.694

[333] Wilhelm Jahnen-Dechentcorresponding author1 and Markus Ketteler2; Magnesium basics; Clin Kidney J. 2012 Feb; 5(Suppl 1): i3–i14. doi: 10.1093/ndtplus/sfr163

[334] Rodríguez-Morán M, Guerrero-Romero F.; Oral magnesium supplementation improves insulin sensitivity and metabolic control in type 2 diabetic subjects: a randomized double-blind controlled trial.; Diabetes Care. 2003 Apr;26(4):1147-52.

[335] Guerrero-Romero F, Tamez-Perez HE, González-González G, Salinas-Martínez AM, Montes-Villarreal J, Treviño-Ortiz JH, Rodríguez-Morán M.; Oral magnesium supplementation improves insulin sensitivity in non-diabetic subjects with insulin resistance. A double-blind placebo-controlled randomized trial.; Diabetes Metab. 2004 Jun;30(3):253-8.

[336] Jinsong Wang,† Gioia Persuitte,† Barbara C. Olendzki, Nicole M. Wedick, Zhiying Zhang, Philip A. Merriam, Hua Fang, James Carmody, Gin-Fei Olendzki, and Yunsheng Ma; Dietary Magnesium Intake Improves Insulin Resistance among Non-Diabetic Individuals with Metabolic Syndrome Participating in a Dietary Trial; Nutrients. 2013 Oct; 5(10): 3910–3919.

[337] Barbagallo M, Dominguez LJ.; Magnesium and aging.; Curr Pharm Des. 2010;16(7):832-9.

[338] R Swaminathan; Magnesium Metabolism and its Disorders; Clin Biochem Rev. 2003 May; 24(2): 47–66.

[339] Kapoor R, Huang YS.; Gamma linolenic acid: an antiinflammatory omega-6 fatty acid.; Curr Pharm Biotechnol. 2006 Dec;7(6):531-4.

[340] Chang CS, Sun HL, Lii CK, Chen HW, Chen PY, Liu KL.; Gamma-linolenic acid inhibits inflammatory responses by regulating NF-kappaB and AP-1 activation

in lipopolysaccharide-induced RAW 264.7 macrophages.; Inflammation. 2010 Feb;33(1):46-57.

[341] Mylonas C, Kouretas D.; Lipid peroxidation and tissue damage.; In Vivo. 1999 May-Jun;13(3):295-309.

[342] Hao W, Wong OY, Liu X, Lee P, Chen Y, Wong KK.; ?-3 fatty acids suppress inflammatory cytokine production by macrophages and hepatocytes.; J Pediatr Surg. 2010 Dec;45(12):2412-8.

[343] Block RC, Dier U, Calderonartero P, Shearer GC, Kakinami L, Larson MK, Harris WS, Georas S, Mousa SA.; The Effects of EPA+DHA and Aspirin on Inflammatory Cytokines and Angiogenesis Factors.; World J Cardiovasc Dis. 2012 Jan 1;2(1):14-19. Epub 2011 Dec 30.

[344] Jeffery L, Fisk HL, Calder PC, Filer A, Raza K, Buckley CD, McInnes I, Taylor PC, Fisher BA.; Plasma Levels of Eicosapentaenoic Acid Are Associated with Anti-TNF Responsiveness in Rheumatoid Arthritis and Inhibit the Etanercept-driven Rise in Th17 Cell Differentiation in Vitro.; J Rheumatol. 2017 Jun;44(6):748-756.

[345] http://www.whfoods.com/genpage.php?tname=george&dbid=75

[346] Alexandra Bulgar, Andreea Brehar, Diana Paun & Constantin Dumitrache; MTHFR mutations in female patients with autoimmune thyroiditis; http://www.endocrine-abstracts.org/ea/0026/ea0026p110.htm

[347] Arakawa Y, Watanabe M, Inoue N, Sarumaru M, Hidaka Y, Iwatani Y.; Association of polymorphisms in DNMT1, DNMT3A, DNMT3B, MTHFR and MTRR genes with global DNA methylation levels and prognosis of autoimmune thyroid disease.; Clin Exp Immunol. 2012 Nov;170(2):194-201.

[348] Agteresch HJ, Dagnelie PC, van den Berg JW, Wilson JH.; Adenosine triphosphate: established and potential clinical applications.; Drugs. 1999 Aug;58(2):211-32.

[349] Ei'Ichiro Nakamura, Yasuhito Uezono, Ken'Ichiro Narusawa, Izumi Shibuya, Yosuke Oishi, Masahiro Tanaka, Nobuyuki Yanagihara, Toshitaka Nakamura, and Futoshi Izumi; ATP activates DNA synthesis by acting on P2X receptors in human osteoblast-like MG-63 cells; Physiology.orgAmerican Journal of Physiology-Cell PhysiologyVol. 279, No. 2

[350] Ames BN.; Mitochondrial decay, a major cause of aging, can be delayed.; J Alzheimers Dis. 2004 Apr;6(2):117-21.

[351] Oduwole KO, Glynn AA, Molony DC, Murray D, Rowe S, Holland LM, McCormack DJ, O'Gara JP.; Anti-biofilm activity of sub-inhibitory povidone-iodine concentrations against Staphylococcus epidermidis and Staphylococcus aureus.; J Orthop Res. 2010 Sep;28(9):1252-6.

[352] Akiyama H, Oono T, Saito M, Iwatsuki K.; Assessment of cadexomer iodine against Staphylococcus aureus biofilm in vivo and in vitro using confocal laser scanning microscopy.; J Dermatol. 2004 Jul;31(7):529-34.

[353] Frederick R. Stoddard II, Ari D. Brooks, Bernard A. Eskin, and Gregg J. Johannes; Iodine Alters Gene Expression in the MCF7 Breast Cancer Cell Line: Evidence for an Anti-Estrogen Effect of Iodine; Int J Med Sci. 2008; 5(4): 189–196.

[354] http://www.optimox.com/iodine-study-8

[355] C. Lynne Burek and Monica V. Talor; Environmental Triggers of Autoimmune Thyroiditis; J Autoimmun. 2009 Nov–Dec; 33(3-4): 183–189.

[356] Pavelka S.; Metabolism of bromide and its interference with the metabolism of iodine.; Physiol Res. 2004;53 Suppl 1:S81-90.

[357] Aruna Dharmasena; Selenium supplementation in thyroid associated ophthalmopathy: an update; Int J Ophthalmol. 2014; 7(2): 365–375.

[358] Ohye H, Sugawara M.; Dual oxidase, hydrogen peroxide and thyroid diseases.; Exp Biol Med (Maywood). 2010 Apr;235(4):424-33.

[359] Roberto Negro; Selenium and thyroid autoimmunity; Biologics. 2008 Jun; 2(2): 265–273.

[360] Turker O, Kumanlioglu K, Karapolat I, Dogan I.; Selenium treatment in autoimmune thyroiditis: 9-month follow-up with variable doses.; J Endocrinol. 2006 Jul;190(1):151-6.

[361] Yaofu Fan, Shuhang Xu, Huifeng Zhang, Wen Cao, Kun Wang, Guofang Chen, Hongjie Di, Meng Cao, and Chao Liu; Selenium Supplementation for Autoimmune Thyroiditis: A Systematic Review and Meta-Analysis; Int J Endocrinol. 2014; 2014: 904573.

[362] Larsen EH, Hansen M, Paulin H, Moesgaard S, Reid M, Rayman M.; Speciation and bioavailability of selenium in yeast-based intervention agents used in cancer chemoprevention studies.; J AOAC Int. 2004 Jan-Feb;87(1):225-32.

[363] Yoshida M, Fukunaga K, Tsuchita H, Yasumoto K.; An evaluation of the bioavailability of selenium in high-selenium yeast.; J Nutr Sci Vitaminol (Tokyo). 1999 Jan;45(1):119-28.

[364] Arranz N1, Haza AI, García A, Delgado E, Rafter J, Morales P.; Effects of organosulfurs, isothiocyanates and vitamin C towards hydrogen peroxide-induced oxidative DNA damage (strand breaks and oxidized purines/pyrimidines) in human hepatoma cells.; Chem Biol Interact. 2007 Aug 15;169(1):63-71. Epub 2007 May 31.

[365] Kontek R, Kontek B, Grzegorczyk K.; Vitamin C modulates DNA damage induced by hydrogen peroxide in human colorectal adenocarcinoma cell lines (HT29) estimated by comet assay in vitro.; Arch Med Sci. 2013 Dec 30;9(6):1006-12. doi: 10.5114/aoms.2013.39791. Epub 2013 Dec 26.

[366] Wu W, Yang N, Feng X, Sun T, Shen P, Sun W.; Effect of vitamin C administration on hydrogen peroxide-induced cytotoxicity in periodontal ligament cells.; Mol Med Rep. 2015 Jan;11(1):242-8.

[367] Guy E. Abraham, M.D., David Brownstein, M.D.; Evidence that the administration of Vitamin C improves a defective cellular transport mechanism for iodine: A Case Report; http://www.optimox.com/iodine-study-11

[368] Rahimifard M, Navaei-Nigjeh M, Baeeri M, Maqbool F, Abdollahi M.; Multiple protective mechanisms of alpha-lipoic acid in oxidation, apoptosis and inflammation against hydrogen peroxide induced toxicity in human lymphocytes.; Mol Cell Biochem. 2015 May;403(1-2):179-86.

[369] Rostami R, Aghasi MR, Mohammadi A, Nourooz-Zadeh J.; Enhanced oxidative stress in Hashimoto's thyroiditis: inter-relationships to biomarkers of thyroid function.; Clin Biochem. 2013 Mar;46(4-5):308-12.

[370] Ates I, Yilmaz FM, Altay M, Yilmaz N, Berker D, Güler S.; The relationship between oxidative stress and autoimmunity in Hashimoto's thyroiditis.; Eur J Endocrinol. 2015 Dec;173(6):791-9.

[371] Shiraev T, Barclay G.; Evidence based exercise - clinical benefits of high intensity interval training.; Aust Fam Physician. 2012 Dec;41(12):960-2.

[372] O Peter Adams; The impact of brief high-intensity exercise on blood glucose levels; Diabetes Metab Syndr Obes. 2013; 6: 113–122.

[373] Boutcher SH.; High-intensity intermittent exercise and fat loss.; J Obes. 2011;2011:868305.

[374] Irving BA, Davis CK, Brock DW, Weltman JY, Swift D, Barrett EJ, Gaesser GA, Weltman A.; Effect of exercise training intensity on abdominal visceral fat and body composition.; Med Sci Sports Exerc. 2008 Nov;40(11):1863-72. doi: 10.1249/MSS.0b013e3181801d40.

[375] Bogdanis GC, Stavrinou P, Fatouros IG, Philippou A, Chatzinikolaou A, Draganidis D, Ermidis G, Maridaki M.; Short-term high-intensity interval exercise training attenuates oxidative stress responses and improves antioxidant status in healthy humans.; Food Chem Toxicol. 2013 Nov;61:171-7.

[376] Haaland DA, Sabljic TF, Baribeau DA, Mukovozov IM, Hart LE.; Is regular exercise a friend or foe of the aging immune system? A systematic review.; Clin J Sport Med. 2008 Nov;18(6):539-48.

[377] Stephen A. Martin, Brandt D. Pence, and Jeffrey A. Woods; Exercise and Respiratory Tract Viral Infections; Exerc Sport Sci Rev. 2009 Oct; 37(4): 157–164.

[378] Lakier Smith L.; Overtraining, excessive exercise, and altered immunity: is this a T helper-1 versus T helper-2 lymphocyte response?; Sports Med. 2003;33(5):347-64.

[379] Corthésy B.; Role of secretory IgA in infection and maintenance of homeostasis.; Autoimmun Rev. 2013 Apr;12(6):661-5. doi: 10.1016/j.autrev.2012.10.012. Epub 2012 Nov 29.

[380] Blaise Corthésy; Multi-Faceted Functions of Secretory IgA at Mucosal Surfaces; Front Immunol. 2013; 4: 185.

[381] Mackinnon LT, Hooper S.; Mucosal (secretory) immune system responses to exercise of varying intensity and during overtraining.; Int J Sports Med. 1994 Oct;15 Suppl 3:S179-83.

[382] Brooks K, Carter J.; Overtraining, Exercise, and Adrenal Insufficiency.; J Nov Physiother. 2013 Feb 16;3(125). pii: 11717.

[383] Stagnaro-Green A.; Postpartum thyroiditis.; Best Pract Res Clin Endocrinol Metab. 2004 Jun;18(2):303-16.

[384] Simon Mills, Kerry Bone; The Essential Guide To Herbal Safety: Page 510

[385] Shelly S, Boaz M, Orbach H.; Prolactin and autoimmunity.; Autoimmun Rev. 2012 May;11(6-7):A465-70.

[386] De Bellis A, Bizzarro A, Pivonello R, Lombardi G, Bellastella A.; Prolactin and autoimmunity.; Pituitary. 2005;8(1):25-30.

[387] Shelly S, Boaz M, Orbach H.; Prolactin and autoimmunity.; Autoimmun Rev. 2012 May;11(6-7):A465-70.

[388] Stagnaro-Green A.; Approach to the patient with postpartum thyroiditis.; J Clin Endocrinol Metab. 2012 Feb;97(2):334-42.

[389] Negro R, Greco G, Mangieri T, Pezzarossa A, Dazzi D, Hassan H.; The influence of selenium supplementation on postpartum thyroid status in pregnant women with thyroid peroxidase autoantibodies.; J Clin Endocrinol Metab. 2007 Apr;92(4):1263-8. Epub 2007 Feb 6.

[390] Güemes M, Rahman SA, Hussain K.; What is a normal blood glucose?; Arch Dis Child. 2016 Jun;101(6):569-74. doi: 10.1136/archdischild-2015-308336. Epub 2015 Sep 14.

[391] Jianping Ye; Mechanisms of insulin resistance in obesity; Front Med. 2013 Mar; 7(1): 14–24.

[392] Ye J1.; Role of insulin in the pathogenesis of free fatty acid-induced insulin resistance in skeletal muscle.; Endocr Metab Immune Disord Drug Targets. 2007 Mar;7(1):65-74.

[393] Wang CH, Wang CC, Huang HC, Wei YH.; Mitochondrial dysfunction leads to impairment of insulin sensitivity and adiponectin secretion in adipocytes.; FEBS J. 2013 Feb;280(4):1039-50.

[394] Weinberg JM.; Lipotoxicity.; Kidney Int. 2006 Nov;70(9):1560-6. Epub 2006 Sep 6.

[395] Schaffer JE.; Lipotoxicity: when tissues overeat.; Curr Opin Lipidol. 2003 Jun;14(3):281-7.

[396] Shen J, Obin MS, Zhao L.; The gut microbiota, obesity and insulin resistance.; Mol Aspects Med. 2013 Feb;34(1):39-58.

[397] Tremellen K, Pearce K.; Dysbiosis of Gut Microbiota (DOGMA)—a novel theory for the development of Polycystic Ovarian Syndrome.; Med Hypotheses. 2012 Jul;79(1):104-12.

[398] Shi SQ, Ansari TS, McGuinness OP, Wasserman DH, Johnson CH.; Circadian disruption leads to insulin resistance and obesity.; Curr Biol. 2013 Mar 4;23(5):372-81.

[399] Fonken LK, Workman JL, Walton JC, Weil ZM, Morris JS, Haim A, Nelson RJ.; Light at night increases body mass by shifting the time of food intake.; Proc Natl Acad Sci U S A. 2010 Oct 26;107(43):18664-9.

[400] Karatsoreos IN, Bhagat S, Bloss EB, Morrison JH, McEwen BS.; Disruption of circadian clocks has ramifications for metabolism, brain, and behavior.; Proc Natl Acad Sci U S A. 2011 Jan 25;108(4):1657-62.

[401] Audrey E. Brown and Mark Walker; Genetics of Insulin Resistance and the Metabolic Syndrome; Curr Cardiol Rep. 2016; 18: 75.

[402] Ling PR, Smith RJ, Bistrian BR.; Hyperglycemia enhances the cytokine production and oxidative responses to a low but not high dose of endotoxin in rats.; Crit Care Med. 2005 May;33(5):1084-9.

[403] de Carvalho Vidigal F, Guedes Cocate P, Gonçalves Pereira L, de Cássia Gonçalves Alfenas R.; The role of hyperglycemia in the induction of oxidative stress and inflammatory process.; Nutr Hosp. 2012 Sep-Oct;27(5):1391-8.

[404] Aronson D.; Hyperglycemia and the pathobiology of diabetic complications.; Adv Cardiol. 2008;45:1-16.

[405] Antonio La Cava; Tregs Are Regulated by Cytokines: Implications for Autoimmunity; Autoimmun Rev. 2008 Oct; 8(1): 83–87.

[406] Wang W, Uzzau S, Goldblum SE, Fasano A.; Human zonulin, a potential modulator of intestinal tight junctions.; J Cell Sci. 2000 Dec;113 Pt 24:4435-40.

[407] Smecuol E, Sugai E, Niveloni S, Vázquez H, Pedreira S, Mazure R, Moreno ML, Label M, Mauriño E, Fasano A, Meddings J, Bai JC.; Permeability, zonulin production, and enteropathy in dermatitis herpetiformis.; Clin Gastroenterol Hepatol. 2005 Apr;3(4):335-41.

[408] Moreno-Navarrete JM1, Sabater M, Ortega F, Ricart W, Fernández-Real JM.; Circulating zonulin, a marker of intestinal permeability, is increased in association with obesity-associated insulin resistance.; PLoS One. 2012;7(5):e37160.

[409] Mokkala K, Pellonperä O2, Röytiö H3, Pussinen P4, Rönnemaa T5, Laitinen K3.; Increased intestinal permeability, measured by serum zonulin, is associated with metabolic risk markers in overweight pregnant women.; Metabolism. 2017 Apr;69:43-50.

[410] Brun P, Castagliuolo I, Di Leo V, Buda A, Pinzani M, Palù G, Martines D.; Increased intestinal permeability in obese mice: new evidence in the pathogenesis of nonalcoholic steatohepatitis.; Am J Physiol Gastrointest Liver Physiol. 2007 Feb;292(2):G518-25. Epub 2006 Oct 5.

[411] Capaldo CT, Nusrat A.; Cytokine regulation of tight junctions.; Biochim Biophys Acta. 2009 Apr;1788(4):864-71.

[412] Schmidt FM, Weschenfelder J, Sander C, Minkwitz J, Thormann J, Chittka T, Mergl R, Kirkby KC, Faßhauer M, Stumvoll M, Holdt LM, Teupser D, Hegerl U, Himmerich H.; Inflammatory cytokines in general and central obesity and modulating effects of physical activity.; PLoS One. 2015 Mar 17;10(3):e0121971.

[413] Kassem Makki, Philippe Froguel, and Isabelle Wolowczuk ; Adipose Tissue in Obesity-Related Inflammation and Insulin Resistance: Cells, Cytokines, and Chemokines; ISRN Inflamm. 2013; 2013: 139239.

[414] Patricia Fernández-Riejos, Souad Najib, Jose Santos-Alvarez, Consuelo Martín-Romero, Antonio Pérez-Pérez, Carmen González-Yanes, and Víctor Sánchez-Margalet; Role of Leptin in the Activation of Immune Cells; Mediators Inflamm. 2010; 2010: 568343.

[415] Lam QL, Lu L.; Role of leptin in immunity.; Cell Mol Immunol. 2007 Feb;4(1):1-13.

[416] Matarese G.; Leptin and the immune system: how nutritional status influences the immune response.; Eur Cytokine Netw. 2000 Mar;11(1):7-14.

[417] Naylor C, Petri WA Jr2.; Leptin Regulation of Immune Responses.; Trends Mol Med. 2016 Feb;22(2):88-98. doi: 10.1016/j.molmed.2015.12.001. Epub 2016 Jan 14.

[418] Reis BS, Lee K, Fanok MH, Mascaraque C, Amoury M, Cohn LB, Rogoz A, Dallner OS, Moraes-Vieira PM, Domingos AI, Mucida D.; Leptin receptor signaling in T cells is required for Th17 differentiation.; J Immunol. 2015 Jun 1;194(11):5253-60.

[419] Manole COJOCARU,a Inimioara Mihaela COJOCARU,b Isabela SILOSI,c and Suzana ROGOZc; Role of Leptin in Autoimmune Diseases; Maedica (Buchar). 2013 Mar; 8(1): 68–74.

[420] Victor L Fulgoni, III,corresponding author1 Mark Dreher,2 and Adrienne J Davenport3; Avocado consumption is associated with better diet quality and nutrient intake, and lower metabolic syndrome risk in US adults: results from the National Health and Nutrition Examination Survey (NHANES) 2001–2008; Nutr J. 2013; 12: 1.

[421] Mark L. Dreher and Adrienne J. Davenport; Hass Avocado Composition and Potential Health Effects; Crit Rev Food Sci Nutr. 2013 May; 53(7): 738–750.

[422] James M. Lattimer and Mark D. Haub; Effects of Dietary Fiber and Its Components on Metabolic Health; Nutrients. 2010 Dec; 2(12): 1266–1289.

[423] Anderson RA; Chromium and polyphenols from cinnamon improve insulin sensitivity.; Proc Nutr Soc. 2008 Feb; 67(1):48-53.

[424] No authors listed; A scientific review: the role of chromium in insulin resistance.; Diabetes Educ. 2004; Suppl:2-14.

[425] Guerrero-Romero F, Tamez-Perez HE, González-González G, Salinas-Martínez AM, Montes-Villarreal J, Treviño-Ortiz JH, Rodríguez-Morán M.; Oral magnesium supplementation improves insulin sensitivity in non-diabetic subjects with insulin resistance. A double-blind placebo-controlled randomized trial.; Diabetes Metab. 2004 Jun;30(3):253-8.

[426] Mooren FC, Krüger K, Völker K, Golf SW, Wadepuhl M, Kraus A.; Oral magnesium supplementation reduces insulin resistance in non-diabetic subjects - a double-blind, placebo-controlled, randomized trial.; Diabetes Obes Metab. 2011 Mar;13(3):281-4.

[427] Kamenova P; Improvement of insulin sensitivity in patients with type 2 diabetes mellitus after oral administration of alpha-lipoic acid.; Hormones (Athens). 2006 Oct-Dec;5(4):251-8.

[428] Ansar H, Mazloom Z, Kazemi F, Hejazi N.; Effect of alpha-lipoic acid on blood glucose, insulin resistance and glutathione peroxidase of type 2 diabetic patients.; Saudi Med J. 2011 Jun;32(6):584-8.

[429] Wang J, Yuen VG, McNeill JH.; Effect of vanadium on insulin sensitivity and appetite.; Metabolism. 2001 Jun;50(6):667-73.

[430] Halberstam M, Cohen N, Shlimovich P, Rossetti L, Shamoon H.; Oral vanadyl sulfate improves insulin sensitivity in NIDDM but not in obese nondiabetic subjects.; Diabetes. 1996 May;45(5):659-66.

[431] Sridhar MG, Vinayagamoorthi R, Arul Suyambunathan V, Bobby Z, Selvaraj N.; Bitter gourd (Momordica charantia) improves insulin sensitivity by increasing skeletal muscle insulin-stimulated IRS-1 tyrosine phosphorylation in high-fat-fed rats.; Br J Nutr. 2008 Apr;99(4):806-12. Epub 2007 Oct 17.

[432] Han J, Lin H, Huang W.; Modulating gut microbiota as an anti-diabetic mechanism of berberine.; Med Sci Monit. 2011 Jul;17(7):RA164-7.

[433] Kumar SN, Mani UV, Mani I.; An open label study on the supplementation of Gymnema sylvestre in type 2 diabetics.; J Diet Suppl. 2010 Sep;7(3):273-82.

[434] Parijat Kanetkar, Rekha Singhal,* and Madhusudan Kamat; Gymnema sylvestre: A Memoir; J Clin Biochem Nutr. 2007 Sep; 41(2): 77–81.

[435] Borghouts LB, Keizer HA.; Exercise and insulin sensitivity: a review.; Int J Sports Med. 2000 Jan;21(1):1-12.

[436] Dubé JJ, Allison KF, Rousson V, Goodpaster BH, Amati F.; Exercise dose and insulin sensitivity: relevance for diabetes prevention.; Med Sci Sports Exerc. 2012 May;44(5):793-9.

[437] Van Cauter E.; Sleep disturbances and insulin resistance.; Diabet Med. 2011 Dec;28(12):1455-62.

[438] Donga E, van Dijk M, van Dijk JG, Biermasz NR, Lammers GJ, van Kralingen KW, Corssmit EP, Romijn JA.; A single night of partial sleep deprivation induces insulin resistance in multiple metabolic pathways in healthy subjects.; J Clin Endocrinol Metab. 2010 Jun;95(6):2963-8.

[439] Patil BS, Patil S, Gururaj TR.; Probable autoimmune causal relationship between periodontitis and Hashimotos thyroidits: a systemic review.; Niger J Clin Pract. 2011 Jul-Sep;14(3):253-61.

[440] Patil BS, Giri GR.; A clinical case report of Hashimoto's thyroiditis and its impact on the treatment of chronic periodontitis.; Niger J Clin Pract. 2012 Jan-Mar;15(1):112-4.

[441] Graves DT.; The potential role of chemokines and inflammatory cytokines in periodontal disease progression.; Clin Infect Dis. 1999 Mar;28(3):482-90.

[442] Okada H, Murakami S.; Cytokine expression in periodontal health and disease.; Crit Rev Oral Biol Med. 1998;9(3):248-66.

[443] Graves D.; Cytokines that promote periodontal tissue destruction.; J Periodontol. 2008 Aug;79(8 Suppl):1585-91.

[444] Cardoso CR, Garlet GP, Crippa GE, Rosa AL, Júnior WM, Rossi MA, Silva JS.; Evidence of the presence of T helper type 17 cells in chronic lesions of human periodontal disease.; Oral Microbiol Immunol. 2009 Feb;24(1):1-6.

[445] George Hajishengallis; Periodontitis: from microbial immune subversion to systemic inflammation; Nature Reviews Immunology 15, 30–44 (2015)

[446] Kisakol G.; Dental amalgam implantation and thyroid autoimmunity.; Bratisl Lek Listy. 2014;115(1):22-4.

[447] Sterzl I1, Prochazkova J, Hrda P, Matucha P, Bartova J, Stejskal V.; Removal of dental amalgam decreases anti-TPO and anti-Tg autoantibodies in patients with autoimmune thyroiditis.; Neuro Endocrinol Lett. 2006 Dec;27 Suppl 1:25-30.

[448] http://www.who.int/mediacentre/factsheets/fs361/en/

[449] Gallagher CM, Meliker JR.; Mercury and thyroid autoantibodies in U.S. women, NHANES 2007-2008.; Environ Int. 2012 Apr;40:39-43.

[450] Chen A, Kim SS, Chung E, Dietrich KN.; Thyroid hormones in relation to lead, mercury, and cadmium exposure in the National Health and Nutrition Examination Survey, 2007-2008.; Environ Health Perspect. 2013 Feb;121(2):181-6.

[451] Ellingsen DG, Efskind J, Haug E, Thomassen Y, Martinsen I, Gaarder PI.; Effects of low mercury vapour exposure on the thyroid function in chloralkali workers.; J Appl Toxicol. 2000 Nov-Dec;20(6):483-9.

[452] Pawel Lukasz Brzewski,1 Magdalena Spalkowska,2 Magdalena Podbielska,2 Joanna Chmielewska,2 Marta Wolek,1 Katarzyna Malec,3 and Anna Wojas-Pelc1; The role of focal infections in the pathogenesis of psoriasis and chronic urticaria; Postepy Dermatol Alergol. 2013 Apr; 30(2): 77–84.

[453] Gergely P.; The role of focal infections in the pathogenesis of diseases.; Orv Hetil. 2002 Jul 21;143(29):1749-53.

[454] Chaturvedi TP.; An overview of the corrosion aspect of dental implants (titanium and its alloys).; Indian J Dent Res. 2009 Jan-Mar;20(1):91-8.

[455] Hensten-Pettersen A.; Casting alloys: side-effects.; Adv Dent Res. 1992 Sep;6:38-43.

[456] Sicilia A, Cuesta S, Coma G, Arregui I, Guisasola C, Ruiz E, Maestro A.; Titanium allergy in dental implant patients: a clinical study on 1500 consecutive patients.; Clin Oral Implants Res. 2008 Aug;19(8):823-35.

[457] Müller K, Valentine-Thon E.; Hypersensitivity to titanium: clinical and laboratory evidence.; Neuro Endocrinol Lett. 2006 Dec;27 Suppl 1:31-5.

[458] Hybenova M, Hrda P, Procházková J, Stejskal V, Sterzl I.; The role of environmental factors in autoimmune thyroiditis.; Neuro Endocrinol Lett. 2010;31(3):283-9.

[459] Sterzl I, Procházková J, Hrdá P, Bártová J, Matucha P, Stejskal VD.; Mercury and nickel allergy: risk factors in fatigue and autoimmunity.; Neuro Endocrinol Lett. 1999;20(3-4):221-228.

[460] Manish Goutam, Chandu Giriyapura, Sunil Kumar Mishra, and Siddharth Gupta; Titanium Allergy: A Literature Review; Indian J Dermatol. 2014 Nov-Dec; 59(6): 630.

[461] Müller K, Valentine-Thon E.; Hypersensitivity to titanium: clinical and laboratory evidence.; Neuro Endocrinol Lett. 2006 Dec;27 Suppl 1:31-5.

[462] https://www.cdc.gov/vaccines/vpd/mmr/public/index.html

[463] Bali Pulendran and Rafi Ahmed; Immunological mechanisms of vaccination; Nat Immunol. 2011 Jun; 12(6): 509–517.

[464] Carolyn R. Casella, Thomas C. Mitchell; Putting endotoxin to work for us: monophosphoryl lipid A as a safe and effective vaccine adjuvant; Cell Mol Life Sci. 2008 Oct; 65(20): 3231–3240.

[465] Exley C; What is the risk of aluminium as a neurotoxin?; Expert Rev Neurother. 2014 Jun;14(6):589-91.

[466] Joshi JG; Aluminum, a neurotoxin which affects diverse metabolic reactions.; Biofactors. 1990 Jul;2(3):163-9.

[467] Masahiro Kawahara, Midori Kato-Negishi; Link between Aluminum and the Pathogenesis of Alzheimer's Disease: The Integration of the Aluminum and Amyloid Cascade Hypotheses; Int J Alzheimers Dis. 2011; 2011: 276393.

[468] Tomljenovic L, Shaw CA.; Mechanisms of aluminum adjuvant toxicity and autoimmunity in pediatric populations.; Lupus. 2012 Feb;21(2):223-30.

[469] Tomljenovic L, Shaw CA.; Aluminum vaccine adjuvants: are they safe?; Curr Med Chem. 2011;18(17):2630-7.

[470] Shaw CA, Li D, Tomljenovic L.; Are there negative CNS impacts of aluminum adjuvants used in vaccines and immunotherapy?; Immunotherapy. 2014;6(10):1055-71.

[471] James T. Li, MD, Matthew A. Rank, MD, Diane L. Squillace, BS, Hirohito Kita, MD; Ovalbumin content of influenza vaccines; J Allergy Clin Immunol. 2010 Jun; 125(6): 1412–1414.

[472] Perdan-Pirkmajer K, Thallinger GG, Snoj N, Cucnik S, Žigon P, Kveder T, Logar D, Praprotnik S, Tomšic M, Sodin-Semrl S, Ambrožic A.; Autoimmune response following influenza vaccination in patients with autoimmune inflammatory rheumatic disease.; Lupus. 2012 Feb;21(2):175-83.

[473] Guimarães LE, Baker B, Perricone C, Shoenfeld Y.; Vaccines, adjuvants and autoimmunity.; Pharmacol Res. 2015 Oct;100:190-209.

[474] Toplak N, Kveder T, Trampus-Bakija A, Subelj V, Cucnik S, Avcin T.; Autoimmune response following annual influenza vaccination in 92 apparently healthy adults.; Autoimmun Rev. 2008 Dec;8(2):134-8.

[475] Abdulla Watad, Paula David, Stav Brown, and Yehuda Shoenfeld; Autoimmune/ Inflammatory Syndrome Induced by Adjuvants and Thyroid Autoimmunity; Front Endocrinol (Lausanne). 2016; 7: 150.

[476] Michael J Rieder, Joan L Robinson; 'Nosodes' are no substitute for vaccines; Paediatr Child Health. 2015 May; 20(4): 219–220.

[477] Cattani D, de Liz Oliveira Cavalli VL, Heinz Rieg CE, Domingues JT, Dal-Cim T, Tasca CI, Mena Barreto Silva FR, Zamoner A; Mechanisms underlying the neurotoxicity induced by glyphosate-based herbicide in immature rat hippocampus: involvement of glutamate excitotoxicity.; Toxicology. 2014 Jun 5;320:34-45.

[478] Chaufan G, Coalova I, Ríos de Molina Mdel C.; Glyphosate commercial formulation causes cytotoxicity, oxidative effects, and apoptosis on human cells: differences with its active ingredient.; Int J Toxicol. 2014 Jan-Feb;33(1):29-38.

[479] Koller VJ, Fürhacker M, Nersesyan A, Mišík M, Eisenbauer M, Knasmueller S.; Cytotoxic and DNA-damaging properties of glyphosate and Roundup in human-derived buccal epithelial cells.; Arch Toxicol. 2012 May;86(5):805-13.

[480] Gress S, Lemoine S, Séralini GE, Puddu PE.; Glyphosate-based herbicides potently affect cardiovascular system in mammals: review of the literature.; Cardiovasc Toxicol. 2015 Apr;15(2):117-26.

[481] Thongprakaisang S, Thiantanawat A, Rangkadilok N, Suriyo T, Satayavivad J.; Glyphosate induces human breast cancer cells growth via estrogen receptors.; Food Chem Toxicol. 2013 Sep;59:129-36.

[482] Lamb DC, Kelly DE, Hanley SZ, Mehmood Z, Kelly SL.; Glyphosate is an inhibitor of plant cytochrome P450: functional expression of Thlaspi arvensae cytochrome P45071B1/reductase fusion protein in Escherichia coli.; Biochem Biophys Res Commun. 1998 Mar 6;244(1):110-4.

[483] Lorbek G, Lewinska M, Rozman D.; Cytochrome P450s in the synthesis of cholesterol and bile acids—from mouse models to human diseases.; FEBS J. 2012 May;279(9):1516-33.

[484] Samsel A, Seneff S.; Glyphosate, pathways to modern diseases III: Manganese, neurological diseases, and associated pathologies.; Surg Neurol Int. 2015 Mar 24;6:45.

[485] Lu W1, Li L, Chen M, Zhou Z, Zhang W, Ping S, Yan Y, Wang J, Lin M.; Genome-wide transcriptional responses of Escherichia coli to glyphosate, a potent inhibitor of the shikimate pathway enzyme 5-enolpyruvylshikimate-3-phosphate synthase.; Mol Biosyst. 2013 Mar;9(3):522-30.

[486] Shehata AA, Schrödl W, Aldin AA, Hafez HM, Krüger M.; The effect of glyphosate on potential pathogens and beneficial members of poultry microbiota in vitro.; Curr Microbiol. 2013 Apr;66(4):350-8.

[487] Ackermann W, Coenen M, Schrödl W, Shehata AA, Krüger M.; The influence of glyphosate on the microbiota and production of botulinum neurotoxin during ruminal fermentation.; Curr Microbiol. 2015 Mar;70(3):374-82.

[488] Stephen O. Duke, John Lydon, William C. Koskinen, Thomas B. Moorman, Rufus L. Chaney, Raymond Hammerschmidt; Glyphosate Effects on Plant Mineral Nutrition, Crop Rhizosphere Microbiota, and Plant Disease in Glyphosate-Resistant Crops; J Agric Food Chem. 2012 Oct 24; 60(42): 10375–10397.

[489] Anthony Samsel, Stephanie Seneff1; Glyphosate, pathways to modern diseases III: Manganese, neurological diseases, and associated pathologies; Surg Neurol Int. 2015; 6: 45.

[490] Herbert LT, Vázquez DE1, Arenas A1, Farina WM2.; Effects of field-realistic doses of glyphosate on honeybee appetitive behaviour.; J Exp Biol. 2014 Oct 1;217(Pt 19):3457-64.

[491] Mesnage R, Bernay B, Séralini GE.; Ethoxylated adjuvants of glyphosate-based herbicides are active principles of human cell toxicity.; Toxicology. 2013 Nov 16;313(2-3):122-8.

[492] Defarge N, Takács E, Lozano VL, Mesnage R, Spiroux de Vendômois J, Séralini GE, Székács A.; Co-Formulants in Glyphosate-Based Herbicides Disrupt Aromatase Activity in Human Cells below Toxic Levels.; Int J Environ Res Public Health. 2016 Feb 26;13(3). pii: E264.

[493] Pessione E.; Lactic acid bacteria contribution to gut microbiota complexity: lights and shadows.; Front Cell Infect Microbiol. 2012 Jun 22;2:86.

[494] Shehata AA, Schrödl W, Aldin AA, Hafez HM, Krüger M.; The effect of glyphosate on potential pathogens and beneficial members of poultry microbiota in vitro.; Curr Microbiol. 2013 Apr;66(4):350-8.

[495] Rayman MP.; The importance of selenium to human health.; Lancet. 2000 Jul 15;356(9225):233-41.

[496] Drutel A, Archambeaud F, Caron P.; Selenium and the thyroid gland: more good news for clinicians.; Clin Endocrinol (Oxf). 2013 Feb;78(2):155-64.

[497] Roberto Negro; Selenium and thyroid autoimmunity; Biologics. 2008 Jun; 2(2): 265–273.

[498] Zhu L, Bai X, Teng WP, Shan ZY, Wang WW, Fan CL, Wang H, Zhang HM.; Effects of selenium supplementation on antibodies of autoimmune thyroiditis.; Zhonghua Yi Xue Za Zhi. 2012 Aug 28;92(32):2256-60.

[499] Vasiluk L, Pinto LJ, Moore MM.; Oral bioavailability of glyphosate: studies using two intestinal cell lines.; Environ Toxicol Chem. 2005 Jan;24(1):153-60.

[500] Charles M. Benbrook; Trends in glyphosate herbicide use in the United States and globally; Environ Sci Eur. 2016; 28(1): 3.

[501] https://www.omicsonline.org/open-access/oral-application-of-charcoal-and-humic-acids-influence-selected-gastrointestinal-microbiota-2161-0525.1000256.php?aid=39228

[502] Andrew C. Dukowicz, MD, Brian E. Lacy, PhD, MD, Gary M. Levine, MD; Small Intestinal Bacterial Overgrowth; Gastroenterol Hepatol (N Y). 2007 Feb; 3(2): 112–122.

[503] Deloose E, Janssen P, Depoortere I, Tack J.; The migrating motor complex: control mechanisms and its role in health and disease.; Nat Rev Gastroenterol Hepatol. 2012 Mar 27;9(5):271-85. doi: 10.1038/nrgastro.2012.57.

[504] Pimentel M, Morales W, Pokkunuri V, Brikos C, Kim SM, Kim SE, Triantafyllou K, Weitsman S, Marsh Z, Marsh E, Chua KS, Srinivasan S, Barlow GM, Chang C.; Autoimmunity Links Vinculin to the Pathophysiology of Chronic Functional Bowel Changes Following Campylobacter jejuni Infection in a Rat Model.; Dig Dis Sci. 2015 May;60(5):1195-205.

[505] Erdogan A, Rao SS.; Small intestinal fungal overgrowth.; Curr Gastroenterol Rep. 2015 Apr;17(4):16. doi: 10.1007/s11894-015-0436-2.

SECTION THREE

[1] Bahram Namjou, R. Hal Scofield, Jennifer A. Kelly, Ellen L. Goodmon, Teresa Aberle, Gail R. Bruner, and John B. Harley; The effects of previous Hysterectomy on Lupus; Lupus. Author manuscript; available in PMC 2009 Oct 28

[2] Cañas CA, Echeverri AF, Ospina FE, Suso JP, Agualimpia A, Echeverri A, Bonilla-Abadía F, Tobón GJ.;Is Bariatric Surgery a Trigger Factor for Systemic Autoimmune Diseases?;J Clin Rheumatol. 2016 Mar;22(2):89-91. doi: 10.1097/RHU.0000000000000363.

[3] Antvorskov JC, Fundova P, Buschard K, Funda DP.;Dietary gluten alters the balance of pro-inflammatory and anti-inflammatory cytokines in T cells of BALB/c mice.;Immunology. 2013 Jan;138(1):23-33.

[4] Ejsing-Duun M, Josephsen J, Aasted B, Buschard K, Hansen AK.; Dietary gluten reduces the number of intestinal regulatory T cells in mice.; Scand J Immunol. 2008 Jun; 67(6):553-9.

[5] Aristo Vojdani; A Potential Link between Environmental Triggers and Autoimmunity; Autoimmune Dis. 2014; 2014: 437231.

6   Carr TF, Saltoun CA.; Chapter 2: Skin testing in allergy.; Allergy Asthma Proc. 2012 May-Jun;33 Suppl 1:6-8. doi: 10.2500/aap.2012.33.3532.

7   Heinzerling L, Mari A, Bergmann KC, Bresciani M, Burbach G, Darsow U, Durham S, Fokkens W, Gjomarkaj M, Haahtela T, Bom AT, Wöhrl S, Maibach H, Lockey R.; The skin prick test - European standards.; Clin Transl Allergy. 2013 Feb 1;3(1):3.

8   Abi Berger, science editor; Skin prick testing; BMJ. 2002 Aug 24; 325(7361): 414.

9   Ortolani C1, Ispano M, Pastorello EA, Ansaloni R, Magri GC.; Comparison of results of skin prick tests (with fresh foods and commercial food extracts) and RAST in 100 patients with oral allergy syndrome.; J Allergy Clin Immunol. 1989 Mar;83(3):683-90.

10 Elizabeth A. Erwin, MD,,* Hayley R. James, BS, Heather M. Gutekunst, MD, John M. Russo, MD, Kelly J. Kelleher, MD, and Thomas A.E. Platts-Mills, MD, PhD2; Serum IgE measurement increases detection of food allergy among pediatric patients with eosinophilic esophagitis; Ann Allergy Asthma Immunol. 2010 Jun; 104(6): 496–502.

11 https://cellsciencesystems.com/providers/alcat-test/

12 Schmitt WH Jr, Leisman G.; Correlation of applied kinesiology muscle testing findings with serum immunoglobulin levels for food allergies.; Int J Neurosci. 1998 Dec;96(3-4):237-44.

13 http://journals.plos.org/plosone/article?id=10.1371/journal.pone.0060726

14 George Yuan, Khalid Z. Al-Shali, and Robert A. Hegele; Hypertriglyceridemia: its etiology, effects and treatment; CMAJ. 2007 Apr 10; 176(8): 1113–1120.

15 By Alan R. Gaby, MD; Vitamin D Deficiency: Irrational Exuberance?; https://www.integrativepractitioner.com/topics/environmental-health/vitamin-d-irrational-exuberance/

16 http://www.aafp.org/afp/recommendations/viewRecommendation. htm?recommendationId=140

17 https://www.vitamindcouncil.org/the-physiology-of-vitamin-d/

18 Selhub J.; Public health significance of elevated homocysteine.; Food Nutr Bull. 2008 Jun;29(2 Suppl):S116-25.

19 Catargi B, Parrot-Roulaud F, Cochet C, Ducassou D, Roger P, Tabarin A.; Homocysteine, hypothyroidism, and effect of thyroid hormone replacement.; Thyroid. 1999 Dec;9(12):1163-6.

20 Perungavur N. Ranganathan, Yan Lu, Lingli Jiang, Changae Kim, and James F. Collinscorresponding author; Serum ceruloplasmin protein expression and activity increases in iron-deficient rats and is further enhanced by higher dietary copper intake; Blood. 2011 Sep 15; 18(11): 3146–3153.

21 Kono S1, Suzuki H, Takahashi K, Takahashi Y, Shirakawa K, Murakawa Y, Yamaguchi S, Miyajima H.; Hepatic iron overload associated with a decreased serum ceruloplasmin level in a novel clinical type of aceruloplasminemia.; Gastroenterology. 2006 Jul;131(1):240-5.

22 Gerald Koenig and Stephanie Seneff; Gamma-Glutamyltransferase: A Predictive Biomarker of Cellular Antioxidant Inadequacy and Disease Risk; Volume 2015 (2015), Disease Markers Article ID 818570, 18 pages

[23] Vining RF, McGinley RA, Maksvytis JJ, Ho KY.; Salivary cortisol: a better measure of adrenal cortical function than serum cortisol.; Ann Clin Biochem. 1983 Nov;20 (Pt 6):329-35.

[24] Aardal-Eriksson E, Karlberg BE, Holm AC.; Salivary cortisol—an alternative to serum cortisol determinations in dynamic function tests.; Clin Chem Lab Med. 1998 Apr;36(4):215-22.

[25] Gozansky WS, Lynn JS, Laudenslager ML, Kohrt WM.; Salivary cortisol determined by enzyme immunoassay is preferable to serum total cortisol for assessment of dynamic hypothalamic—pituitary—adrenal axis activity.; Clin Endocrinol (Oxf). 2005 Sep;63(3):336-41.

[26] Kiang-Tech J.Yeo, PhD, Nikolina Babic, PhD, Zeina Hannoush, MD, and Roy E Weiss, M.D., PhD.; Endocrine Testing Protocols: Hypothalamic Pituitary Adrenal Axis; https://www.ncbi.nlm.nih.gov/books/NBK278940/

[27] Dastych M, Dastych M Jr, Novotná H, Číhalová J.; Lactulose/mannitol test and specificity, sensitivity, and area under curve of intestinal permeability parameters in patients with liver cirrhosis and Crohn's disease.; Dig Dis Sci. 2008 Oct;53(10):2789-92.

[28] Johnston SD, Smye M, Watson RG, McMillan SA, Trimble ER, Love AH.; Lactulose-mannitol intestinal permeability test: a useful screening test for adult coeliac disease.; Ann Clin Biochem. 2000 Jul;37 (Pt 4):512-9.

[29] Guo S, Al-Sadi R, Said HM, Ma TY.; Lipopolysaccharide causes an increase in intestinal tight junction permeability in vitro and in vivo by inducing enterocyte membrane expression and localization of TLR-4 and CD14.; Am J Pathol. 2013 Feb;182(2):375-87.

[30] O'Dwyer ST, Michie HR, Ziegler TR, Revhaug A, Smith RJ, Wilmore DW.; A single dose of endotoxin increases intestinal permeability in healthy humans.; Arch Surg. 1988 Dec;123(12):1459-64.

[31] http://www.mayomedicallaboratories.com/test-catalog/Clinical+and+Interpretive/84421

[32] Hamed Samavat, MS and Mindy S Kurzer, PhD; Estrogen Metabolism and Breast Cancer; Cancer Lett. 2015 Jan 28; 356(2 0 0): 231–243.

[33] Swaran J.S. Flora and Vidhu Pachauri; Chelation in Metal Intoxication; Int J Environ Res Public Health. 2010 Jul; 7(7): 2745–2788.

[34] Ishihara N, Matsushiro T.; Biliary and urinary excretion of metals in humans.; Arch Environ Health. 1986 Sep-Oct;41(5):324-30.

[35] Ma ZF1, Skeaff SA.; Thyroglobulin as a biomarker of iodine deficiency: a review.; Thyroid. 2014 Aug;24(8):1195-209. doi: 10.1089/thy.2014.0052. Epub 2014 Jun 12.

[36] Krejbjerg A1, Bjergved L, Bülow Pedersen I, Carlé A, Knudsen N, Perrild H, Ovesen L, Banke Rasmussen L, Laurberg P.; Serum thyroglobulin as a biomarker of iodine deficiency in adult populations.; Clin Endocrinol (Oxf). 2016 Sep;85(3):475-82.

[37] Ji Hye Yim, Eui Young Kim, Won Bae Kim,corresponding author Won Gu Kim, Tae Yong Kim, Jin-Sook Ryu, Gyungyub Gong, Suck Joon Hong, Jong Ho Yoon, and Young Kee Shong; Long-Term Consequence of Elevated Thyroglobulin in Differentiated Thyroid Cancer; Thyroid. 2013 Jan; 23(1): 58–63.

[38] Evans C, Tennant S, Perros P.; Thyroglobulin in differentiated thyroid cancer.; Clin Chim Acta. 2015 Apr 15;444:310-7.

[39] Sampson HA.; Food allergy. Part 1: immunopathogenesis and clinical disorders.; J Allergy Clin Immunol. 1999 May;103(5 Pt 1):717-28.

[40] Julie Wangcorresponding author and Hugh A Sampson; Food allergy: recent advances in pathophysiology and treatment; Allergy Asthma Immunol Res. 2009 Oct; 1(1): 19–29.

[41] Sicherer SH, Sampson HA.; Food allergy: Epidemiology, pathogenesis, diagnosis, and treatment.; J Allergy Clin Immunol. 2014 Feb;133(2):291-307; quiz 308.

[42] Perrier C, Corthésy B.; Gut permeability and food allergies.; Clin Exp Allergy. 2011 Jan;41(1):20-8.

[43] Ortolani C, Pastorello EA.; Food allergies and food intolerances.; Best Pract Res Clin Gastroenterol. 2006;20(3):467-83.

[44] Hanusková E, Plevková J.; Histamine intolerance.; Cesk Fysiol. 2013;62(1):26-33.

[45] Rejane Mattar, Daniel Ferraz de Campos Mazo, and Flair José Carrilho; Lactose intolerance: diagnosis, genetic, and clinical factors; Clin Exp Gastroenterol. 2012; 5: 113–121.

[46] Kaukinen K, Partanen J, Mäki M, Collin P.; HLA-DQ typing in the diagnosis of celiac disease.; Am J Gastroenterol. 2002 Mar;97(3):695-9.

[47] Welker MJ1, Orlov D. ; Thyroid nodules.; Am Fam Physician. 2003 Feb 1;67(3):559-66.

[48] Dean DS, Gharib H.; Epidemiology of thyroid nodules.; Best Pract Res Clin Endocrinol Metab. 2008 Dec;22(6):901-11.

[49] Xu S, Chen G, Peng W, Renko K, Derwahl M.; Oestrogen action on thyroid progenitor cells: relevant for the pathogenesis of thyroid nodules?; J Endocrinol. 2013 Jun 1;218(1):125-33.

[50] Kim MH, Park YR, Lim DJ, Yoon KH, Kang MI, Cha BY, Lee KW, Son HY.; The relationship between thyroid nodules and uterine fibroids.; Endocr J. 2010;57(7):615-21. Epub 2010 May 13.

[51] Geanina Popoveniuc, MD, Jacqueline Jonklaas, MD, PhD; Thyroid Nodules; Med Clin North Am. 2012 Mar; 96(2): 329–349.

[52] Rebecca Smith-Bindman, MD, Rebecca Smith-Bindman, MD, Paulette Lebda, MD; Risk of Thyroid Cancer Based on Thyroid Ultrasound Imaging Characteristics; JAMA Intern Med. 2013;173(19):1788-1795.

SECTION FOUR:

[1] Thérèse Truong, Dominique Baron-Dubourdieu, Yannick Rougier,3 and Pascal Guénel1,; Role of dietary iodine and cruciferous vegetables in thyroid cancer: a countrywide case-control study in New Caledonia; Cancer Causes Control. 2010 Aug; 21(8): 1183–1192.

[2] Busker RW, van Helden HP.; Toxicologic evaluation of pepper spray as a possible weapon for the Dutch police force: risk assessment and efficacy.; Am J Forensic Med Pathol. 1998 Dec;19(4):309-16.

[3] Miller JJ, Skolnick J.; Inhalation injury after capsaicin exposure.; J Ky Med Assoc. 2006 Mar;104(3):103-5.

[4] Steffee CH, Lantz PE, Flannagan LM, Thompson RL, Jason DR.; Oleoresin capsicum (pepper) spray and "in-custody deaths".; Am J Forensic Med Pathol. 1995 Sep;16(3):185-92.

[5] Wierenga JM, Hollingworth RM.; Inhibition of insect acetylcholinesterase by the potato glycoalkaloid alpha-chaconine.; Nat Toxins. 1992;1(2):96-9.

[6] A.Tajner-CzopekM.Jarych-SzyszkaG.Lisinska; Changes in glycoalkaloids content of potatoes destined for consumption; Food Chemistry Volume 106, Issue 2, 15 January 2008, Pages 706-711

[7] Joseph SV, Edirisinghe I, Burton-Freeman BM.; Fruit Polyphenols: A Review of Anti-inflammatory Effects in Humans.; Crit Rev Food Sci Nutr. 2016;56(3):419-44.

[8] González-Gallego J, García-Mediavilla MV, Sánchez-Campos S, Tuñón MJ.; Fruit polyphenols, immunity and inflammation.; Br J Nutr. 2010 Oct;104 Suppl 3:S15-27.

[9] Christensen AS, Viggers L, Hasselström K, Gregersen S.; Effect of fruit restriction on glycemic control in patients with type 2 diabetes—a randomized trial.; Nutr J. 2013 Mar 5;12:29.

[10] V Persky, M Turyk, H A Anderson, L P Hanrahan, C Falk, D N Steenport, R Chatterton, Jr, S Freels, and Great Lakes Consortium; The effects of PCB exposure and fish consumption on endogenous hormones.; Environ Health Perspect. 2001 Dec; 109(12): 1275–1283.

[11] Fitzgerald EF, Hwang SA, Langguth K, Cayo M, Yang BZ, Bush B, Worswick P, Lauzon T.; Fish consumption and other environmental exposures and their associations with serum PCB concentrations among Mohawk women at Akwesasne.; Environ Res. 2004 Feb;94(2):160-70.

[12] Judd N, Griffith WC, Faustman EM.; Contribution of PCB exposure from fish consumption to total dioxin-like dietary exposure.; Regul Toxicol Pharmacol. 2004 Oct;40(2):125-35.

[13] Raj Kishor Gupta, Shivraj Singh Gangoliya, and Nand Kumar Singhcorresponding author; Reduction of phytic acid and enhancement of bioavailable micronutrients in food grains; J Food Sci Technol. 2015 Feb; 52(2): 676–684.

[14] McWilliam V, Koplin J, Lodge C, Tang M, Dharmage S, Allen K.; The Prevalence of Tree Nut Allergy: A Systematic Review.; Curr Allergy Asthma Rep. 2015 Sep;15(9):54.

[15] Mark J Messina; Legumes and soybeans: overview of their nutritional profiles and health effects1,2; http://ajcn.nutrition.org/content/70/3/439s.full

[16] Bouchenak M, Lamri-Senhadji M.;Nutritional quality of legumes, and their role in cardiometabolic risk prevention: a review.; J Med Food. 2013 Mar;16(3):185-98.

[17] Goebel-Stengel M, Mönnikes H.; [Malabsorption of fermentable oligo-, di-, or monosaccharides and polyols (FODMAP) as a common cause of unclear abdominal discomfort].; Dtsch Med Wochenschr. 2014 Jun;139(24):1310-4.

[18] Melis MS.; Effects of chronic administration of Stevia rebaudiana on fertility in rats.; J Ethnopharmacol. 1999 Nov 1;67(2):157-61.

[19] Denina I, Semjonovs P, Fomina A, Treimane R, Linde R.; The influence of stevia glycosides on the growth of Lactobacillus reuteri strains.; Lett Appl Microbiol. 2014 Mar;58(3):278-84.

[20] Zheng Y, Liu Z, Ebersole J, Huang CB.; A new antibacterial compound from Luo Han Kuo fruit extract (Siraitia grosvenori).; J Asian Nat Prod Res. 2009 Aug;11(8):761-5.

[21] Allouche Y, Jiménez A, Gaforio JJ, Uceda M, Beltrán G.; How heating affects extra virgin olive oil quality indexes and chemical composition.; J Agric Food Chem. 2007 Nov 14;55(23):9646-54. Epub 2007 Oct 13.

[22] Casal S, Malheiro R, Sendas A, Oliveira BP, Pereira JA.; Olive oil stability under deep-frying conditions.;Food Chem Toxicol. 2010 Oct;48(10):2972-9.

[23] Ding LA, Li JS.; Effects of glutamine on intestinal permeability and bacterial translocation in TPN-rats with endotoxemia.; World J Gastroenterol. 2003 Jun;9(6):1327-32.

[24] Hond ED, Peeters M, Hiele M, Bulteel V, Ghoos Y, Rutgeerts P.; Effect of glutamine on the intestinal permeability changes induced by indomethacin in humans.; Aliment Pharmacol Ther. 1999 May;13(5):679-85.

[25] dos Santos Rd, Viana ML, Generoso SV, Arantes RE, Davisson Correia MI, Cardoso VN.; Glutamine supplementation decreases intestinal permeability and preserves gut mucosa integrity in an experimental mouse model.; JPEN J Parenter Enteral Nutr. 2010 Jul-Aug;34(4):408-13.

[26] Afriyanti D, Kroeze C, Saad A.; Indonesia palm oil production without deforestation and peat conversion by 2050.; Sci Total Environ. 2016 Jul 1;557-558:562-70.

[27] https://nccih.nih.gov/health/meditation/overview.htm

[28] Davidson RJ, Kabat-Zinn J, Schumacher J, Rosenkranz M, Muller D, Santorelli SF, Urbanowski F, Harrington A, Bonus K, Sheridan JF.; Alterations in brain and immune function produced by mindfulness meditation.; Psychosom Med. 2003 Jul-Aug;65(4):564-70.

[29] Jain S, Shapiro SL, Swanick S, Roesch SC, Mills PJ, Bell I, Schwartz GE.; A randomized controlled trial of mindfulness meditation versus relaxation training: effects on distress, positive states of mind, rumination, and distraction.; Ann Behav Med. 2007 Feb;33(1):11-21.

[30] Singh Y, Sharma R, Talwar A.; Immediate and long-term effects of meditation on acute stress reactivity, cognitive functions, and intelligence.; Altern Ther Health Med. 2012 Nov-Dec;18(6):46-53.

[31] https://nccih.nih.gov/health/yoga

[32] Riley KE, Park CL.; How does yoga reduce stress? A systematic review of mechanisms of change and guide to future inquiry.; Health Psychol Rev. 2015;9(3):379-96.

[33] Dana L Frank, BS, Lamees Khorshid, PsyD, Jerome F Kiffer, MA, Christine S Moravec, PhD,corresponding author and Michael G McKee, PhD; Biofeedback in medicine: who, when, why and how?; Ment Health Fam Med. 2010 Jun; 7(2): 85–91.

[34] Jane B Lemaire, Jean E Wallace, Adriane M Lewin, Jill de Grood, and Jeffrey P Schaefer; The effect of a biofeedback-based stress management tool on physician stress: a randomized controlled clinical trial; Open Med. 2011; 5(4): e154–e165.

[35] Cutshall SM, Wentworth LJ, Wahner-Roedler DL, Vincent A, Schmidt JE, Loehrer LL, Cha SS, Bauer BA.; Evaluation of a biofeedback-assisted meditation program as a stress management tool for hospital nurses: a pilot study.; Explore (NY). 2011 Mar-Apr;7(2):110-2.

[36] Lin G, Xiang Q, Fu X, Wang S, Wang S, Chen S, Shao L, Zhao Y, Wang T.; Heart rate variability biofeedback decreases blood pressure in prehypertensive subjects by improving autonomic function and baroreflex.; J Altern Complement Med. 2012 Feb;18(2):143-52.

[37] Tan G, Dao TK, Farmer L, Sutherland RJ, Gevirtz R.; Heart rate variability (HRV) and posttraumatic stress disorder (PTSD): a pilot study.; Appl Psychophysiol Biofeedback. 2011 Mar;36(1):27-35.

[38] Vanderlei LC, Pastre CM, Hoshi RA, Carvalho TD, Godoy MF.; Basic notions of heart rate variability and its clinical applicability.; Rev Bras Cir Cardiovasc. 2009 Apr-Jun;24(2):205-17.

[39] Faye S Routledge, PhD RN, Tavis S Campbell, PhD, Judith A McFetridge-Durdle, PhD RN, and Simon L Bacon, PhD; Improvements in heart rate variability with exercise therapy; Can J Cardiol. 2010 Jun-Jul; 26(6): 303–312.

[40] Lynn SJ, Malakataris A, Condon L, Maxwell R, Cleere C.; Post-traumatic stress disorder: cognitive hypnotherapy, mindfulness, and acceptance-based treatment approaches.; Am J Clin Hypn. 2012 Apr;54(4):311-30.

[41] Hammond DC.; Hypnosis in the treatment of anxiety- and stress-related disorders.; Expert Rev Neurother. 2010 Feb;10(2):263-73.

[42] Alladin A.; Evidence-based hypnotherapy for depression.; Int J Clin Exp Hypn. 2010 Apr;58(2):165-85.

[43] Ng BY, Lee TS.; Hypnotherapy for sleep disorders.; Ann Acad Med Singapore. 2008 Aug;37(8):683-8.

[44] Whorwell PJ.; Review article: The history of hypnotherapy and its role in the irritable bowel syndrome.; Aliment Pharmacol Ther. 2005 Dec;22(11-12):1061-7.

[45] Lindfors P, Unge P, Arvidsson P, Nyhlin H, Björnsson E, Abrahamsson H, Simrén M.; Effects of gut-directed hypnotherapy on IBS in different clinical settings-results from two randomized, controlled trials.; Am J Gastroenterol. 2012 Feb;107(2):276-85.

[46] Weber C, Arck P, Mazurek B, Klapp BF.; Impact of a relaxation training on psychometric and immunologic parameters in tinnitus sufferers.; J Psychosom Res. 2002 Jan;52(1):29-33.

[47] Wood GJ, Bughi S, Morrison J, Tanavoli S, Tanavoli S, Zadeh HH.; Hypnosis, differential expression of cytokines by T-cell subsets, and the hypothalamo-pituitary-adrenal axis.; Am J Clin Hypn. 2003 Jan;45(3):179-96.

[48] Gruzelier J, Clow A, Evans P, Lazar I, Walker L.; Mind-body influences on immunity: lateralized control, stress, individual differences predictors, and prophylaxis.; Ann N Y Acad Sci. 1998 Jun 30;851:487-94.

[49] Dorothy Long Parma, Daniel C Hughes, Sagar Ghosh, Rong Li, Rose A Treviño-Whitaker, Susan M Ogden, and Amelie G Ramirezcorresponding author; Effects of

six months of Yoga on inflammatory serum markers prognostic of recurrence risk in breast cancer survivors; Springerplus. 2015; 4: 143.

[50] Arora S, Bhattacharjee J.; Modulation of immune responses in stress by Yoga.; Int J Yoga. 2008 Jul;1(2):45-55. doi: 10.4103/0973-6131.43541.

[51] Black DS, Cole SW, Irwin MR, Breen E, St Cyr NM, Nazarian N, Khalsa DS, Lavretsky H.; Yogic meditation reverses NF-?B and IRF-related transcriptome dynamics in leukocytes of family dementia caregivers in a randomized controlled trial.; Psychoneuroendocrinology. 2013 Mar;38(3):348-55.

[52] Patak P, Willenberg HS, Bornstein SR.; Vitamin C is an important cofactor for both adrenal cortex and adrenal medulla.; Endocr Res. 2004 Nov;30(4):871-5.

[53] Brody S, Preut R, Schommer K, Schürmeyer TH.; A randomized controlled trial of high dose ascorbic acid for reduction of blood pressure, cortisol, and subjective responses to psychological stress.; Psychopharmacology (Berl). 2002 Jan;159(3):319-24. Epub 2001 Nov 20.

[54] Jaroenporn S, Yamamoto T, Itabashi A, Nakamura K, Azumano I, Watanabe G, Taya K.; Effects of pantothenic acid supplementation on adrenal steroid secretion from male rats.; Biol Pharm Bull. 2008 Jun;31(6):1205-8.

[55] David A. Camfield, Mark A. Wetherell,Andrew B. Scholey, Katherine H. M. Cox, Erin Fogg, David J. White, Jerome Sarris, Marni Kras, Con Stough, Avni Sali, and Andrew Pipingas,; The Effects of Multivitamin Supplementation on Diurnal Cortisol Secretion and Perceived Stress; Nutrients. 2013 Nov; 5(11): 4429–4450.

[56] Elena Diaz, Fatima Ruiz, Itziar Hoyos, Jaime Zubero, Leyre Gravina, Javier Gil, Jon Irazusta, and Susana Maria Gil,; Cell Damage, Antioxidant Status, and Cortisol Levels Related to Nutrition in Ski Mountaineering During a Two-Day Race; J Sports Sci Med. 2010 Jun; 9(2): 338–346.

[57] Hesham R. Omar,corresponding author Irina Komarova, Mohamed El-Ghonemi, Ahmed Fathy, Rania Rashad, Hany D. Abdelmalak, Muralidhar Reddy Yerramadha, Yaseen Ali, Engy Helal, and Enrico M. Camporesi; Licorice abuse: time to send a warning message; Ther Adv Endocrinol Metab. 2012 Aug; 3(4): 125–138.

[58] Kelly GS.; Rhodiola rosea: a possible plant adaptogen.; Altern Med Rev. 2001 Jun;6(3):293-302.

[59] Wang SM1, Lee LJ, Lin WW, Chang CM.; Effects of a water-soluble extract of Cordyceps sinensis on steroidogenesis and capsular morphology of lipid droplets in cultured rat adrenocortical cells.; J Cell Biochem. 1998 Jun 15;69(4):483-9.

[60] Monteleone P, Beinat L, Tanzillo C, Maj M, Kemali D.; Effects of phosphatidylserine on the neuroendocrine response to physical stress in humans.; Neuroendocrinology. 1990 Sep;52(3):243-8.

[61] Michael A Starks, Stacy L Starks, Michael Kingsley, Martin Purpura, and Ralf Jäger; The effects of phosphatidylserine on endocrine response to moderate intensity exercise; J Int Soc Sports Nutr. 2008; 5: 11.

[62] https://www.livestrong.com/article/289824-foods-that-contain-phosphatidylserine/

[63] Douglas S Kalman,corresponding author Samantha Feldman, Robert Feldman, Howard I Schwartz, Diane R Krieger, and Robert Garrison; Effect of a proprietary

Magnolia and Phellodendron extract on stress levels in healthy women: a pilot, double-blind, placebo-controlled clinical trial; Nutr J. 2008; 7: 11.

[64] Michael A Starks, Stacy L Starks, Michael Kingsley, Martin Purpura, and Ralf Jägercorresponding; The effects of phosphatidylserine on endocrine response to moderate intensity exercise; J Int Soc Sports Nutr. 2008; 5: 11.

[65] Mishra LC1, Singh BB, Dagenais S.; Scientific basis for the therapeutic use of Withania somnifera (ashwagandha): a review.; Altern Med Rev. 2000 Aug;5(4):334-46.

[66] Khan MK1, Jalil MA, Khan MS.; Oral contraceptives in gall stone diseases.; Mymensingh Med J. 2007 Jul;16(2 Suppl):S40-45.

[67] Palmery M, Saraceno A, Vaiarelli A, Carlomagno G.; Oral contraceptives and changes in nutritional requirements.; Eur Rev Med Pharmacol Sci. 2013 Jul;17(13):1804-13.

[68] Kossman DA, Williams NI, Domchek SM, Kurzer MS, Stopfer JE, Schmitz KH.; Exercise lowers estrogen and progesterone levels in premenopausal women at high risk of breast cancer.; J Appl Physiol (1985). 2011 Dec;111(6):1687-93. doi: 10.1152/japplphysiol.00319.2011. Epub 2011 Sep 8.

[69] Smith AJ, Phipps WR, Thomas W, Schmitz KH, Kurzer MS.; The effects of aerobic exercise on estrogen metabolism in healthy premenopausal women.; Cancer Epidemiol Biomarkers Prev. 2013 May;22(5):756-64.

[70] Laura Mulvey, Alamelu Chandrasekaran,1 Kai Liu,1 Sarah Lombardi,1 Xue-Ping Wang,1 Karen J Auborn,1,2,3 and Leslie Goodwin; Interplay of Genes Regulated by Estrogen and Diindolylmethane in Breast Cancer Cell Lines; Mol Med. 2007 Jan-Feb; 13(1-2): 69–78.

[71] Dalessandri KM, Firestone GL, Fitch MD, Bradlow HL, Bjeldanes LF; Pilot study: effect of 3,3'-diindolylmethane supplements on urinary hormone metabolites in postmenopausal women with a history of early-stage breast cancer.; Nutr Cancer. 2004;50(2):161-7.

[72] Döll M.; The premenstrual syndrome: effectiveness of Vitex agnus castus.; Med Monatsschr Pharm. 2009 May;32(5):186-91.

[73] Wuttke W, Jarry H, Christoffel V, Spengler B, Seidlová-Wuttke D.; Chaste tree (Vitex agnus-castus)—pharmacology and clinical indications.; Phytomedicine. 2003 May;10(4):348-57.

[74] Fukuda Y, Bamba H, Okui M, Tamura K, Tanida N, Satomi M, Shimoyama T, Nishigami T.; Helicobacter pylori infection increases mucosal permeability of the stomach and intestine.; Digestion. 2001;63 Suppl 1:93-6.

[75] Mei Xing Lim,a,b Chin Wen Png,a,b Crispina Yan Bing Tay,a,b Joshua Ding Wei Teo,a Huipeng Jiao,a,b Norbert Lehming,a Kevin Shyong Wei Tan,corresponding authora and Yongliang Zhangcorresponding authora,b; Differential Regulation of Proinflammatory Cytokine Expression by Mitogen-Activated Protein Kinases in Macrophages in Response to Intestinal Parasite Infection; Infect Immun. 2014 Nov; 82(11): 4789–4801.

[76] De Magistris L, Secondulfo M, Sapone A, Carratù R, Iafusco D, Prisco F, Generoso M, Cartenì M, Mezzogiorno A, Esposito V.; Infection with Giardia and intestinal permeability in humans.; Gastroenterology. 2003 Jul;125(1):277-9; author reply 279.

[77] Yan L, Yang C, Tang J.; Disruption of the intestinal mucosal barrier in Candida albicans infections.; Microbiol Res. 2013 Aug 25;168(7):389-95.

[78] Carol A. Kumamoto*; Inflammation and gastrointestinal Candida colonization; Curr Opin Microbiol. 2011 Aug; 14(4): 386–391.

[79] S M Riordan, V M Duncombe, M C Thomas, A Nagree, T D Bolin, C J McIver, and R Williams; Small intestinal bacterial overgrowth, intestinal permeability, and non-alcoholic steatohepatitis; Gut. 2002 Jan; 50(1): 136–138.

[80] Yean Jung Choi, Melissa J. Seelbach, Hong Pu, Sung Yong Eum, Lei Chen, Bei Zhang, Bernhard Hennig, and Michal Toborek; Polychlorinated Biphenyls Disrupt Intestinal Integrity via NADPH Oxidase-Induced Alterations of Tight Junction Protein Expression; Environ Health Perspect. 2010 Jul; 118(7): 976–981.

[81] Vázquez M, Vélez D, Devesa V.; In vitro evaluation of inorganic mercury and methylmercury effects on the intestinal epithelium permeability.; Food Chem Toxicol. 2014 Dec;74:349-59.

[82] Jeong CH, Seok JS, Petriello MC, Han SG.; Arsenic downregulates tight junction claudin proteins through p38 and NF-?B in intestinal epithelial cell line, HT-29.; Toxicology. 2017 Mar 15;379:31-39.

[83] G Sigthorsson, J Tibble, J Hayllar, I Menzies, A Macpherson, R Moots, D Scott, M Gumpel, and I Bjarnason; Intestinal permeability and inflammation in patients on NSAIDs; Gut. 1998 Oct; 43(4): 506–511.

[84] Tulstrup MV, Christensen EG, Carvalho V, Linninge C2, Ahrné S, Højberg O, Licht TR, Bahl MI.; Antibiotic Treatment Affects Intestinal Permeability and Gut Microbial Composition in Wistar Rats Dependent on Antibiotic Class.; PLoS One. 2015 Dec 21;10(12):e0144854.

[85] Julia König, Jerry Wells, Patrice D Cani, Clara L García-Ródenas, Tom MacDonald, Annick Mercenier, Jacqueline Whyte, Freddy Troost, and Robert-Jan Brummer; Human Intestinal Barrier Function in Health and Disease; Clin Transl Gastroenterol. 2016 Oct; 7(10): e196.

[86] Imhann F, Bonder MJ, Vich Vila A, Fu J, Mujagic Z, Vork L, Tigchelaar EF, Jankipersadsing SA, Cenit MC, Harmsen HJ, Dijkstra G, Franke L, Xavier RJ, Jonkers D, Wijmenga C, Weersma RK, Zhernakova A.; Proton pump inhibitors affect the gut microbiome.; Gut. 2016 May;65(5):740-8.

[87] Shunji Fujimori; What are the effects of proton pump inhibitors on the small intestine?; World J Gastroenterol. 2015 Jun 14; 21(22): 6817–6819.

[88] Lo WK, Chan WW.; Proton pump inhibitor use and the risk of small intestinal bacterial overgrowth: a meta-analysis.; Clin Gastroenterol Hepatol. 2013 May;11(5):483-90.

[89] Vanuytsel T, van Wanrooy S, Vanheel H, Vanormelingen C, Verschueren S, Houben E, Salim Rasoel S, T?th J, Holvoet L, Farré R, Van Oudenhove L, Boeckxstaens G, Verbeke K, Tack J.; Psychological stress and corticotropin-releasing hormone increase intestinal permeability in humans by a mast cell-dependent mechanism.; Gut. 2014 Aug;63(8):1293-9.

[90] Zheng G, Wu SP, Hu Y, Smith DE, Wiley JW, Hong S.; Corticosterone mediates stress-related increased intestinal permeability in a region-specific manner.; Neurogastroenterol Motil. 2013 Feb;25(2):e127-39.

[91] Rana Al-Sadi, Michel Boivin, and Thomas Ma, Mechanism of cytokine modulation of epithelial tight junction barrier; Front Biosci. 2009 Jan 1; 14: 2765–2778.

[92] A. H. M. Viswanatha Swamy and P A. Patil; Effect of Some Clinically Used Proteolytic Enzymes on Inflammation in Rats; Indian J Pharm Sci. 2008 Jan-Feb; 70(1): 114–117.

[93] Mecikoglu M, Saygi B, Yildirim Y, Karadag-Saygi E, Ramadan SS, Esemenli T.; The effect of proteolytic enzyme serratiopeptidase in the treatment of experimental implant-related infection.; J Bone Joint Surg Am. 2006 Jun;88(6):1208-14.

[94] Anderson JW, Baird P, Davis RH Jr, Ferreri S, Knudtson M, Koraym A, Waters V, Williams Health benefits of dietary fiber.; Nutr Rev. 2009 Apr;67(4):188-205.

[95] Eaton The ancestral human diet: what was it and should it be a paradigm for contemporary nutrition?; Proc Nutr Soc. 2006 Feb;65(1):1-6.

[96] Joanne Slavin; Fiber and Prebiotics: Mechanisms and Health Benefits; Nutrients. 2013 Apr; 5(4): 1417–1435.

[97] Mingming Zhang, Qian Zhou, Robert G. Dorfman, Xiaoli Huang, Tingting Fan, Hao Zhang, Jun Zhang,corresponding author2 and Chenggong Yucorresponding author1; Butyrate inhibits interleukin-17 and generates Tregs to ameliorate colorectal colitis in rats; BMC Gastroenterol. 2016; 16: 84.

[98] Grazul H, Kanda LL, Gondek D.; Impact of probiotic supplements on microbiome diversity following antibiotic treatment of mice; Gut Microbes. 2016;7(2):101-14.

[99] Jin JS, Touyama M, Hisada T, Benno Y.; Effects of green tea consumption on human fecal microbiota with special reference to Bifidobacterium species.; Microbiol Immunol. 2012 Nov;56(11):729-39.

[100] Dan C Vodnar and Carmen Socaciu; Green tea increases the survival yield of Bifidobacteria in simulated gastrointestinal environment and during refrigerated conditions; Chem Cent J. 2012; 6: 61.

[101] Zeinhom M, Tellez AM, Delcenserie V, El-Kholy AM, El-Shinawy SH, Griffiths MW.; Yogurt containing bioactive molecules produced by Lactobacillus acidophilus La-5 exerts a protective effect against enterohemorrhagic Escherichia coli in mice.; J Food Prot. 2012 Oct;75(10):1796-805.

[102] Todorov SD, Furtado DN, Saad SM, Gombossy de Melo Franco BD.; Bacteriocin production and resistance to drugs are advantageous features for Lactobacillus acidophilus La-14, a potential probiotic strain.; New Microbiol. 2011 Oct;34(4):357-70. Epub 2011 Oct 31.

[103] Sanders ME.; Summary of probiotic activities of Bifidobacterium lactis HN019.; J Clin Gastroenterol. 2006 Oct;40(9):776-83.

[104] Shu Q, Lin H, Rutherfurd KJ, Fenwick SG, Prasad J, Gopal PK, Gill HS.; Dietary Bifidobacterium lactis (HN019) enhances resistance to oral Salmonella typhimurium infection in mice.; Microbiol Immunol. 2000;44(4):213-22.

[105] Holscher HD, Czerkies LA, Cekola P, Litov R, Benbow M, Santema S, Alexander DD, Perez V, Sun S, Saavedra JM, Tappenden KA.; Bifidobacterium lactis Bb12 enhances

intestinal antibody response in formula-fed infants: a randomized, double-blind, controlled trial.; JPEN J Parenter Enteral Nutr. 2012 Jan;36(1 Suppl):106S-17S.

[106] Sgouras D, Maragkoudakis P, Petraki K, Martinez-Gonzalez B, Eriotou E, Michopoulos S, Kalantzopoulos G, Tsakalidou E, Mentis A.; In vitro and in vivo inhibition of Helicobacter pylori by Lactobacillus casei strain Shirota.; Appl Environ Microbiol. 2004 Jan;70(1):518-26.

[107] Villena J, Salva S, Agüero G, Alvarez S.; Immunomodulatory and protective effect of probiotic Lactobacillus casei against Candida albicans infection in malnourihed mice.; Microbiol Immunol. 2011 Jun;55(6):434-45.

[108] Bueno DJ, Silva JO, Oliver G, González SN.; Lactobacillus casei CRL 431 and Lactobacillus rhamnosus CRL 1224 as biological controls for Aspergillus flavus J Food Prot. 2006 Oct;69(10):2544-8.

[109] Philippe Ducrotté, Prabha Sawant, and Venkataraman Jayanthi; Clinical trial: Lactobacillus plantarum 299v (DSM 9843) improves symptoms of irritable bowel syndrome; World J Gastroenterol. 2012 Aug 14; 18(30): 4012–4018.

[110] Sen S, Mullan MM, Parker TJ, Woolner JT, Tarry SA, Hunter JO.; Effect of Lactobacillus plantarum 299v on colonic fermentation and symptoms of irritable bowel syndrome.; Dig Dis Sci. 2002 Nov;47(11):2615-20.;

[111] Giselle Nobre Costa, Francismar Corrêa Marcelino-Guimarães, Gislayne Trindade Vilas-Bôas, Tiemi Matsuo, and Lucia Helena S. Miglioranzaa; Potential Fate of Ingested Lactobacillus plantarum and Its Occurrence in Human Feces; Appl Environ Microbiol. 2014 Feb; 80(3): 1013–1019.

[112] Liu S, Hu P, Du X, Zhou T, Pei X.; Lactobacillus rhamnosus GG supplementation for preventing respiratory infections in children: a meta-analysis of randomized, placebo-controlled trials.; Indian Pediatr. 2013 Apr;50(4):377-81.

[113] Szajewska H, Kolodziej M.; Systematic review with meta-analysis: Lactobacillus rhamnosus GG in the prevention of antibiotic-associated diarrhoea in children and adults.; Aliment Pharmacol Ther. 2015 Nov;42(10):1149-57.

[114] Marco Toscano, Roberta De Grandi, Laura Stronati, Elena De Vecchi, and Lorenzo Drago; Effect of Lactobacillus rhamnosus HN001 and Bifidobacterium longum BB536 on the healthy gut microbiota composition at phyla and species level: A preliminary study; World J Gastroenterol. 2017 Apr 21; 23(15): 2696–2704.

[115] Wickens KL, Barthow CA, Murphy R, Abels PR, Maude RM, Stone PR, Mitchell EA, Stanley TV, Purdie GL, Kang JM, Hood FE, Rowden JL, Barnes PK, Fitzharris PF, Crane J.; Early pregnancy probiotic supplementation with Lactobacillus rhamnosus HN001 may reduce the prevalence of gestational diabetes mellitus: a randomised controlled trial.; Br J Nutr. 2017 Mar;117(6):804-813.

[116] Krasowska A, Murzyn A, Dyjankiewicz A, Lukaszewicz M, Dziadkowiec D.; The antagonistic effect of Saccharomyces boulardii on Candida albicans filamentation, adhesion and biofilm formation.; FEMS Yeast Res. 2009 Dec;9(8):1312-21.

[117] Jawhara S, Poulain D.; Saccharomyces boulardii decreases inflammation and intestinal colonization by Candida albicans in a mouse model of chemically-induced colitis.; Med Mycol. 2007 Dec;45(8):691-700.

[118] Guslandi M, Mezzi G, Sorghi M, Testoni PA.; Saccharomyces boulardii in maintenance treatment of Crohn's disease.; Dig Dis Sci. 2000 Jul;45(7):1462-4.

[119] Garcia Vilela E, De Lourdes De Abreu Ferrari M, Oswaldo Da Gama Torres H, Guerra Pinto A, Carolina Carneiro Aguirre A, Paiva Martins F, Marcos Andrade Goulart E, Sales Da Cunha A.; Influence of Saccharomyces boulardii on the intestinal permeability of patients with Crohn's disease in remission.; Scand J Gastroenterol. 2008;43(7):842-8.

[120] Justino PF, Melo LF, Nogueira AF, Costa JV, Silva LM, Santos CM, Mendes WO, Costa MR, Franco AX, Lima AA, Ribeiro RA, Souza MH, Soares PM.; Treatment with Saccharomyces boulardii reduces the inflammation and dysfunction of the gastrointestinal tract in 5-fluorouracil-induced intestinal mucositis in mice.; Br J Nutr. 2014 May;111(9):1611-21.

[121] Bader J, Albin A, Stahl U.; Spore-forming bacteria and their utilisation as probiotics.; Benef Microbes. 2012 Mar 1;3(1):67-75. doi: 10.3920/BM2011.0039.

[122] McFarlin BK, Henning AL, Bowman EM, Gary MA, Carbajal KM.; Oral spore-based probiotic supplementation was associated with reduced incidence of post-prandial dietary endotoxin, triglycerides, and disease risk biomarkers.; World J Gastrointest Pathophysiol. 2017 Aug 15;8(3):117-126. doi: 10.4291/wjgp.v8.i3.117.

[123] Lübbert C, Salzberger B, Mössner J.; Fecal microbiota transplantation.; Internist (Berl). 2017 May;58(5):456-468. doi: 10.1007/s00108-017-0203-6.

[124] Seon Ho Bak, Hyun Ho Choi, Jinhee Lee, Mi Hee Kim, Youn Hee Lee, Jin Su Kim, and Young-Seok Cho; Fecal microbiota transplantation for refractory Crohn's disease; Intest Res. 2017 Apr; 15(2): 244–248.

[125] Ahmet Uygun, MD,a Kadir Ozturk, MD,a,* Hakan Demirci, MD,a Cem Oger, MD,a Ismail Yasar Avci, MD,b Turker Turker, MD, PhD,c and Mustafa Gulsen, MDa, Fecal microbiota transplantation is a rescue treatment modality for refractory ulcerative colitis; Medicine (Baltimore). 2017 Apr; 96(16): e6479.

[126] Meng-Que Xu, Hai-Long Cao, Wei-Qiang Wang, Shan Wang, Xiao-Cang Cao, Fang Yan, and Bang-Mao Wang; Fecal microbiota transplantation broadening its application beyond intestinal disorders; World J Gastroenterol. 2015 Jan 7; 21(1): 102–111.

[127] Bergström J, Fürst P, Norée LO, Vinnars E.; Intracellular free amino acid concentration in human muscle tissue.; J Appl Physiol. 1974 Jun;36(6):693-7.

[128] Yang H, Söderholm JD, Larsson J, Permert J, Lindgren J, Wirén M.; Bidirectional supply of glutamine maintains enterocyte ATP content in the in vitro using chamber model.; Int J Colorectal Dis. 2000 Nov;15(5-6):291-6.

[129] Ding LA, Li JS.; Effects of glutamine on intestinal permeability and bacterial translocation in TPN-rats with endotoxemia.; World J Gastroenterol. 2003 Jun;9(6):1327-32.

[130] Hond ED, Peeters M, Hiele M, Bulteel V, Ghoos Y, Rutgeerts P.; Effect of glutamine on the intestinal permeability changes induced by indomethacin in humans.; Aliment Pharmacol Ther. 1999 May;13(5):679-85.

[131] dos Santos Rd, Viana ML, Generoso SV, Arantes RE, Davisson Correia MI, Cardoso VN.; Glutamine supplementation decreases intestinal permeability and preserves

gut mucosa integrity in an experimental mouse model.; JPEN J Parenter Enteral Nutr. 2010 Jul-Aug;34(4):408-13.

[132] Sonja Skrovanek, Katherine DiGuilio, Robert Bailey, William Huntington, Ryan Urbas, Barani Mayilvaganan, Giancarlo Mercogliano, and James M Mullin; Zinc and gastrointestinal disease; World J Gastrointest Pathophysiol. 2014 Nov 15; 5(4): 496–513.

[133] Chen P, Soares AM, Lima AA, Gamble MV, Schorling JB, Conway M, Barrett LJ, Blaner WS, Guerrant RL.; Association of vitamin A and zinc status with altered intestinal permeability: analyses of cohort data from northeastern Brazil.; J Health Popul Nutr. 2003 Dec;21(4):309-15.

[134] A Mahmood, A J FitzGerald, T Marchbank, E Ntatsaki, D Murray, S Ghosh, and R J Playford; Zinc carnosine, a health food supplement that stabilises small bowel integrity and stimulates gut repair processes; Gut. 2007 Feb; 56(2): 168–175.

[135] Amit-Romach E, Uni Z, Cheled S, Berkovich Z, Reifen Bacterial population and innate immunity-related genes in rat gastrointestinal tract are altered by vitamin A-deficient diet.; J Nutr Biochem. 2009 Jan;20(1):70-7.

[136] Teff KL.; Visceral nerves: vagal and sympathetic innervation.; JPEN J Parenter Enteral Nutr. 2008 Sep-Oct;32(5):569-71.

[137] Innes KE, Bourguignon C, Taylor AG.; Risk indices associated with the insulin resistance syndrome, cardiovascular disease, and possible protection with yoga: a systematic review.; J Am Board Fam Pract. 2005 Nov-Dec;18(6):491-519.

[138] Abe C, Uchida T, Ohta M, Ichikawa T, Yamashita K, Ikeda S.; Cytochrome P450-dependent metabolism of vitamin E isoforms is a critical determinant of their tissue concentrations in rats.; Lipids. 2007 Jul;42(7):637-45. Epub 2007 May 23.

[139] Tsuchiya Y, Nakajima M, Yokoi T.; Cytochrome P450-mediated metabolism of estrogens and its regulation in human.; Cancer Lett. 2005 Sep 28;227(2):115-24. Epub 2004 Nov 19.

[140] Jones G, Prosser DE, Kaufmann M.; Cytochrome P450-mediated metabolism of vitamin D.; J Lipid Res. 2014 Jan;55(1):13-31.

[141] Zhou SF, Liu JP, Chowbay B.; Polymorphism of human cytochrome P450 enzymes and its clinical impact.; Drug Metab Rev. 2009;41(2):89-295.

[142] Park YJ, Lee EK, Lee YK, Park DJ, Jang HC, Moore DD.; Opposing regulation of cytochrome P450 expression by CAR and PXR in hypothyroid mice.; Toxicol Appl Pharmacol. 2012 Sep 1;263(2):131-7.

[143] O'Leary KA, Li HC, Ram PA, McQuiddy P, Waxman DJ, Kasper CB.; Thyroid regulation of NADPH:cytochrome P450 oxidoreductase: identification of a thyroid-responsive element in the 5'-flank of the oxidoreductase gene.; Mol Pharmacol. 1997 Jul;52(1):46-53.

[144] Brtko J, Dvorak Z.; Role of retinoids, rexinoids and thyroid hormone in the expression of cytochrome p450 enzymes.; Curr Drug Metab. 2011 Feb;12(2):71-88.

[145] Liu D, Waxman DJ.; Post-transcriptional regulation of hepatic NADPH-cytochrome P450 reductase by thyroid hormone: independent effects on poly(A) tail length and mRNA stability.; Mol Pharmacol. 2002 May;61(5):1089-96.

[146] Lee SA, Fowke JH, Lu W, Ye C, Zheng Y, Cai Q, Gu K, Gao YT, Shu XO, Zheng W.; Cruciferous vegetables, the GSTP1 Ile105Val genetic polymorphism, and breast cancer risk.; Am J Clin Nutr. 2008 Mar;87(3):753-60.

[147] Shaw WD, Walker M, Benson M.; Treating and drinking well water in the presence of health risks from arsenic contamination: results from a U.S. hot spot.; Risk Anal. 2005 Dec;25(6):1531-43.

[148] Wasserman GA, Liu X, Loiacono NJ, Kline J, Factor-Litvak P, van Geen A, Mey JL, Levy D, Abramson R, Schwartz A, Graziano JH.; A cross-sectional study of well water arsenic and child IQ in Maine schoolchildren.; Environ Health. 2014 Apr 1;13(1):23.

[149] Kurttio P, Pukkala E, Kahelin H, Auvinen A, Pekkanen J.; Arsenic concentrations in well water and risk of bladder and kidney cancer in Finland.; Environ Health Perspect. 1999 Sep;107(9):705-10.

[150] Lynge E, Tinnerberg H, Rylander L, Romundstad P, Johansen K, Lindbohm ML, Heikkilä P, Westberg H, Clausen LB, Piombino A, Thorsted BL.; Exposure to tetrachloroethylene in dry cleaning shops in the Nordic countries.; Ann Occup Hyg. 2011 May;55(4):387-96.

[151] Guha N, Loomis D, Grosse Y, Lauby-Secretan B, El Ghissassi F, Bouvard V, Benbrahim-Tallaa L, Baan R, Mattock H, Straif K; International Agency for Research on Cancer Monograph Working Group.; Carcinogenicity of trichloroethylene, tetrachloroethylene, some other chlorinated solvents, and their metabolites.; Lancet Oncol. 2012 Dec;13(12):1192-3.

[152] Azimi Pirsaraei SR, Khavanin A, Asilian H, Soleimanian A.; Occupational exposure to perchloroethylene in dry-cleaning shops in Tehran, Iran.; Ind Health. 2009 Apr;47(2):155-9.

[153] http://www.epa.gov/drycleaningrule/basic.html

[154] Ceballos DM, Whittaker SG, Lee EG, Roberts J, Streicher R, Nourian F, Gong W, Broadwater K.; Occupational exposures to new dry cleaning solvents: High-flashpoint hydrocarbons and butylal.; J Occup Environ Hyg. 2016 Oct 2;13(10):759-69.

[155] Sinsheimer P, Grout C, Namkoong A, Gottlieb R.; The viability of professional wet cleaning as a pollution prevention alternative to perchloroethylene dry cleaning.; J Air Waste Manag Assoc. 2007 Feb;57(2):172-8.

[156] Carolina Barragán-Martínez,1 Cesar A. Speck-Hernández,1 Gladis Montoya-Ortiz,1 Rubén D. Mantilla,1 Juan-Manuel Anaya,1 and Adriana Rojas-Villarraga1,; Organic Solvents as Risk Factor for Autoimmune Diseases: A Systematic Review and Meta-Analysis; PLoS One. 2012; 7(12): e51506.

[157] Tanya Tillett, MA; Formaldehyde Exposure among Children: A Potential Building Block of Asthma; Environ Health Perspect. 2010 Mar; 118(3): A131.

[158] Chang JC, Fortmann R, Roache N, Lao HC.; Evaluation of low-VOC latex paints.; Indoor Air. 1999 Dec;9(4):253-8.

[159] Anderson RC, Anderson JH.; Respiratory toxicity of mattress emissions in mice.; Arch Environ Health. 2000 Jan-Feb;55(1):38-43.

[160] Rajwanshi P, Singh V, Gupta MK, Kumari V, Shrivastav R, Ramanamurthy M, Dass S.; Studies on aluminium leaching from cookware in tea and coffee and estimation

of aluminium content in toothpaste, baking powder and paan masala.; Sci Total Environ. 1997 Jan 30;193(3):243-9.

[161] Kristin L. Kamerud, Kevin A. Hobbie, and Kim A. Anderson; Stainless Steel Leaches Nickel and Chromium into Foods During Cooking; J Agric Food Chem. 2013 Oct 2; 61(39): 9495–9501.

[162] Geerligs PD, Brabin BJ, Omari AA.; Food prepared in iron cooking pots as an intervention for reducing iron deficiency anaemia in developing countries: a systematic review.; J Hum Nutr Diet. 2003 Aug;16(4):275-81.

[163] Sokal P, Sokal K.; The neuromodulative role of earthing.; Med Hypotheses. 2011 Nov;77(5):824-6.

[164] Chevalier G.; The effect of grounding the human body on mood.; Psychol Rep. 2015 Apr;116(2):534-42.

[165] Omura Y, Shimotsuura Y, Fukuoka A, Fukuoka H, Nomoto T.; Significant mercury deposits in internal organs following the removal of dental amalgam, & development of pre-cancer on the gingiva and the sides of the tongue and their represented organs as a result of inadvertent exposure to strong curing light (used to solidify synthetic dental filling material) & effective treatment: a clinical case report, along with organ representation areas for each tooth.; Acupunct Electrother Res. 1996 Apr-Jun;21(2):133-60.

[166] Aga M, Iwaki K, Ueda Y, Ushio S, Masaki N, Fukuda S, Kimoto T, Ikeda M, Kurimoto M.; Preventive effect of Coriandrum sativum (Chinese parsley) on localized lead deposition in ICR mice.; J Ethnopharmacol. 2001 Oct;77(2-3):203-8.

[167] Nicholas Eriksson, Shirley Wu, Chuong B Do, Amy K Kiefer, Joyce Y Tung, Joanna L Mountain, David A Hinds and Uta Francke; A genetic variant near olfactory receptor genes influences cilantro preference; Flavour 2012 1:22

[168] Post-White J, Ladas EJ, Kelly KM.; Advances in the use of milk thistle (Silybum marianum).; Integr Cancer Ther. 2007 Jun;6(2):104-9.

[169] Pradhan SC, Girish C.; Hepatoprotective herbal drug, silymarin from experimental pharmacology to clinical medicine.; Indian J Med Res. 2006 Nov;124(5):491-504.

[170] Shalan MG, Mostafa MS, Hassouna MM, El-Nabi SE, El-Refaie A.; Amelioration of lead toxicity on rat liver with Vitamin C and silymarin supplements.; Toxicology. 2005 Jan 5;206(1):1-15.

[171] Jain A, Yadav A, Bozhkov AI, Padalko VI, Flora SJ.; Therapeutic efficacy of silymarin and naringenin in reducing arsenic-induced hepatic damage in young rats.; Ecotoxicol Environ Saf. 2011 May;74(4):607-14.

[172] N Ballatori, M W Lieberman, and W Wang; N-acetylcysteine as an antidote in methylmercury poisoning.; Environ Health Perspect. 1998 May; 106(5): 267–271.

[173] Reddy PS, Rani GP, Sainath SB, Meena R, Supriya Ch.; Protective effects of N-acetylcysteine against arsenic-induced oxidative stress and reprotoxicity in male mice.; J Trace Elem Med Biol. 2011 Dec;25(4):247-53.

[174] Martin DS, Willis SE, Cline DM.; N-acetylcysteine in the treatment of human arsenic poisoning.; J Am Board Fam Pract. 1990 Oct-Dec;3(4):293-6.

[175] Kannan GM, Flora SJ.; Combined administration of N-acetylcysteine and monoisoamyl DMSA on tissue oxidative stress during arsenic chelation therapy.; Biol Trace Elem Res. 2006 Apr;110(1):43-59.

[176] Kate Petersen Shay,1 Régis F. Moreau,1 Eric J. Smith,1,2 Anthony R. Smith,1 and Tory M. Hagen1,2; Alpha-lipoic acid as a dietary supplement: Molecular mechanisms and therapeutic potential; Biochim Biophys Acta. 2009 Oct; 1790(10): 1149–1160.

[177] Patrick L.; Mercury toxicity and antioxidants: Part 1: role of glutathione and alpha-lipoic acid in the treatment of mercury toxicity.; Altern Med Rev. 2002 Dec;7(6):456-71.

[178] Gurer H, Ozgunes H, Oztezcan S, Ercal N.; Antioxidant role of alpha-lipoic acid in lead toxicity.; Free Radic Biol Med. 1999 Jul;27(1-2):75-81.

[179] Pande M, Flora SJ.; Lead induced oxidative damage and its response to combined administration of alpha-lipoic acid and succimers in rats.; Toxicology. 2002 Aug 15;177(2-3):187-96.

[180] Margaret E. Sears; Chelation: Harnessing and Enhancing Heavy Metal Detoxification—A Review; ScientificWorldJournal. 2013; 2013: 219840.

[181] Patrick L; Mercury toxicity and antioxidants: Part 1: role of glutathione and alpha-lipoic acid in the treatment of mercury toxicity; Altern Med Rev. 2002 Dec;7(6):456-71.

[182] Singhal RK, Anderson ME, Meister A.; Glutathione, a first line of defense against cadmium toxicity.; FASEB J. 1987 Sep;1(3):220-3.

[183] Struzynska L, Sulkowski G, Lenkiewicz A, Rafalowska U.; Lead stimulates the glutathione system in selective regions of rat brain.; Folia Neuropathol. 2002;40(4):203-9.

[184] Merchant RE, Andre CA.; A review of recent clinical trials of the nutritional supplement Chlorella pyrenoidosa in the treatment of fibromyalgia, hypertension, and ulcerative colitis.; Altern Ther Health Med. 2001 May-Jun;7(3):79-91.

[185] Uchikawa T, Maruyama I, Kumamoto S, Ando Y, Yasutake A.; Chlorella suppresses methylmercury transfer to the fetus in pregnant mice.; J Toxicol Sci. 2011 Oct;36(5):675-80.

[186] Shim JA, Son YA, Park JM, Kim MK.; Effect of Chlorella intake on Cadmium metabolism in rats.; Nutr Res Pract. 2009 Spring;3(1):15-22.

[187] Bae MJ, Shin HS, Chai OH, Han JG, Shon DH.; Inhibitory effect of unicellular green algae (Chlorella vulgaris) water extract on allergic immune response.; J Sci Food Agric. 2013 Sep;93(12):3133-6.

[188] Jung Hyun Kwak, Seung Han Baek, Yongje Woo, Jae Kab Han, Byung Gon Kim, Oh Yoen Kim,corresponding author and Jong Ho Leecorresponding author; Beneficial immunostimulatory effect of short-term Chlorella supplementation: enhancement of Natural Killer cell activity and early inflammatory response (Randomized, double-blinded, placebo-controlled trial); Nutr J. 2012; 11: 53.

[189] Fatma Vatansever and Michael R. Hamblin; Far infrared radiation (FIR): its biological effects and medical applications; Photonics Lasers Med. 2012 Nov 1; 4: 255–266.

[190] Sheppard AR, Swicord ML, Balzano Q.; Quantitative evaluations of mechanisms of radiofrequency interactions with biological molecules and processes.; Health Phys. 2008 Oct;95(4):365-96.

[191] Margaret E. Sears, Kathleen J. Kerr, and Riina I. Bray; Arsenic, Cadmium, Lead, and Mercury in Sweat: A Systematic Review; J Environ Public Health. 2012; 2012: 184745.

[192] Minshall C, Nadal J, Exley C.; Aluminium in human sweat.; J Trace Elem Med Biol. 2014 Jan;28(1):87-8.

[193] Genuis SJ, Beesoon S, Birkholz D, Lobo RA.; Human excretion of bisphenol A: blood, urine, and sweat (BUS) study.; J Environ Public Health. 2012;2012:185731.

[194] Stephen J. Genuis, Sanjay Beesoon, Rebecca A. Lobo, and Detlef Birkholz; Human Elimination of Phthalate Compounds: Blood, Urine, and Sweat (BUS) Study; ScientificWorldJournal. 2012; 2012: 615068.

[195] Saat M, Singh R, Sirisinghe RG, Nawawi M.; Rehydration after exercise with fresh young coconut water, carbohydrate-electrolyte beverage and plain water.; J Physiol Anthropol Appl Human Sci. 2002 Mar;21(2):93-104.

[196] Oosterveld FG, Rasker JJ, Floors M, Landkroon R, van Rennes B, Zwijnenberg J, van de Laar MA, Koel GJ.; Infrared sauna in patients with rheumatoid arthritis and ankylosing spondylitis. A pilot study showing good tolerance, short-term improvement of pain and stiffness, and a trend towards long-term beneficial effects.; Clin Rheumatol. 2009 Jan;28(1):29-34. doi: 10.1007/s10067-008-0977-y. Epub 2008 Aug 7.

[197] Flora SJ, Mittal M, Mehta A.; Heavy metal induced oxidative stress & its possible reversal by chelation therapy.; Indian J Med Res. 2008 Oct;128(4):501-23.

[198] Crinnion WJ; EDTA Redistribution of Lead and Cadmium Into the Soft Tissues in a Human With a High Lead Burden – Should DMSA Always Be Used to Follow EDTA in Such Cases; http://www.altmedrev.com/publications/16/2/109.pdf

[199] Margaret E. Sears; Chelation: Harnessing and Enhancing Heavy Metal Detoxification—A Review; ScientificWorldJournal. 2013; 2013: 219840.

[200] Torres-Alanís O, Garza-Ocañas L, Bernal MA, Piñeyro-López A.; Urinary excretion of trace elements in humans after sodium 2,3-dimercaptopropane-1-sulfonate challenge test.; J Toxicol Clin Toxicol. 2000;38(7):697-700.

[201] James B Adams, Matthew Baral, Elizabeth Geis, Jessica Mitchell, Julie Ingram, Andrea Hensley, Irene Zappia, Sanford Newmark, Eva Gehn, Robert A Rubin, Ken Mitchell, Jeff Bradstreet, and Jane El-Dahr; Safety and efficacy of oral DMSA therapy for children with autism spectrum disorders: Part A - Medical results; BMC Clin Pharmacol. 2009; 9: 16.

[202] Cabañero AI, Carvalho C, Madrid Y, Batoréu C, Cámara C.; Quantification and speciation of mercury and selenium in fish samples of high consumption in Spain and Portugal.; Biol Trace Elem Res. 2005 Jan;103(1):17-35.

[203] Mazokopakis EE, Papadakis JA, Papadomanolaki MG, Batistakis AG, Giannakopoulos TG, Protopapadakis EE, Ganotakis ES.; Effects of 12 months treatment with L-selenomethionine on serum anti-TPO Levels in Patients with Hashimoto's thyroiditis.; Thyroid. 2007 Jul;17(7):609-12.

[204] Omer Turker, Kamil Kumanlioglu1, Inanc Karapolat2 and Ismail Dogan; Selenium treatment in autoimmune thyroiditis: 9-month follow-up with variable doses; http://joe.endocrinology-journals.org/content/190/1/151.full

[205] Hill MJ.; Intestinal flora and endogenous vitamin synthesis.; Eur J Cancer Prev. 1997 Mar;6 Suppl 1:S43-5.

[206] Palmery M, Saraceno A, Vaiarelli A, Carlomagno G.; Oral contraceptives and changes in nutritional requirements.; Eur Rev Med Pharmacol Sci. 2013 Jul;17(13):1804-13.

[207] Joel J. Heidelbaugh; Proton pump inhibitors and risk of vitamin and mineral deficiency: evidence and clinical implications; Ther Adv Drug Saf. 2013 Jun; 4(3): 125–133.

[208] Richard Deichmann, MD,* Carl Lavie, MD,† and Samuel Andrews, MD‡; Coenzyme Q10 and Statin-Induced Mitochondrial Dysfunction; Ochsner J. 2010 Spring; 10(1): 16–21.

[209] Sun-Hye Ko, Sun-Hee Ko,1 Yu-Bae Ahn,1 Ki-Ho Song,1 Kyung-Do Han,2 Yong-Moon Park,3,4 Seung-Hyun Ko,1 and Hye-Soo Kim,1; Association of Vitamin B12 Deficiency and Metformin Use in Patients with Type 2 Diabetes; J Korean Med Sci. 2014 Jul; 29(7): 965–972.

[210] Guntram Bezold, M.D., Monika Lange, M.D., Ralf Uwe Peter, M.D; Homozygous Methylenetetrahydrofolate Reductase C677T Mutation and Male Infertility; N Engl J Med 2001; 344:1172-1173

[211] Lara Pizzorno, MDiv, MA, LMT; Nothing Boring About Boron; Integr Med (Encinitas). 2015 Aug; 14(4): 35–48.

[212] Cimino JA, Jhangiani S, Schwartz E, Cooperman JM.; Riboflavin metabolism in the hypothyroid human adult.; Proc Soc Exp Biol Med. 1987 Feb;184(2):151-3.

[213] Amin Talebi Bezmin Abadi; Helicobacter pylori: A Beneficial Gastric Pathogen?; Front Med (Lausanne). 2014; 1: 26.

[214] Graham DY.; The changing epidemiology of GERD: geography and Helicobacter pylori.; Am J Gastroenterol. 2003 Jul;98(7):1462-70.

[215] Falk GW.; Evaluating the Association of Helicobacter pylori to GERD.; Gastroenterol Hepatol (N Y). 2008 Sep;4(9):631-2.

[216] Junod C.; Blastocystis hominis: a common commensal in the colon. Study of prevalence in different populations of Paris.; Presse Med. 1995 Nov 25;24(36):1684-8.

[217] Senay H, MacPherson D.; Blastocystis hominis: epidemiology and natural history.; J Infect Dis. 1990 Oct;162(4):987-90.

[218] Reinthaler FF, Mascher F, Marth E.; Blastocystis hominis—intestinal parasite or commensal?.; Wien Med Wochenschr. 1988 Nov 15;138(21):545-7.

[219] R R Babb and S Wagener; Blastocystis hominis—a potential intestinal pathogen.; West J Med. 1989 Nov; 151(5): 518–519.

[220] Duda A, Kosik-Bogacka D, Lanocha N, Szymanski S.; Blastocystis hominis-parasites or commensals?.; Ann Acad Med Stetin. 2014;60(1):23-8.

221 Christina M. Coyle, Julie Varughese, Louis M. Weiss, Herbert B. Tanowitz; Blastocystis: To Treat or Not to Treat... ; Clinical Infectious Diseases, Volume 54, Issue 1, 1 January 2012, Pages 105–110, https://doi.org/10.1093/cid/cir810

222 Aydin A, Ersöz G, Tekesin O, Akçiçek E, Tuncyürek M.; Garlic oil and Helicobacter pylori infection.; Am J Gastroenterol. 2000 Feb;95(2):563-4.

223 Ankri S, Mirelman D.; Antimicrobial properties of allicin from garlic.; Microbes Infect. 1999 Feb;1(2):125-9.

224 Ross ZM, O'Gara EA, Hill DJ, Sleightholme HV, Maslin DJ.; Antimicrobial properties of garlic oil against human enteric bacteria: evaluation of methodologies and comparisons with garlic oil sulfides and garlic powder.; Appl Environ Microbiol. 2001 Jan;67(1):475-80.

225 Guo NL, Lu DP, Woods GL, Reed E, Zhou GZ, Zhang LB, Waldman RH.; Demonstration of the anti-viral activity of garlic extract against human cytomegalovirus in vitro.; Chin Med J (Engl). 1993 Feb;106(2):93-6.

226 Weber ND, Andersen DO, North JA, Murray BK, Lawson LD, Hughes BG.; In vitro virucidal effects of Allium sativum (garlic) extract and compounds.; Planta Med. 1992 Oct;58(5):417-23.

227 Pozzatti P, Scheid LA, Spader TB, Atayde ML, Santurio JM, Alves SH.; In vitro activity of essential oils extracted from plants used as spices against fluconazole-resistant and fluconazole-susceptible Candida spp.; Can J Microbiol. 2008 Nov;54(11):950-6.

228 Soylu S, Yigitbas H, Soylu EM, Kurt S.; Antifungal effects of essential oils from oregano and fennel on Sclerotinia sclerotiorum.; J Appl Microbiol. 2007 Oct;103(4):1021-30.

229 Force M, Sparks WS, Ronzio RA.; Inhibition of enteric parasites by emulsified oil of oregano in vivo.; Phytother Res. 2000 May;14(3):213-4.

230 Ettefagh KA, Burns JT, Junio HA, Kaatz GW, Cech NB.; Goldenseal (Hydrastis canadensis L.) extracts synergistically enhance the antibacterial activity of berberine via efflux pump inhibition.; Planta Med. 2011 May;77(8):835-40.

231 Zhang LJ, Zhang LJ, Quan W, Wang BB, Shen BL, Zhang TT, Kang Y.; Berberine inhibits HEp-2 cell invasion induced by Chlamydophila pneumoniae infection.; J Microbiol. 2011 Oct;49(5):834-40.

232 Sun D, Abraham SN, Beachey EH.; Influence of berberine sulfate on synthesis and expression of Pap fimbrial adhesin in uropathogenic Escherichia coli.; Antimicrob Agents Chemother. 1988 Aug;32(8):1274-7.

233 Dabos KJ, Sfika E, Vlatta LJ, Giannikopoulos G.; The effect of mastic gum on Helicobacter pylori: a randomized pilot study.; Phytomedicine. 2010 Mar;17(3-4):296-9. doi: 10.1016/j.phymed.2009.09.010. Epub 2009 Oct 29.

234 Farhad U. Huwez, M.R.C.P., Ph.D., Debbie Thirlwell, B.Sc., Alan Cockayne, Ph.D., Dlawer A.A. Ala'Aldeen, Ph.D., M.R.C.Path.; Mastic Gum Kills Helicobacter pylori; N Engl J Med 1998; 339:1946

235 Reis SR, Valente LM, Sampaio AL, Siani AC, Gandini M, Azeredo EL, D'Avila LA, Mazzei JL, Henriques Md, Kubelka CF.; Immunomodulating and antiviral activities

of Uncaria tomentosa on human monocytes infected with Dengue Virus-2.; Int Immunopharmacol. 2008 Mar;8(3):468-76.

[236] Herrera DR, Tay LY, Rezende EC, Kozlowski VA Jr, Santos EB.; In vitro antimicrobial activity of phytotherapic Uncaria tomentosa against endodontic pathogens.;J Oral Sci. 2010 Sep;52(3):473-6.

[237] Medina AL, Lucero ME, Holguin FO, Estell RE, Posakony JJ, Simon J, O'Connell MA.; Composition and Antimicrobial Activity of Anemopsis californica leaf oil.; J Agric Food Chem. 2005 Nov 2;53(22):8694-8.

[238] Valipe SR, Nadeau JA, Annamali T, Venkitanarayanan K, Hoagland T.; In vitro antimicrobial properties of caprylic acid, monocaprylin, and sodium caprylate against Dermatophilus congolensis.; Am J Vet Res. 2011 Mar;72(3):331-5.

[239] Nair MK, Joy J, Vasudevan P, Hinckley L, Hoagland TA, Venkitanarayanan KS.; Antibacterial effect of caprylic acid and monocaprylin on major bacterial mastitis pathogens.; J Dairy Sci. 2005 Oct;88(10):3488-95.

[240] Omura Y, O'Young B, Jones M, Pallos A, Duvvi H, Shimotsuura Y.; Caprylic acid in the effective treatment of intractable medical problems of frequent urination, incontinence, chronic upper respiratory infection, root canalled tooth infection, ALS, etc., caused by asbestos & mixed infections of Candida albicans, Helicobacter pylori & cytomegalovirus with or without other microorganisms & mercury.; Acupunct Electrother Res. 2011;36(1-2):19-64.

[241] Eliezer Menezes Pereira, Thelma de Barros Machado, Ivana Correa Ramos Leal, Desyreé Murta Jesus, Clarissa Rosa de Almeida Damaso, Antonio Ventura Pinto, Marcia Giambiagi-deMarval, Ricardo Machado Kuster, and Kátia Regina Netto dos Santos; Tabebuia avellanedae naphthoquinones: activity against methicillin-resistant staphylococcal strains, cytotoxic activity and in vivo dermal irritability analysis; Ann Clin Microbiol Antimicrob. 2006; 5: 5.

[242] Morrill K, May K, Leek D, Langland N, Jeane LD, Ventura J, Skubisz C, Scherer S, Lopez E, Crocker E, Peters R, Oertle J, Nguyen K, Just S, Orian M, Humphrey M, Payne D, Jacobs B, Waters R, Langland J.; Spectrum of antimicrobial activity associated with ionic colloidal silver.; J Altern Complement Med. 2013 Mar;19(3):224-31.

[243] van Hasselt P, Gashe BA, Ahmad J.; Colloidal silver as an antimicrobial agent: fact or fiction?; J Wound Care. 2004 Apr;13(4):154-5.

[244] Gulbranson SH, Hud JA, Hansen RC.; Argyria following the use of dietary supplements containing colloidal silver protein.; Cutis. 2000 Nov;66(5):373-4.

[245] Chang AL, Khosravi V, Egbert B.; A case of argyria after colloidal silver ingestion.; J Cutan Pathol. 2006 Dec;33(12):809-11.

[246] Yildiz K, Basalan M, Duru O, Gökpinar S.; Antiparasitic efficiency of Artemisia absinthium on Toxocara cati in naturally infected cats.; Turkiye Parazitol Derg. 2011;35(1):10-4.

[247] Tariq KA, Chishti MZ, Ahmad F, Shawl AS.; Anthelmintic activity of extracts of Artemisia absinthium against ovine nematodes.; Vet Parasitol. 2009 Mar 9;160(1-2):83-8.

[248] Faramarz Zakavi, Leila Golpasand Hagh, Arash Daraeighadikolaei, Ahmad Farajzadeh Sheikh, Arsham Daraeighadikolaei, and Zahra Leilavi Shooshtari;

Antibacterial Effect of Juglans Regia Bark against Oral Pathologic Bacteria; Int J Dent. 2013; 2013: 854765.

[249] Head KA.; Natural approaches to prevention and treatment of infections of the lower urinary tract.; Altern Med Rev. 2008 Sep;13(3):227-44.

[250] Lin JC, Cherng JM, Hung MS, Baltina LA, Baltina L, Kondratenko R.; Inhibitory effects of some derivatives of glycyrrhizic acid against Epstein-Barr virus infection: structure-activity relationships.; Antiviral Res. 2008 Jul;79(1):6-11.

[251] Lin JC.; Mechanism of action of glycyrrhizic acid in inhibition of Epstein-Barr virus replication in vitro.; Antiviral Res. 2003 Jun;59(1):41-7.

[252] Griffith RS, DeLong DC, Nelson JD.; Relation of arginine-lysine antagonism to herpes simplex growth in tissue culture.; Chemotherapy. 1981;27(3):209-13.

[253] Griffith RS, Norins AL, Kagan C.; A multicentered study of lysine therapy in Herpes simplex infection.; Dermatologica. 1978;156(5):257-67.

[254] Minjung Lee, Myoungki Son, Eunhyun Ryu, Yu Su Shin, Jong Gwang Kim, Byung Woog Kang, Gi-Ho Sung, Hyosun Cho, and Hyojeung Kang; Quercetin-induced apoptosis prevents EBV infection; Oncotarget. 2015 May 20; 6(14): 12603–12624.

[255] Na X, Kelly C.; Probiotics in clostridium difficile Infection.; J Clin Gastroenterol. 2011 Nov;45 Suppl:S154-8.

[256] Krasowska A, Murzyn A, Dyjankiewicz A, Lukaszewicz M, Dziadkowiec D.; The antagonistic effect of Saccharomyces boulardii on Candida albicans filamentation, adhesion and biofilm formation.; FEMS Yeast Res. 2009 Dec;9(8):1312-21.

[257] Jawhara S, Poulain D.; Saccharomyces boulardii decreases inflammation and intestinal colonization by Candida albicans in a mouse model of chemically-induced colitis.; Med Mycol. 2007 Dec;45(8):691-700.

[258] Dinleyici EC, Eren M, Dogan N, Reyhanioglu S, Yargic ZA, Vandenplas Y.; Clinical efficacy of Saccharomyces boulardii or metronidazole in symptomatic children with Blastocystis hominis infection.; Parasitol Res. 2011 Mar;108(3):541-5.

[259] Ouoba LI, Diawara B, Jespersen L, Jakobsen M.; Antimicrobial activity of Bacillus subtilis and Bacillus pumilus during the fermentation of African locust bean (Parkia biglobosa) for Soumbala production.; J Appl Microbiol. 2007 Apr;102(4):963-70.

[260] Heggers JP, Cottingham J, Gusman J, Reagor L, McCoy L, Carino E, Cox R, Zhao JG.; The effectiveness of processed grapefruit-seed extract as an antibacterial agent: II. Mechanism of action and in vitro toxicity.; J Altern Complement Med. 2002 Jun;8(3):333-40.

[261] Høiby N, Ciofu O, Johansen HK, Song ZJ, Moser C, Jensen PØ, Molin S, Givskov M, Tolker-Nielsen T, Bjarnsholt T.; The clinical impact of bacterial biofilms.; Int J Oral Sci. 2011 Apr;3(2):55-65.

[262] Douglas LJ.; Candida biofilms and their role in infection.; Trends Microbiol. 2003 Jan;11(1):30-6.

[263] Reffuveille F, de la Fuente-Núñez C, Mansour S, Hancock RE.; A broad-spectrum antibiofilm peptide enhances antibiotic action against bacterial biofilms.; Antimicrob Agents Chemother. 2014 Sep;58(9):5363-71.

[264] Cammarota G, Sanguinetti M, Gallo A, Posteraro B.; Review article: biofilm formation by Helicobacter pylori as a target for eradication of resistant infection.; Aliment Pharmacol Ther. 2012 Aug;36(3):222-30.

[265] Coticchia JM, Sugawa C, Tran VR, Gurrola J, Kowalski E, Carron MA.; Presence and density of Helicobacter pylori biofilms in human gastric mucosa in patients with peptic ulcer disease.; J Gastrointest Surg. 2006 Jun;10(6):883-9.

[266] Grande R, Di Campli E, Di Bartolomeo S, Verginelli F, Di Giulio M, Baffoni M, Bessa LJ, Cellini L.; Helicobacter pylori biofilm: a protective environment for bacterial recombination.; J Appl Microbiol. 2012 Sep;113(3):669-76.

[267] Sapi E, Bastian SL, Mpoy CM, Scott S, Rattelle A, Pabbati N, Poruri A, Burugu D, Theophilus PA, Pham TV, Datar A, Dhaliwal NK, MacDonald A, Rossi MJ, Sinha SK, Luecke DF.; Characterization of biofilm formation by Borrelia burgdorferi in vitro.; PLoS One. 2012;7(10):e48277.

[268] Ioannidis A, Kyratsa A, Ioannidou V, Bersimis S, Chatzipanagiotou S.; Detection of biofilm production of Yersinia enterocolitica strains isolated from infected children and comparative antimicrobial susceptibility of biofilm versus planktonic forms.; Mol Diagn Ther. 2014 Jun;18(3):309-14.

[269] Wood TK.; Insights on Escherichia coli biofilm formation and inhibition from whole-transcriptome profiling.; Environ Microbiol. 2009 Jan;11(1):1-15.

[270] Beloin C, Roux A, Ghigo JM.; Escherichia coli biofilms.; Curr Top Microbiol Immunol. 2008;322:249-89.

[271] Stahlhut SG, Struve C, Krogfelt KA, Reisner A.; Biofilm formation of Klebsiella pneumoniae on urethral catheters requires either type 1 or type 3 fimbriae.; FEMS Immunol Med Microbiol. 2012 Jul;65(2):350-9.

[272] Warren L. Simmons and Kevin Dybvig; Mycoplasma Biofilms Ex Vivo and In Vivo; FEMS Microbiol Lett. 2009 Jun; 295(1): 77–81.

[273] McAuliffe L, Ellis RJ, Miles K, Ayling RD, Nicholas RA.; Biofilm formation by mycoplasma species and its role in environmental persistence and survival.; Microbiology. 2006 Apr;152(Pt 4):913-22.

[274] Kornspan JD, Tarshis M, Rottem Adhesion and biofilm formation of Mycoplasma pneumoniae on an abiotic surface.; Arch Microbiol. 2011 Nov;193(11):833-6.

[275] Desai JV, Mitchell AP.; Candida albicans Biofilm Development and Its Genetic Control.; Microbiol Spectr. 2015 Jun;3(3).

[276] Lotte Mathé and Patrick Van Dijck; Recent insights into Candida albicans biofilm resistance mechanisms; Curr Genet. 2013; 59(4): 251–264.

[277] Seneviratne CJ, Wang Y, Jin L, Abiko Y, Samaranayake LP.; Candida albicans biofilm formation is associated with increased anti-oxidative capacities.; Proteomics. 2008 Jul;8(14):2936-47.

[278] Chandra J, Kuhn DM, Mukherjee PK, Hoyer LL, McCormick T, Ghannoum MA.; Biofilm formation by the fungal pathogen Candida albicans: development, architecture, and drug resistance.; J Bacteriol. 2001 Sep;183(18):5385-94.

[279] Ann-Cathrin Olofsson,1, Malte Hermansson,2 and Hans Elwing1; N-Acetyl-l-Cysteine Affects Growth, Extracellular Polysaccharide Production, and Bacterial

Biofilm Formation on Solid Surfaces; Appl Environ Microbiol. 2003 Aug; 69(8): 4814–4822.

[280] Dinicola S, De Grazia S, Carlomagno G, Pintucci JP.; N-acetylcysteine as powerful molecule to destroy bacterial biofilms. A systematic review.; Eur Rev Med Pharmacol Sci. 2014 Oct;18(19):2942-8.

[281] Quah SY, Wu S, Lui JN, Sum CP, Tan KS.; N-acetylcysteine inhibits growth and eradicates biofilm of Enterococcus faecalis.; J Endod. 2012 Jan;38(1):81-5.

[282] El-Feky MA, El-Rehewy MS, Hassan MA, Abolella HA, Abd El-Baky RM, Gad GF.; Effect of ciprofloxacin and N-acetylcysteine on bacterial adherence and biofilm formation on ureteral stent surfaces.; Pol J Microbiol. 2009;58(3):261-7.

[283] Cammarota G, Sanguinetti M, Gallo A, Posteraro B.; Review article: biofilm formation by Helicobacter pylori as a target for eradication of resistant infection.; Aliment Pharmacol Ther. 2012 Aug;36(3):222-30.

[284] El-Baky Rehab Mahmoud Abd, Dalia Mohamed Mohamed Abo El Ela, Gamal Fad Mamoud Gad; N-acetylcysteine Inhibits and Eradicates Candida albicans Biofilms; http://pubs.sciepub.com/ajidm/2/5/5/ - AJIDM» Archive» Volume 2» Issue 5»Research Article

[285] Kaplan JB.; Biofilm matrix-degrading enzymes.; Methods Mol Biol. 2014;1147:203-13.

[286] Kaplan JB.; Therapeutic potential of biofilm-dispersing enzymes.; Int J Artif Organs. 2009 Sep;32(9):545-54.

[287] Thallinger B, Prasetyo EN, Nyanhongo GS, Guebitz GM.; Antimicrobial enzymes: an emerging strategy to fight microbes and microbial biofilms.; Biotechnol J. 2013 Jan;8(1):97-109.

[288] Monteiro DR, Takamiya AS2, Feresin LP2, Gorup LF3, de Camargo ER3, Delbem AC2, Henriques M4, Barbosa DB5.; Silver colloidal nanoparticle stability: influence on Candida biofilms formed on denture acrylic.; Med Mycol. 2014 Aug;52(6):627-35.

[289] Monteiro DR, Silva S, Negri M, Gorup LF, de Camargo ER, Oliveira R, Barbosa DB, Henriques M.; Silver colloidal nanoparticles: effect on matrix composition and structure of Candida albicans and Candida glabrata biofilms.; J Appl Microbiol. 2013 Apr;114(4):1175-83.

[290] Monteiro DR, Gorup LF, Silva S, Negri M, de Camargo ER, Oliveira R, Barbosa DB, Henriques M.; Silver colloidal nanoparticles: antifungal effect against adhered cells and biofilms of Candida albicans and Candida glabrata.; Biofouling. 2011 Aug;27(7):711-9.

[291] Goggin R, Jardeleza C, Wormald PJ, Vreugde S.; Colloidal silver: a novel treatment for Staphylococcus aureus biofilms?; Int Forum Allergy Rhinol. 2014 Mar;4(3):171-5.

[292] Rajiv S, Drilling A, Bassiouni A, James C, Vreugde S, Wormald PJ.; Topical colloidal silver as an anti-biofilm agent in a Staphylococcus aureus chronic rhinosinusitis sheep model.; Int Forum Allergy Rhinol. 2015 Apr;5(4):283-8.

[293] Berlutti F, Pantanella F, Natalizi T, Frioni A, Paesano R, Polimeni A, Valenti P.; Antiviral properties of lactoferrin—a natural immunity molecule.; Molecules. 2011 Aug 16;16(8):6992-7018.

[294] Hiroyuki Wakabayashi, Koji Yamauchi, Tetsuo Kobayashi, Tomoko Yaeshima, Keiji Iwatsuki, and Hiromasa Yoshie; Inhibitory Effects of Lactoferrin on Growth and Biofilm Formation of Porphyromonas gingivalis and Prevotella intermedia; Antimicrob Agents Chemother. 2009 Aug; 53(8): 3308–3316.

[295] Psaltis AJ, Wormald PJ, Ha KR, Tan LW.; Reduced levels of lactoferrin in biofilm-associated chronic rhinosinusitis.; Laryngoscope. 2008 May;118(5):895-901.

[296] M.C. Ammons, and V. Copié1; Lactoferrin: A bioinspired, anti-biofilm therapeutic; Biofouling. 2013 Apr; 29(4): 443–455.

[297] Oduwole KO, Glynn AA, Molony DC, Murray D, Rowe S, Holland LM, McCormack DJ, O'Gara JP.; Anti-biofilm activity of sub-inhibitory povidone-iodine concentrations against Staphylococcus epidermidis and Staphylococcus aureus.; J Orthop Res. 2010 Sep;28(9):1252-6.

[298] Thorn RM, Austin AJ, Greenman J, Wilkins JP, Davis PJ.; In vitro comparison of antimicrobial activity of iodine and silver dressings against biofilms.; J Wound Care. 2009 Aug;18(8):343-6.

[299] Vaidya B, Cho SY, Oh KS, Kim SH, Kim YO, Jeong EH, Nguyen TT, Kim SH, Kim IS, Kwon J, Kim D.; Effectiveness of Periodic Treatment of Quercetin against Influenza A Virus H1N1 through Modulation of Protein Expression.; J Agric Food Chem. 2016 Jun 1;64(21):4416-25.

[300] Haruno Nishimuro, Hirofumi Ohnishi, Midori Sato, Mayumi Ohnishi-Kameyama, Izumi Matsunaga, Shigehiro Naito, Katsunari Ippoushi, Hideaki Oike, Tadahiro Nagata, Hiroshi Akasaka, Shigeyuki Saitoh, Kazuaki Shimamoto, and Masuko Kobori,; Estimated Daily Intake and Seasonal Food Sources of Quercetin in Japan; Nutrients. 2015 Apr; 7(4): 2345–2358.

[301] Vgontzas A1, Bixler EO, Lin HM, Prolo P, Mastorakos G, Vela-Bueno A, Kales A, Chrousos GP.; Chronic insomnia is associated with nyctohemeral activation of the hypothalamic-pituitary-adrenal axis: clinical implications.; J Clin Endocrinol Metab. 2001 Aug;86(8):3787-94.

[302] Maria Basta, M.D., George P Chrousos, M.D, Antonio Vela-Bueno, M.D, and Alexandros N Vgontzas, M.D.; CHRONIC INSOMNIA AND STRESS SYSTEM; Sleep Med Clin. 2007 Jun; 2(2): 279–291.

[303] Healey ES, Kales A, Monroe LJ, Bixler EO, Chamberlin K, Soldatos CR.; Onset of insomnia: role of life-stress events.; Psychosom Med. 1981 Oct;43(5):439-51.

[304] Sanjay Kalra, Ambika Gopalakrishnan Unnikrishnan,1 and Rakesh Sahay2; The hypoglycemic side of hypothyroidism; Indian J Endocrinol Metab. 2014 Jan-Feb; 18(1): 1–3.

[305] Schultes B, Oltmanns KM, Kern W, Born J, Fehm HL, Peters A.; Acute and prolonged effects of insulin-induced hypoglycemia on the pituitary-thyroid axis in humans.; Metabolism. 2002 Oct;51(10):1370-4.

[306] Lange J, Arends J, Willms B.; Alcohol-induced hypoglycemia in type I diabetic patients.; Med Klin (Munich). 1991 Nov 15;86(11):551-4.

[307] H. A. Krebs, R. A. Freedland, R. Hems, and Marion Stubbs; Inhibition of hepatic gluconeogenesis by ethanol; Inhibition of hepatic gluconeogenesis by ethanol

[308] Lynnette K Nieman, MD; http://www.uptodate.com/contents/clinical-manifestations-of-adrenal-insufficiency-in-adults

[309] Debreceni L, Mészáros I.; Persistent hypoglycemia due to hyperinsulinemia, hypoglucagonemia and mild adrenal insufficiency.; Exp Clin Endocrinol. 1987 Sep;90(2):221-6.

[310] Zhdanova IV, Wurtman RJ, Regan MM, Taylor JA, Shi JP, Leclair OU.; Melatonin treatment for age-related insomnia.; J Clin Endocrinol Metab. 2001 Oct;86(10):4727-30.

[311] Halgamuge MN.; Pineal melatonin level disruption in humans due to electromagnetic fields and ICNIRP limits.; Radiat Prot Dosimetry. 2013 May;154(4):405-16.

[312] Joshua J. Gooley, Kyle Chamberlain, Kurt A. Smith, Sat Bir S. Khalsa, Shantha M. W. Rajaratnam, Eliza Van Reen, Jamie M. Zeitzer, Charles A. Czeisler, and Steven W. Lockley; Exposure to Room Light before Bedtime Suppresses Melatonin Onset and Shortens Melatonin Duration in Humans; J Clin Endocrinol Metab. 2011 Mar; 96(3): E463–E472.

[313] Figueiro MG, Wood B, Plitnick B, Rea MS.; The impact of light from computer monitors on melatonin levels in college students.; Neuro Endocrinol Lett. 2011;32(2):158-63.

[314] Andersen ML, Bittencourt LR, Antunes IB, Tufik S.; Effects of progesterone on sleep: a possible pharmacological treatment for sleep-breathing disorders?; Curr Med Chem. 2006;13(29):3575-82.

[315] Shazia Jehan, Alina Masters-Isarilov, Idoko Salifu, Ferdinand Zizi, Girardin Jean-Louis, Seithikurippu R Pandi-Perumal, Ravi Gupta, Amnon Brzezinski, and Samy I McFarlane,; Sleep Disorders in Postmenopausal Women; J Sleep Disord Ther. 2015 Aug; 4(5): 1000212.

[316] Samüel Deurveilher, PhD,1 Benjamin Rusak, PhD,2,3,4 and Kazue Semba, PhD1,2; Estradiol and Progesterone Modulate Spontaneous Sleep Patterns and Recovery from Sleep Deprivation in Ovariectomized Rats; Sleep. 2009 Jul 1; 32(7): 865–877.

[317] Rondanelli M, Opizzi A, Monteferrario F, Antoniello N, Manni R, Klersy C.; The effect of melatonin, magnesium, and zinc on primary insomnia in long-term care facility residents in Italy: a double-blind, placebo-controlled clinical trial.; J Am Geriatr Soc. 2011 Jan;59(1):82-90.

[318] Xiaopeng Ji and Jianghong Liu; Associations between Blood Zinc Concentrations and Sleep Quality in Childhood: A Cohort Study; Nutrients. 2015 Jul; 7(7): 5684–5696.

[319] Ursin R.; Serotonin and sleep.; Sleep Med Rev. 2002 Feb;6(1):55-69.

[320] Byrne EM, Johnson J, McRae AF, Nyholt DR, Medland SE, Gehrman PR, Heath AC, Madden PA, Montgomery GW, Chenevix-Trench G, Martin NG.; A genome-wide association study of caffeine-related sleep disturbance: confirmation of a role for a common variant in the adenosine receptor.; Sleep. 2012 Jul 1;35(7):967-75.

[321] Amy Yang, Abraham A. Palmer, and Harriet de Wit; Genetics of caffeine consumption and responses to caffeine; Psychopharmacology (Berl). 2010 Aug; 211(3): 245–257.

[322] Humphries P, Pretorius E, Naudé H.; Direct and indirect cellular effects of aspartame on the brain.; Eur J Clin Nutr. 2008 Apr;62(4):451-62. Epub 2007 Aug 8.

[323] Ebrahim IO, Shapiro CM, Williams AJ, Fenwick PB.; Alcohol and sleep I: effects on normal sleep.; Alcohol Clin Exp Res. 2013 Apr;37(4):539-49.

[324] Michael D. Stein, MD and Peter D. Friedmann, MD, MPH; Disturbed Sleep and Its Relationship to Alcohol Use; Subst Abus. 2005 Mar; 26(1): 1–13.

[325] Gottesmann C.; GABA mechanisms and sleep.; Neuroscience. 2002;111(2):231-9.

[326] Winkelman JW, Buxton OM, Jensen JE, Benson KL, O'Connor SP, Wang W, Renshaw PF.; Reduced brain GABA in primary insomnia: preliminary data from 4T proton magnetic resonance spectroscopy (1H-MRS).; Sleep. 2008 Nov;31(11):1499-506.

[327] Plante DT, Jensen JE, Schoerning L, Winkelman JW.; Reduced ?-aminobutyric acid in occipital and anterior cingulate cortices in primary insomnia: a link to major depressive disorder?; Neuropsychopharmacology. 2012 May;37(6):1548-57.

[328] Yuan CS, Mehendale S, Xiao Y, Aung HH, Xie JT, Ang-Lee MK.; The gamma-aminobutyric acidergic effects of valerian and valerenic acid on rat brainstem neuronal activity.; Anesth Analg. 2004 Feb;98(2):353-8, table of contents.

[329] Becker A, Felgentreff F, Schröder H, Meier B, Brattström A1.; The anxiolytic effects of a Valerian extract is based on valerenic acid.; BMC Complement Altern Med. 2014 Jul 28;14:267.

[330] Yuan Shi,a Jing-Wen Dong,a Jiang-He Zhao,b Li-Na Tang,a and Jian-Jun Zhanga,; Herbal Insomnia Medications that Target GABAergic Systems: A Review of the Psychopharmacological Evidence; Curr Neuropharmacol. 2014 May; 12(3): 289–302.

[331] Ibarra-Coronado EG1, Pantaleón-Martínez AM1, Velazquéz-Moctezuma J2, Prospéro-García O3, Méndez-Díaz M3, Pérez-Tapia M4, Pavón L5, Morales-Montor J1.; The Bidirectional Relationship between Sleep and Immunity against Infections.; J Immunol Res. 2015;2015:678164.

[332] Luca Imeri and Mark R. Opp; How (and why) the immune system makes us sleep; Nat Rev Neurosci. 2009 Mar; 10(3): 199–210.

[333] Buguet A, Bourdon L, Bouteille B, Cespuglio R, Vincendeau P, Radomski MW, Dumas M.; The duality of sleeping sickness: focusing on sleep; Sleep Med Rev. 2001 Apr;5(2):139-153.

[334] Drake CL, Roehrs TA, Royer H, Koshorek G, Turner RB, Roth T.; Effects of an experimentally induced rhinovirus cold on sleep, performance, and daytime alertness.; Physiol Behav. 2000 Oct 1-15;71(1-2):75-81.

[335] Tesoriero C, Codita A2, Zhang MD3, Cherninsky A4, Karlsson H5, Grassi-Zucconi G6, Bertini G6, Harkany T7, Ljungberg K8, Liljeström P8, Hökfelt TG9, Bentivoglio M6, Kristensson K9.; H1N1 influenza virus induces narcolepsy-like sleep disruption and targets sleep-wake regulatory neurons in mice.; Proc Natl Acad Sci U S A. 2016 Jan 19;113(3):E368-77.

[336] Alexandre Sasseville,Nathalie Paquet,Jean Sévigny,Marc Hébert; Blue blocker glasses impede the capacity of bright light to suppress melatonin production; Journal of Pineal Research May 18, 2006

[337] Burkhart K, Phelps JR.; Amber lenses to block blue light and improve sleep: a randomized trial.; Chronobiol Int. 2009 Dec;26(8):1602-12.

[338] Dugas EN, Sylvestre MP2, O'Loughlin EK3, Brunet J4, Kakinami L5, Constantin E6, O'Loughlin J7.; Nicotine dependence and sleep quality in young adults.; Addict Behav. 2017 Feb;65:154-160.

[339] Karadag E, Samancioglu S2, Ozden D3, Bakir E4.; Effects of aromatherapy on sleep quality and anxiety of patients.; Nurs Crit Care. 2017 Mar;22(2):105-112.

[340] Hwang E, Shin S.; The effects of aromatherapy on sleep improvement: a systematic literature review and metaanalysis.; J Altern Complement Med. 2015 Feb;21(2):61-8.

[341] Mi-Yeon Cho, 1 Eun Sil Min, 2 Myung-Haeng Hur, 2 ,* and Myeong Soo Lee 3; Effects of Aromatherapy on the Anxiety, Vital Signs, and Sleep Quality of Percutaneous Coronary Intervention Patients in Intensive Care Units; Evid Based Complement Alternat Med. 2013; 2013: 381381.

[342] Janmejai K Srivastava,* Eswar Shankar,1,2 and Sanjay Gupta1,2,3; Chamomile: A herbal medicine of the past with bright future; Mol Med Report. 2010 Nov 1; 3(6): 895–901.

[343] New link between pollution, temperature and sleep-disordered breathing; Science News June 21 2010 http://www.sciencedaily.com/releases/2010/06/100614141346.htm

[344] Dorsey CM, Teicher MH, Cohen-Zion M, Stefanovic L, Satlin A, Tartarini W, Harper D, Lukas SE.; Core body temperature and sleep of older female insomniacs before and after passive body heating.; Sleep. 1999 Nov 1;22(7):891-8.

[345] Kanda K, Tochihara Y, Ohnaka T.; Bathing before sleep in the young and in the elderly.; Eur J Appl Physiol Occup Physiol. 1999 Jul;80(2):71-5.

[346] Forrest CM, Mackay GM, Stoy N, Stone TW, Darlington LG.; Inflammatory status and kynurenine metabolism in rheumatoid arthritis treated with melatonin.; Br J Clin Pharmacol. 2007 Oct;64(4):517-26. Epub 2007 May 15.

[347] Hong YG, Riegler JL.; Is melatonin associated with the development of autoimmune hepatitis?; J Clin Gastroenterol. 1997 Jul;25(1):376-8.

[348] Gu-Jiun Lin, Shing-Hwa Huang, Shyi-Jou Chen, Chih-Hung Wang, Deh-Ming Chang, and Huey-Kang Sytwu,; Modulation by Melatonin of the Pathogenesis of Inflammatory Autoimmune Diseases; Int J Mol Sci. 2013 Jun; 14(6): 11742–11766.

[349] McCarty MF; Complementary vascular-protective actions of magnesium and taurine: a rationale for magnesium taurate.; Med Hypotheses. 1996 Feb;46(2):89-100.

[350] Morais JBS, Severo JS, de Alencar GRR, de Oliveira ARS, Cruz KJC, Marreiro DDN, Freitas BJESA, de Carvalho CMR, Martins MDCCE, Frota KMG.; Effect of magnesium supplementation on insulin resistance in humans: A systematic review.; Nutrition. 2017 Jun;38:54-60.

[351] Kimura K, Ozeki M, Juneja LR, Ohira H.; L-Theanine reduces psychological and physiological stress responses.; Biol Psychol. 2007 Jan;74(1):39-45. Epub 2006 Aug 22.

[352] Nathan PJ, Lu K, Gray M, Oliver C.; The neuropharmacology of L-theanine(N-ethyl-L-glutamine): a possible neuroprotective and cognitive enhancing agent.; J Herb Pharmacother. 2006;6(2):21-30.

[353] Hidese S, Ota M, Wakabayashi C, Noda T, Ozawa H, Okubo T, Kunugi H.; Effects of chronic l-theanine administration in patients with major depressive disorder: an open-label study.; Acta Neuropsychiatr. 2017 Apr;29(2):72-79. doi: 10.1017/neu.2016.33. Epub 2016 Jul 11.

[354] Lyon MR, Kapoor MP, Juneja LR.; The effects of L-theanine (Suntheanine®) on objective sleep quality in boys with attention deficit hyperactivity disorder (ADHD): a randomized, double-blind, placebo-controlled clinical trial.; Altern Med Rev. 2011 Dec;16(4):348-54.

[355] Glade MJ, Smith K.; Phosphatidylserine and the human brain.; Nutrition. 2015 Jun;31(6):781-6. doi: 10.1016/j.nut.2014.10.014. Epub 2014 Nov 4.

[356] Juliane Hellhammer, Dominic Vogt,1 Nadin Franz,1 Ulla Freitas,2 and David Rutenberg3, A soy-based phosphatidylserine/ phosphatidic acid complex (PAS) normalizes the stress reactivity of hypothalamus-pituitary-adrenal-axis in chronically stressed male subjects: a randomized, placebo-controlled study; Lipids Health Dis. 2014; 13: 121.

[357] A. Kumar and H. Kalonia; Effect of Withania somnifera on Sleep-Wake Cycle in Sleep-Disturbed Rats: Possible GABAergic Mechanism; Indian J Pharm Sci. 2008 Nov-Dec; 70(6): 806–810.

[358] Shawn M Talbott, Julie A Talbott,1 and Mike Pugh2; Effect of Magnolia officinalis and Phellodendron amurense (Relora®) on cortisol and psychological mood state in moderately stressed subjects; J Int Soc Sports Nutr. 2013; 10: 37.

[359] [No authors listed]; A scientific review: the role of chromium in insulin resistance; Diabetes Educ. 2004;Suppl:2-14.

[360] Parijat Kanetkar, Rekha Singhal, and Madhusudan Kamat; Gymnema sylvestre: A Memoir; J Clin Biochem Nutr. 2007 Sep; 41(2): 77–81.

[361] Xiaoyun Wei, Chunyan Wang, Shijun Hao, Haiyan Song, and Lili Yang; The Therapeutic Effect of Berberine in the Treatment of Nonalcoholic Fatty Liver Disease: A Meta-Analysis; Evid Based Complement Alternat Med. 2016; 2016: 3593951.

[362] Yang Y, Li W, Liu Y, Li Y, Gao L, Zhao JJ; Alpha-lipoic acid attenuates insulin resistance and improves glucose metabolism in high fat diet-fed mice; Acta Pharmacol Sin. 2014 Oct;35(10):1285-92.

[363] Susanta Mondal and Kalipada Pahan; Cinnamon Ameliorates Experimental Allergic Encephalomyelitis in Mice via Regulatory T Cells: Implications for Multiple Sclerosis Therapy; PLoS One. 2015; 10(1): e0116566.

[364] Diaz DE, Hagler WM Jr, Hopkins BA, Whitlow LW; Aflatoxin binders I: in vitro binding assay for aflatoxin B1 by several potential sequestering agents; Mycopathologia. 2002;156(3):223-6.

[365] Freitas-Silva O, Venâncio A; Ozone applications to prevent and degrade mycotoxins: a review; Drug Metab Rev. 2010 Nov;42(4):612-20.

366 Young JC, Zhu H, Zhou T; Degradation of trichothecene mycotoxins by aqueous ozone; Food Chem Toxicol. 2006 Mar;44(3):417-24. Epub 2005 Sep 23.

367 Maccaferri S, Vitali B, Klinder A, Kolida S, Ndagijimana M, Laghi L, Calanni F, Brigidi P, Gibson GR, Costabile A; Rifaximin modulates the colonic microbiota of patients with Crohn's disease: an in vitro approach using a continuous culture colonic model system; J Antimicrob Chemother. 2010 Dec;65(12):2556-65.

368 Furnari M, Parodi A, Gemignani L, Giannini EG, Marenco S, Savarino E, Assandri L, Fazio V, Bonfanti D, Inferrera S, Savarino V; Clinical trial: the combination of rifaximin with partially hydrolysed guar gum is more effective than rifaximin alone in eradicating small intestinal bacterial overgrowth; Aliment Pharmacol Ther. 2010 Oct;32(8):1000-6.

369 Victor Chedid, MD, Sameer Dhalla, MD, John O. Clarke, MD, Bani Chander Roland, MD, Kerry B. Dunbar, MD, Joyce Koh, MD, Edmundo Justino, MD, Eric Tomakin, RN, and Gerard E. Mullin, MD; Herbal Therapy Is Equivalent to Rifaximin for the Treatment of Small Intestinal Bacterial Overgrowth; Glob Adv Health Med. 2014 May; 3(3): 16–24.

370 Guo Y, Chen Y, Tan ZR, Klaassen CD, Zhou HH; Repeated administration of berberine inhibits cytochromes P450 in humans; Eur J Clin Pharmacol. 2012 Feb;68(2):213-7.

371 Amit H. Sachdev and Mark Pimentel; Gastrointestinal bacterial overgrowth: pathogenesis and clinical significance; Ther Adv Chronic Dis. 2013 Sep; 4(5): 223–231.

SECTION FIVE

1 Hewagalamulage SD, Lee TK, Clarke IJ, Henry BA; Stress, cortisol, and obesity: a role for cortisol responsiveness in identifying individuals prone to obesity; Domest Anim Endocrinol. 2016 Jul;56 Suppl:S112-20.

2 Mousumi Bose, Blanca Oliván, and Blandine Laferrère; Stress and obesity: the role of the hypothalamic–pituitary–adrenal axis in metabolic disease; Curr Opin Endocrinol Diabetes Obes. 2009 Oct; 16(5): 340–346.

3 Coughlin JW, Smith MT; Sleep, obesity, and weight loss in adults: is there a rationale for providing sleep interventions in the treatment of obesity?; Int Rev Psychiatry. 2014 Apr;26(2):177-88.

4 Beccuti G, Pannain S; Sleep and obesity; Curr Opin Clin Nutr Metab Care. 2011 Jul;14(4):402-12.

5 Giuseppe Latini,corresponding author Francesco Gallo, and Lorenzo Iughetti; Toxic environment and obesity pandemia: Is there a relationship?; Published online 2010 Jan 22.

6 Michalopoulos GK; Liver regeneration; J Cell Physiol. 2007 Nov;213(2):286-300.

7 Shioko Kimura; Thyroid Regeneration: How Stem Cells Play a Role?; Front Endocrinol (Lausanne). 2014; 5: 55.

8 Höfling DB, Chavantes MC, Juliano AG, Cerri GG, Knobel M, Yoshimura EM, Chammas MC; Low-level laser in the treatment of patients with hypothyroidism

induced by chronic autoimmune thyroiditis: a randomized, placebo-controlled clinical trial; Lasers Med Sci. 2013 May;28(3):743-53.

[9] Höfling DB, Chavantes MC, Juliano AG, Cerri GG, Romão R, Yoshimura EM, Chammas MC; Low-level laser therapy in chronic autoimmune thyroiditis: a pilot study; Lasers Surg Med. 2010 Aug;42(6):589-96.

[10] Kaya M, Kalayci R, Arican N, Küçük M, Elmas I; Effect of aluminum on the blood-brain barrier permeability during nitric oxide-blockade-induced chronic hypertension in rats; Biol Trace Elem Res. 2003 Jun;92(3):221-30.

[11] Banks WA, Kastin AJ; The aluminum-induced increase in blood-brain barrier permeability to delta-sleep-inducing peptide occurs throughout the brain and is independent of phosphorus and acetylcholinesterase levels; Psychopharmacology (Berl). 1985;86(1-2):84-9.

[12] Peterson EW, Cardoso ER; The blood-brain barrier following experimental subarachnoid hemorrhage. Part 2: Response to mercuric chloride infusion; J Neurosurg. 1983 Mar;58(3):345-51.

[13] Shukla A1, Shukla GS, Srimal RC; Cadmium-induced alterations in blood-brain barrier permeability and its possible correlation with decreased microvessel antioxidant potential in rat; Hum Exp Toxicol. 1996 May;15(5):400-5.

[14] Melissa Seelbach Lei Chen, Anita Powell, Yean Jung Choi, Bei Zhang,1 Bernhard Hennig, and Michal Toborek; Polychlorinated Biphenyls Disrupt Blood–Brain Barrier Integrity and Promote Brain Metastasis Formation; Environ Health Perspect. 2010 Apr; 118(4): 479–484.

[15] Selvakumar K, Prabha RL, Saranya K, Bavithra S, Krishnamoorthy G, Arunakaran J; Polychlorinated biphenyls impair blood-brain barrier integrity via disruption of tight junction proteins in cerebrum, cerebellum and hippocampus of female Wistar rats: neuropotential role of quercetin; Hum Exp Toxicol. 2013 Jul;32(7):706-20.

[16] Tang J, Zhang Y, Yang L, Chen Q, Tan L, Zuo S, Feng H, Chen Z, Zhu G; Exposure to 900 MHz electromagnetic fields activates the mkp-1/ERK pathway and causes blood-brain barrier damage and cognitive impairment in rats; Brain Res. 2015 Mar 19;1601:92-101.

[17] Esposito P, Gheorghe D, Kandere K, Pang X, Connolly R, Jacobson S, Theoharides TC; Acute stress increases permeability of the blood-brain-barrier through activation of brain mast cells; Brain Res. 2001 Jan 5;888(1):117-127.

[18] Chaudhuri JD; Blood brain barrier and infection; Med Sci Monit. 2000 Nov-Dec;6(6):1213-22.

[19] Nicola G. Cascella,* Debby Santora, Patricia Gregory, Deanna L. Kelly, Alessio Fasano, and William W. Eaton; Increased Prevalence of Transglutaminase 6 Antibodies in Sera From Schizophrenia Patients; Schizophr Bull. 2013 Jul; 39(4): 867–871.

[20] Haorah J, Knipe B, Gorantla S, Zheng J, Persidsky Y; Alcohol-induced blood-brain barrier dysfunction is mediated via inositol 1,4,5-triphosphate receptor (IP3R)-gated intracellular calcium release; J Neurochem. 2007 Jan;100(2):324-36.

[21] Singh AK, Jiang Y, Gupta S, Benlhabib E; Effects of chronic ethanol drinking on the blood brain barrier and ensuing neuronal toxicity in alcohol-preferring

rats subjected to intraperitoneal LPS injection; Alcohol Alcohol. 2007 Sep-Oct;42(5):385-99. Epub 2007 Mar 6.

22 Chaudhuri JD; Blood brain barrier and infection; Med Sci Monit. 2000 Nov-Dec;6(6):1213-22.

23 Köhrle J; The deiodinase family: selenoenzymes regulating thyroid hormone availability and action; Cell Mol Life Sci. 2000 Dec;57(13-14):1853-63.

24 Huang SA, Dorfman DM, Genest DR, Salvatore D, Larsen PR; Type 3 iodothyronine deiodinase is highly expressed in the human uteroplacental unit and in fetal epithelium; J Clin Endocrinol Metab. 2003 Mar;88(3):1384-8.

25 Brtko J, Macejová D, Knopp J, Kvetnanský R; Stress is associated with inhibition of type I iodothyronine 5'-deiodinase activity in rat liver; Ann N Y Acad Sci. 2004 Jun;1018:219-23.

26 Hidal JT, Kaplan MM; Inhibition of thyroxine 5'-deiodination type II in cultured human placental cells by cortisol, insulin, 3', 5'-cyclic adenosine monophosphate, and butyrate; Metabolism. 1988 Jul;37(7):664-8.

27 Song S, Oka T; Regulation of type II deiodinase expression by EGF and glucocorticoid in HC11 mouse mammary epithelium; Am J Physiol Endocrinol Metab. 2003 Jun;284(6):E1119-24. Epub 2003 Feb 11.

28 Arthur JR, Nicol F, Beckett GJ; Selenium deficiency, thyroid hormone metabolism, and thyroid hormone deiodinases; Am J Clin Nutr. 1993 Feb;57(2 Suppl):236S-239S.

29 DePalo D, Kinlaw WB, Zhao C, Engelberg-Kulka H, St Germain DL; Effect of selenium deficiency on type I 5'-deiodinase; J Biol Chem. 1994 Jun 10;269(23):16223-8.

30 Perrild H, Hansen JM, Skovsted L, Christensen LK; Different effects of propranolol, alprenolol, sotalol, atenolol and metoprolol on serum T3 and serum rT3 in hyperthyroidism; Clin Endocrinol (Oxf). 1983 Feb;18(2):139-42.

31 Molnár I, Balázs C, Szegedi G, Sipka S; Inhibition of type 2,5'-deiodinase by tumor necrosis factor alpha, interleukin-6 and interferon gamma in human thyroid tissue; Immunol Lett. 2002 Jan 1;80(1):3-7.

32 Rushton DH, Norris MJ, Dover R, Busuttil N; Causes of hair loss and the developments in hair rejuvenation; Int J Cosmet Sci. 2002 Feb;24(1):17-23.

33 Riedel-Baima B, Riedel A; Female pattern hair loss may be triggered by low oestrogen to androgen ratio; Endocr Regul. 2008 Mar;42(1):13-6.

34 Wallace ML, Smoller BR; Estrogen and progesterone receptors in androgenic alopecia versus alopecia areata; Am J Dermatopathol. 1998 Apr;20(2):160-3.

35 Camacho-Martínez FM; Hair loss in women; Semin Cutan Med Surg. 2009 Mar;28(1):19-32.

36 Izabela Urysiak-Czubatka, Małgorzata L. Kmieć,corresponding author and Grażyna Broniarczyk-Dyła; Assessment of the usefulness of dihydrotestosterone in the diagnostics of patients with androgenetic alopecia; Postepy Dermatol Alergol. 2014 Aug; 31(4): 207–215.

[37] Lutz G; Hair loss and hyperprolactinemia in women; Dermatoendocrinol. 2012 Jan 1;4(1):65-71.

[38] Vladimir A. Botchkarev; Stress and the Hair Follicle; Am J Pathol. 2003 Mar; 162(3): 709–712.

[39] Paus R, Botchkarev VA, Botchkareva NV, Mecklenburg L, Luger T, Slominski A; The skin POMC system (SPS). Leads and lessons from the hair follicle; Ann N Y Acad Sci. 1999 Oct 20;885:350-63.

[40] Paus R, Peters EM, Eichmüller S, Botchkarev VA; Neural mechanisms of hair growth control; J Investig Dermatol Symp Proc. 1997 Aug;2(1):61-8.

[41] Katsarou-Katsari A, Singh LK, Theoharides TC; Alopecia areata and affected skin CRH receptor upregulation induced by acute emotional stress; Dermatology. 2001;203(2):157-61.

[42] Alopecia Areata https://www.ncbi.nlm.nih.gov/pubmedhealth/PMHT0025278/

[43] Garg S, Messenger AG; Alopecia areata: evidence-based treatments; Semin Cutan Med Surg. 2009 Mar;28(1):15-8.

[44] Vayssairat M, Mimoun M, Houot B, Abuaf N, Rouquette AM, Chaouat M; Hashimoto's thyroiditis and silicone breast implants: 2 cases; J Mal Vasc. 1997 Jul;22(3):198-9.

[45] Brown SL, Langone JJ, Brinton LA; Silicone breast implants and autoimmune disease; J Am Med Womens Assoc (1972). 1998 Winter;53(1):21-4, 40.

[46] Wolfram D, Rabensteiner E, Grundtman C, Böck G, Mayerl C, Parson W, Almanzar G, Hasenöhrl C, Piza-Katzer H, Wick G; T regulatory cells and TH17 cells in peri-silicone implant capsular fibrosis; Plast Reconstr Surg. 2012 Feb;129(2):327e-337e.

[47] Ashry KM, El-Sayed YS, Khamiss RM, El-Ashmawy IM; Oxidative stress and immunotoxic effects of lead and their amelioration with myrrh (Commiphora molmol) emulsion; Food Chem Toxicol. 2010 Jan;48(1):236-41.

[48] Al-Said A. Haffor; Effect of myrrh (Commiphora molmol) on leukocyte levels before and during healing from gastric ulcer or skin injury; Journal of Immunotoxicology Volume 7, 2010 - Issue 1

[49] Ammon HP; Boswellic acids (components of frankincense) as the active principle in treatment of chronic inflammatory diseases; Wien Med Wochenschr. 2002;152(15-16):373-8.

[50] Roller S, Ernest N, Buckle J; The antimicrobial activity of high-necrodane and other lavender oils on methicillin-sensitive and -resistant Staphylococcus aureus (MSSA and MRSA); J Altern Complement Med. 2009 Mar;15(3):275-9.

[51] Schneider E, Leite-de-moraes M, Dy M; Histamine, immune cells and autoimmunity; Adv Exp Med Biol. 2010;709:81-94.

[52] Nielsen HJ, Hammer JH; Possible role of histamine in pathogenesis of autoimmune diseases: implications for immunotherapy with histamine-2 receptor antagonists; Med Hypotheses. 1992 Dec;39(4):349-55.

[53] Packard KA, Khan MM; Effects of histamine on Th1/Th2 cytokine balance; Int Immunopharmacol. 2003 Jul;3(7):909-20.

INDEX

About the Author

Dr. Eric Osansky is a licensed chiropractor, clinical nutritionist, and certified functional medicine practitioner through the Institute for Functional Medicine. He graduated summa cum laude from Life Chiropractic College in March of 1999, and like most other chiropractors he initially focused on musculoskeletal conditions, and did so for 7 1/2 years. But he was diagnosed with the autoimmune thyroid condition Graves' disease in 2008, and restored his health back to normal through natural treatment methods. Since then he has helped thousands of people with the autoimmune thyroid conditions Graves' disease and Hashimoto's thyroiditis.

Dr. Osansky lives in Matthews, NC, with his wife Cindy, and his two daughters, Marissa and Jaylee.

Thank You For Reading My Book

I hope you enjoyed reading my book on Hashimoto's Triggers. I really do appreciate receiving feedback from others, and I'd love to hear what you have to say about my book.

In addition, I need your input to make my future books better.

Please leave me an honest review on Amazon letting me know what you thought of the book. Not only will you be helping me, but you'll also be helping others who have Hashimoto's.

Thank you so much!

Dr. Eric

Don't Forget Your Free Bonus Gifts!

As a small token of thanks for buying this book, I'd like to offer two free bonus gifts exclusive to my readers:

- Bonus #1: The Hashimoto's Triggers FREE Video Training Series
- Bonus #2: The Hashimoto's Triggers FREE Action Plan Checklist

You can download your free gifts here:
http://www.naturalendocrinesolutions.com/freegift

Made in United States
North Haven, CT
07 April 2024

51031099R00310